Health and Well-Being in Islamic Societies

Harold G. Koenig • Saad Al Shohaib

Health and Well-Being in Islamic Societies

Background, Research, and Applications

Springer

Harold G. Koenig
Duke University Medical Center
Durham, NC, USA

King Abdulaziz University
Jeddah, Saudi Arabia

Saad Al Shohaib
King Abdulaziz University
Jeddah, Saudi Arabia

ISBN 978-3-319-05872-6 ISBN 978-3-319-05873-3 (eBook)
DOI 10.1007/978-3-319-05873-3
Springer Cham Heidelberg New York Dordrecht London

Library of Congress Control Number: 2014936169

Printed on acid-free paper

Springer is part of Springer Science+Business Media (www.springer.com)

Introduction

The central question asked in this book is whether religious involvement is related to better health in Muslims. We seek to examine and understand the relationships between Islam and health from a historical, theological, and scientific perspective, based in part on what we know about religion and health in Christian populations. There are many books that compare Christianity and Islam in various ways, although few provide a balanced evenhanded approach that we seek to do here. There is usually an unspoken agenda by the authors that favors one religion over the other. To our knowledge, no attempt has yet been made to understand the important contributions that Muslim beliefs and practices make to health and well-being in Islamic societies, or explain why and how such influences occur. We—a Christian (or follower of Jesus) and a Muslim (or follower of the Prophet Muhammad)—seek to do this by directly examining the findings from research on religion and health in Muslim populations, and comparing the results to those from a much larger research literature in Christian populations. We take particular care in documenting the information presented here with citations from original sources, i.e., reputable English translations of the Qur'an, the Hadith, and the Bible, and writings of recognized religious and health experts familiar with these sources. When discussing the research, we focus on original quantitative research reports published in mainstream peer-reviewed health journals. Our goal is to *objectively* present the beliefs and practices of these two great monotheistic religions and determine their relationships with health, while showing the utmost respect for both traditions.

The primary audiences for this volume are Muslim and Christian health professionals and religious professionals with health interests. This includes physicians, nurses, social workers, counselors, psychologists, psychiatrists, chaplains, pastoral counselors, community clergy, sociologists, epidemiologists, and public policy experts, as well as undergraduate and graduate students in these fields. The secondary audience for this book, however, is a much broader one. The content here is designed to capture the interest of professionals and nonprofessionals in many other areas. This includes those wanting to know more about the role that Muslim beliefs and practices play in health, why such effects occur, and how this information can be used to maximize health. Everyone has an interest in their own health and well-being, and this book in the end is really about that.

We begin by providing a historical background to set the stage for what is to come. The history that lies behind the development of Islamic beliefs, cultures, and healthcare practices is key to understanding relationships with health today. We then carefully examine present-day Muslim beliefs, practices, and values, and explore Muslim attitudes toward health and healing. Many Christians (and even some Muslims) may not be fully aware of the core teachings of Islam or how these relate to attitudes toward health. We next carefully examine Christian beliefs, practices, and values in detail. Many Muslims (and even some Christians) may not be aware of the beliefs and practices of Christians or their views on ethical issues that are also dear to the hearts of Muslims. We then describe the differences and similarities between Islam and Christianity, and discuss how these might influence health and impact relationships between Muslims and Christians, which will likely affect global health.

In the second section of this book, we summarize research on religion, spirituality, and health in Christian populations. Given that 90 % of the published research on religion and health comes from Christian-majority samples, this review provides a baseline from which we can then examine research on religion and health in Muslim populations. After this review, we turn our focus to the heart of this book—a systematic review of research on religiosity and the mental, social, behavioral, and physical health of Muslim-majority populations and a comparison of health outcomes in Muslims and non-Muslims. This review and update is based on scientific research published from around the world during the past 50 years. We conclude this research summary with a discussion of pathways that might explain how and why Islamic beliefs and practices might influence physical health and longevity.

The final section of this book focuses on applications. How might the knowledge gained from this research review be used to improve the delivery of healthcare to Muslims and enhance the health and well-being of Islamic societies more generally. Our goal throughout is to identify and discuss aspects of Islamic faith and practice that influence health, and determine how these are similar to or different from the ways that Christian beliefs and practices affect health. Over one-half of the world's population is now Muslim or Christian, yet the forces of modernization and secularization are rapidly encroaching on and devaluing the traditions that people of faith hold sacred. Depending on the impact that religion has on health (including social health), such forces could influence not only the physical and emotional well-being but also the economic growth of Islamic societies. While considerable information has accumulated on the relationships between religion and health within Christianity, much less is known about how these factors relate in Islam. This book is intended to change that and utilize the information identified from systematic research to improve healthcare, promote health practices, prevent disease, and foster healthy human relationships in Muslim populations worldwide.

Durham, NC, USA Harold G. Koenig
Jeddah, Saudi Arabia Saad Al Shohaib

Contents

Part I Background

1 Historical Background 3
Ancient Empires and Their Religions 3
Religion and Early Medicine 4
Pre-Islamic Times 6
Early Islamic Period 7
Medicine of the Prophet 9
Spiritual Medicine 10
Golden Age of Islam 11
Islamic Medicine 12
Islamic Physicians 15
Period of Decline 21
Summary and Conclusions 24
References 24

2 Muslim Beliefs, Practices, and Values 27
Islamic Beliefs 28
Islamic Practices 34
Islamic Values and Attitudes 38
Summary and Conclusions 40
References 40

3 Beliefs About Health, Healing, and Healthcare 43
Sayings on Health and Healing in the Qur'an and Hadith 43
The Body 46
Sickness 47
Healing 47
Health and Medical Care 48
Supernatural Beliefs 49
Ethical Issues in Medicine 50

Miscellaneous Health Practices 52
Summary and Conclusions 54
References 54

4 Christian Beliefs, Practices, and Values 57
Christian Beliefs 57
Christian Practices 67
Christian Values 70
Attitudes on Health and Healing 73
Range of Belief and Practice 77
Summary and Conclusions 77
References 78

5 Differences and Similarities 81
Differences 81
Beliefs 81
Practices 87
Values 89
Similarities 90
Beliefs 90
Practices 98
Values 101
Similarities Acknowledged in the Qur'an 104
Differences Acknowledged 104
Summary and Conclusions 105
References 106

Part II Research

6 Religion and Health in Christian Populations 111
Definitions 111
Mental Health 113
Negative Mental Health 113
Positive Mental Health 114
Personality Traits 116
Social Health 117
Health Behaviors 118
Physical Health 118
Mechanisms and Pathways 121
Summary and Conclusions 122
References 124

7 Religion and Negative Emotions in Muslims 125
Introduction to Review 125
Religious Coping 126
Descriptive Reports 127
Quantitative 128

Depression 130
Suicide 135
Anxiety 141
Psychosis 150
Alcohol Use/Abuse 155
Drug Use/Abuse 158
Summary and Conclusions 160
References 160

8 Religion and Positive Emotions in Muslims 167
Well-Being 167
Hope 171
Optimism 173
Meaning and Purpose 177
Self-Esteem 177
Sense of Control 181
Personality Traits 185
Extraversion 185
Neuroticism 189
Conscientiousness 190
Agreeableness 191
Openness to Experience 192
Other Personality Traits 193
Summary and Conclusions 193
References 193

9 Religion and Social Health in Muslims 197
Social Support 197
Marital Stability 199
Delinquency and Crime 204
Social Capital 209
Summary and Conclusions 213
References 214

10 Religiosity and Behavioral Health in Muslims 217
Cigarette Smoking 217
Physical Activity/Exercise 224
Diet 226
Weight 228
Sexual Behavior 231
Summary and Conclusions 237
References 237

11 Religion and Physical Health in Muslims 243
Heart Disease 243
Hypertension/Blood Pressure 252
Cerebrovascular Disease 257
Dementia/Alzheimer's Disease 258

Diabetes 260
Cholesterol and Triglycerides 264
Immune Function 269
Endocrine Function 271
Cancer 273
Self-Rated Health 278
Mortality 282
Summary and Conclusions 286
References 287

12 Understanding How Islam Influences Health 295
Mental and Social Health 295
Negative Influences on Mental and Social Health 301
Behavioral Health 303
Physical Health 304
Summary and Conclusions 308
References 308

13 Future Research Needs on Islam and Health 311
Mental Health 311
Social Health 314
Behavioral Health 314
Physical Health 315
Summary and Conclusions 320
References 320

Part III Applications

14 Applications in Clinical Practice 325
The Language of Spirituality 325
Why Integrate Spirituality 326
How to Integrate Spirituality 328
Limitations 331
Summary and Conclusions 333
References 334

15 Implications for Public Health 335
Positive Implications 335
Negative Implications 336
Faith-Based Initiatives 337
Implications for Muslim–Christian Relations 339
Summary and Conclusions 341
References 342

16 Summary and Conclusions 343

Index 349

Part I
Background

To fully appreciate how religious involvement relates to health in Islamic societies, it is important to recognize the cultures and religions in the Middle East that preceded Islam, the sudden emergence of Islam and explosive spread across half of the known world, and the influence that Islam had on scientific advancements and, in particular, the development of medicine. Furthermore, a deeper understanding of the specific beliefs, behaviors, traditions, and values of Muslims will help readers appreciate why Muslims believe what they do and why devout Islamic beliefs might be related to health in one way or another. Likewise, a better understanding of exactly what Christians believe, the religious behaviors they engage in, and the values they hold dear will give readers a deeper appreciation of why they believe as they do and how this could affect their health. Although there are important differences in what Muslims and Christians believe, and this has often served as grounds for conflict and division, there are also striking similarities that bind these two religions together like no other religions anywhere in the world. These similarities in belief, behavior, and values may also help to explain the connections found between devout belief and practice in these faith traditions and the health and well-being of their members.

Chapter 1
Historical Background

We begin by reviewing the history of Islam and the development of medicine and healthcare in this context. The story begins long before the emergence of Islam and extends through several distinct periods: the beginning and rise of Islam, the Islamic Golden Age, the decline of the Golden Age, and the tumultuous transition to modern times.

Ancient Empires and Their Religions

Human civilization has its origin in the Middle East and North Africa. Religion, medicine, and healthcare were intimately connected from the beginning. This relationship, however, waxed and waned depending in part on the attitudes and influences of the rulers who controlled the region. The Sumerian (4000–2550 BCE), Akkadian (2400–2200 BCE), Babylonian (1800–1500 BCE), and Assyrian (1400–800 BCE) empires fought to take control over the rich and fertile land between the Tigris and Euphrates rivers (Mesopotamia) and surrounding areas. The Sumerians are thought to have first settled southern Mesopotamia between 4500 and 4000 BCE after migrating there from Eastern Europe (present-day Hungary) to escape the bitter cold of the Ice Age. Ancient Sumerian texts describe the Epic of Creation—which, secular historians speculate, may be a source for the Biblical book of Genesis (Heidel 1963).

The Sumerian city/state of Ur is where the patriarch Abraham was born, raised, and lived much of his adult life. What we know about him comes primarily from Biblical sources, which suggest that Abraham was born around the year 1976 BCE and left the region around 1901 (Thompson 2002). However, information contained in the Book of Jubilees and Mesoretic Torah puts his birth about a hundred years later between 1884 and 1812 BCE and his departure from Ur between 1809 and 1737 BCE. Other sources (the Samaritan Pentateuch, for example) place Abraham's birth even later (around 1513 BCE). Regardless of the exact date, Abraham lived during

H.G. Koenig and S. Al Shohaib, *Health and Well-Being in Islamic Societies: Background, Research, and Applications*, DOI 10.1007/978-3-319-05873-3_1,

the period when the Akkadian and Babylonian empires dominated the region. The primary religion of these empires during that time was Ashurism. The word Assyrian comes from Ashur, the chief Assyrian god (Van Der Toorn et al. 1999). According to mythology, Ashur was the god of war who replaced Marduk (the son of the Sumerian god Enki) as king of the pantheon (gods and goddesses of the ancient world).

The Egyptian and Persian empires would also have strong influences on this region. The Egyptian empire to the south and west of Mesopotamia dates back to 3100 BCE, reaching its peak between 1600 and 1100 BCE, when it covered much of North Africa around present-day Egypt and regions next to the Mediterranean Sea in the Middle East. The Egyptian empire had many gods and deities (e.g., Horus, Ra, Isis), although formal religious practice centered around the Pharaoh, who acted as an intermediary between the people and the gods (and was often worshiped as a god). A renaissance man who lived around 2600 BCE, Imhotep, is considered by some to be the world's first physician and was himself ultimately deified.

The first Persian empire reached its height between 550 and 300 BCE and spanned from Egypt on the west to Turkey on the north, and from Mesopotamia to the Indus River on the east. It was the largest empire the world had ever known, exceeding even the Assyrian empire before it. The religion of the empire was Zoroastrianism, one of the first monotheistic religions which emerged out of ancient Iran in 1200–1500 BCE (Foltz 2011). By the sixth century BCE, Zoroastrianism had become the established religion of the region and would have strong influences on Judaism, gnostic Christianity, and later Islam. Zoroastrianism emphasized the constant struggle between good and evil, a battle in which good would eventually triumph. It continues to have many followers in Iran and India today.

The Persian empire would not be seriously threatened until the Roman empire began spreading eastward, beginning in the third century BCE. The Roman empire continued to advance eastward, peaking in 90–120 CE, when it controlled large portions of North Africa and the Middle East. It was not until the fall of the Roman empire in 275–475 CE that its influence began to diminish. The Roman empire was polytheistic, with many gods and goddesses. The Roman leaders negotiated with the gods and were themselves worshiped as gods similar to pharaohs in the Egyptian empire. It was not until the Edict of Milan in 313 CE that Christianity became the official religion of the Holy Roman empire (as it came to be called).

Around the third century CE, the Sassanid empire (Neo-Persian or the second Persian empire) began to take control over the Middle Eastern lands previously held by the Holy Roman empire. The Sassanid empire would dominate the region until the armies of Islam conquered it in 651. The state religion of the Sassanid empire was again Zoroastrianism, as in the first Persian empire.

Religion and Early Medicine

All diseases in ancient Egypt and Mesopotamia were thought to result from religious forces, either evil spirits or the actions of the gods. During this period of history, the healing art of medicine was considered a religious practice.

Early Egyptians believed a person consisted of a physical body ("khat") and a soul. The soul consisted of three parts: the ka, the ba, and the ahk. The "ka" was thought to be an exact double of the person and was the life force that animated the body. It was expelled when the person died, but remained close to the physical body. The "ba" was how a person acted (their personality) and was thought to be unique for each individual. The ba was separate from the life force (ka), and survived after the body died. The ba was symbolized by a bird, often a falcon. After a person died, the ba would roam around on the earth during the daytime with the living and return to the underworld at night with the dead. Given the right circumstances, the ka and ba would unite after death to form the "akh." The akh "was the transfigured spirit that survived death and mingled with the gods" (Wisseman 2003). It was thought to survive in the afterlife only if the person had lived a good and worthy life.

For those with financial resources, physical healing in ancient Egypt was performed through the "temple sleep," where a person would take drugs to induce sleep and dreaming. During the sleep, priests would whisper suggestions into the sleeping person's ears. This worked well for the wealthy. A different system was in place for the unwealthy. For the common people, the specific healer depended on the type of ailment causing the suffering. If the condition was due to accidents or fighting, the *sunu* (regular physician) dealt with the problem. If the condition resulted from a scorpion sting or snakebite, the *kherep serqet* or priest of Serqet (the scorpion goddess) was sought. This healer made pleas and performed rituals to the goddess. For physical illnesses or those with unknown causes, an exorcist (physician-priest) was consulted. The exorcist prescribed the appropriate spells, incantations, or prayers to various gods to rid the body of evil spirits. These prayers were often made to Sekhmet, the Egyptian goddess of healing. The exorcist would also administer unpleasant strong smelling, nasty tasting medicines either by mouth or via other body orifices.

The situation was similar in early Mesopotamia. Treatments for illness were both spiritual and physical. The *Treatise of Medical Diagnosis and Prognoses* is the oldest surviving medical text from ancient Mesopotamia and dates back to around 1600 BCE (Avalos 1995). The document, recorded on 40 cuneiform tablets, conveys centuries of Mesopotamian medical knowledge. There were two kinds of healers in early Mesopotamian medicine. The first was the Ashipu who was a type of sorcerer and member of the clergy. This healer determined whether the illness was due to sin (i.e., error in behavior on the person's part) or was caused by a spirit, demon or god, and which spirit was responsible for the illness. Depending on the diagnosis, the Ashipu could either drive out the spirit through charms or spells, or send the sick person for physical treatment to an Ashu, the second type of healer. The Ashu was a craftsman and specialist in herbal medicine (physician) (Paulissian 1991). The Ashu would refer to medical texts for knowledge on how to treat a disease using bandages, massage, and salves, but would occasionally resort to incantations and supernatural methods as well. Physicians (Ashu) themselves worshiped several healing dieties (Ninazu, Ninib, and Gula, in particular), and both physician and patient were likely to invoke them for healing. The emblem of Ningishzida (son of the god Ninazu) was a double-headed snake, from which today's medical symbol may have come from.

Medicine in ancient Persia was also practiced by religious and nonreligious specialists, with considerable overlap between the two (like in Egypt and Mesopotamia). There was the *ravan-pezeshk* (priest) who treated the mind, psyche, or soul, and the *tan-pezeshk* (physician) who treated the physical body. One of the early Iranian medical texts, the *Vendidad*, written around the eighth century BCE, distinguished three types of medicine: surgery, healing by herbs, and healing by divine words. Centuries later, a registration for physicians was developed in Persia that separated them from quacks and charlatans. While medicine became more distinctly separated from the priesthood over time, students at the medical school in Jundishapur in the third century CE were trained in both medicine and theology. After graduation, they had to chose whether to become a priest (called magi) or a physician.

Thus, religion and medicine in ancient times were closely related and their specialists often worked hand in hand.

Pre-Islamic Times

During the centuries preceding the emergence of Islam, Arabia was a large area covered primarily by desert and roamed by nomadic Bedouin tribes. Towns were established at locations where water was available and trade routes intersected. One of these places was Mecca (Makkah). Here there was a natural spring where the Damascus-Yemen trade routes crossed. Located in Mecca was the Kaaba or *al-Ka'bah* ("The Cube" or "The Sacred/Forbidden House"), which contained many idols representing the gods of different Bedouin tribes. This was a polytheistic and primitive society characterized by frequent wars and feuds between tribes, attacks on caravans traveling along the trade routes, and many different religions (including those that buried female children alive to appease blood-thirsty gods). This period before the emergence of Islam has been called the "age of ignorance" (Nagamia 2003).

In 76 CE, with the destruction of Jerusalem by the Romans, many Jews fled to Arabia carrying with them their Greco-Roman medical knowledge. In 271 CE, the second Sassanid King Shapur I of the Persian empire founded the city of Jundishapur (or Gondeshapur) in Khuzistan located in present-day southwestern Iran. Soon after Shapur I captured the city, Syrian Christians came to Jundishapur from Antioch (Turkey). Among them were a group of Syrian physicians trained in Damascus. Centuries later, in 489 CE, Nestorian Christians (supporters of Nestorius, the Archbishop of Constantinople) came to Jundishapur from Edessa, Mesopotamia, after the Roman emperor Nero plundered the city. Among the Nestorians was a large community of physicians and medical scholars from the medical school in Edessa before Nero closed it. Thus, a critical mass of Jews and Christians began to accumulate in Jundishapur. Soon after arriving there, Nestorian physicians began building a hospital, medical school, pharmacology laboratory, library, and began translating medical texts into Arabic (Taylor 2010). When the

Roman emperor Justinian closed the Academy of Athens medical school in 529 CE, many Greek physicians with their medical knowledge also came to Jundishapur. Not long afterward, several well-known physicians from India (including Mankah and Sustura) also came to the city.

The result of this migration of physicians from Southeastern Europe, southern Asia, and North Africa to Jundishapur was the development of a center of Greek, Syrian, and Indian Medicine that had no match anywhere in the world at the time. The medical school in Jundishapur was modeled after training programs in Alexandria (Egypt) and Athens (Greece). When Muslims took over Jundishapur in 638 CE, the hospital and medical school were already well established. This would become the model for Islamic hospitals and medical schools in the Middle East for centuries to come.

Early Islamic Period

When Islam emerged in the early seventh century, the major powers were the Persians and Byzantines (eastern Christians), although disorganized government structures and rampant corruption led to a weakening of these powers. Christianity, Judaism, and Zoroastrianism, as well as many tribal religions, were practiced in different parts of the Middle East at this time. It was into this environment that on April 26, 570 CE, the Prophet Muhammad was born in Mecca. As noted above, the region at this time was characterized by widespread polytheism. There was a great socioeconomic gap between the rich and the poor. "Allah" was considered the chief God, but there were many smaller gods that mediated between Allah and humans. Even the Kaaba in Mecca had become polytheistic. Statues of hundreds of idols were housed within the Kaaba (one for every day of the year) (Armstrong 2002). According to a well-known Hadith, the Kaaba was built as a place of worship to the one and only God by Abraham and Ishmael (Bukhari 4/55/583).[1] The custom of the time was for people of the region to make a pilgrimage to Mecca once yearly to perform the *Hajj*, whether Christian, Jew, or pagan.

Much took place during the 60-year period between 570 and 632 CE. The Prophet Muhammad's life did not start out easy. He lost his father before he was born and his mother died when he was only 6 years old. After living a couple of years with his grandfather, his grandfather also died and he was then forced to live with his uncle, Abu Talib, who took care of him for the rest of his childhood. The Prophet belonged to the Banu Hashim clan, which was part of the Quraysh tribe, a powerful group of merchants that controlled Mecca and the Kaaba. In his 20s, the Prophet Muhammad worked as a trader for a wealthy widow, Khadijah.

[1] Citations to *Sahih Bukhari* (the most respected of all Sunni Hadiths) is based on a 2009 translation by M. Muhain Khan (2009). We list the reference by volume, book, and number (vol/book/no). See http://d1.islamhouse.com/data/en/ih_books/single/en_Sahih_Al-Bukhari.pdf (last accessed October 3, 2013).

Although 15 years older than he was, Khadijah and the Prophet married and remained together for over 25 years until her death in 619 CE.

In 609, during deep prayer in a cave on mount Hira, the Prophet at the age of 39 began to receive revelations from God through the angel Gabriel. The revelations would continue for the next 23 years until his death. The angel told the Prophet to tell the revelations to others, so he dictated them to those who could write. They recorded his words verbatim (as he had heard them) on tablets, bones, flat rocks, and the wide flat ends of date palm leaves. These writings were eventually compiled into a book called the Qur'an (Koran), the text which Muslims believe is the Word of God. Although it is not clear when the writings were compiled into a single volume, this was done some time within 20 years of the Prophet's death. Scholars agree that the third caliph Uthman ibn Affan canonized the Qu'ran around 653–656 CE to produce the present-day Qur'an. All other copies of the Qur'an existing at the time were burned, as this version became authoritative. The longest suras (chapters) at the beginning of the Qur'an are actually the last revelations to the Prophet (called "Medinan" suras), whereas the shorter chapters toward the end were the first messages (called "Meccan" suras). The revelations focused on the oneness of God (monotheism) contrasting with the polytheism of the day, and emphasized the importance of giving to the poor to reset the economic imbalance so prevalent at that time.

The revelations received by the Prophet Muhammad were not initially met with open arms by the Meccan community; they saw the Prophet as a threat to their religions and economic well-being. Many Arabs came to the Kaaba to worship their gods and engage in trade along the way. The Prophet underwent great persecution during this time. By his late 40s, not only were his teachings rejected and his entire clan boycotted and almost starved to death, but his wife died and his uncle and protector Abu Talib also died. To avoid persecution and probably assassination, he and his followers escaped to Medina in 621 (the start of the Muslim calendar, AH or *anno hegirae* in Latin). Over the next 10 years, the Prophet led a number of battles both against the Meccans and against the Jewish tribes in Medina to solidify his reputation and protect his followers. He died on June 8, 632 (AH 11) in Medina.

The Prophet Muhammad was not only a religious leader, but also a warrior and a statesman. He was the first to bring the warring tribes in Arabia into a unified Islamic state. During a period of about 20 years after the revelations began, Islam would spread over most of Arabia, and during the 30 years after the Prophet's death, under the leadership of Abu Bakr (close friend and father-in-law of the Prophet) and the three caliphs ("successors") that followed, Islam would spread rapidly far beyond Arabia. Within 100 years, the influence of Islam had reached as far as Spain and parts of France on the west, to China on the east, to Africa and Egypt on the south, to India, Turkey, and central Asia on the north, to Syria and the entire Middle East, nearly one-quarter of the known world. The spread of Islam would give rise to three Muslim dynasties (rulers from the same family): Umayyad dynasty (661–750 CE) (that continued to rule the Western Islamic empire from Cordoba, Spain from 756 to 1031), the Abbasid dynasty (750–1258 CE) with Baghdad (Iraq) as its center, and later the Fatimid dynasty (909–1171 CE) based in Cairo (Egypt).

The conquest and assimilation of many different people groups by Islamic rulers influenced health practices in each region. The health beliefs and practices in the region, however, could not conflict with Islamic law. Islamic law (*shari'ah*) directed life from birth to death, including health practices. Islamic law did not distinguish secular from religious law, and covered all aspects of religious, political, and civil life (Savage-Smith 1995). It was derived from the Qur'an, the sayings and traditions of the Prophet Muhammad (Hadith), and the practices of the early Muslim community (Sunnah). Islamic law was interpreted during the first century of Islam by judges (qadis), appointed by the governors of the provinces, who were appointed by the caliphs (during the early *Umayyad* caliphate between 661 and 700 CE, in particular).

During the early eighth century, a separate group called Traditionists began recording the traditions and sayings of the Prophet Muhammad (Hadith), which included decisions made by the early Umayyad qadis along with the sayings and traditions of the Prophet. The Traditionists believed that the law should be based on the traditions and sayings of the Prophet alone (along with decisions of the early qadis mixed in), and that there should be no further interpretation. Islamic law, however, was not systematized or "codified" as law was in the West, but instead relied on the legal opinions of muftis (Islamic scholars) based on the previous sources (Qur'an, Hadith, Sunnah, and early qadis interpretations). By the end of the eleventh century, this gave rise to four schools of law: the Hanafi, the Maliki, the Hanbali, and the Shafii, where the Hanbali and Shafii schools were the most conservative, and the Hanbali school was the more conservative of the latter two. The Shafii school of law, which held that the Hadith had overriding authority but also relied on legal reasoning that depended on analogy, was the law most often applied to medicine. We will come back to these schools of Islamic law in future chapters.

Medicine of the Prophet

The first type of medicine before Islam emerged was pre-Islamic Arabic Medicine, which was practiced by the Bedouin tribes and was based on Arab customs and natural treatments found in the desert environment. With the rise of Islam came other approaches to medical treatment. According to Nagamia (2003), the Qur'an does not say much directly about medicine, except for the benefits of honey and the need to avoid alcohol and other intoxicating substances. Nagamia notes, however, that the Hadith referred to a number of health practices that eventually became known as *Al-Tibb Al-Nabawi* (Prophetic Medicine). Prophetic Medicine focused on eating a healthy diet, avoidance of alcohol, treatments involving natural products, and practices such as "cupping" for symptoms of fever, headache, pain, or eye problems. Some practices, however, were more substantial—such as separating those with conditions such as leprosy or plague from healthy individuals. Despite its name, however, Prophetic Medicine was not based on revelations from God to the Prophet in the Qur'an, but more on the customs that had been approved by the

Prophet Muhammad. One reason for the rise of Prophet Medicine was that the Islamic orthodoxy wanted to counter the increasing influence that the teachings of Galen (a pagan of Greek and Roman descent) was having on Islamic Medicine (Rahman 1998, p. 42).

This approach to medicine reached its greatest influence during the fourteenth and fifteenth centuries with the writings of Al-Jauziyah, As-Suyuti, and Az-Zahabi, who were religious scholars, not physicians. Of particular interest for our purposes, these writers stressed the emotional aspects of illness and the need for patients to use their faith for healing. For example, Al-Jauziyah encouraged physicians to ask patients about aspects of their life besides their physical symptoms. This included exploring the patient's emotional state, their lifestyle, and diet (Abdullah 2003). They stressed that Muslim physicians should consider the effects of the patient's emotional state on their physical illness, and instructed patients to recite positive statements from the Qur'an and the Sunnahs to speed the healing process. They urged physicians to prescribe moral behaviors such as love, courage, patience, kindness, and provide for the needs of others, along with prayer (Ayad 2008). Patients were to engage in these activities to build their faith and mobilize psychological and spiritual resources for combating illness. Summing it all up, As-Suyuti advised physicians to be "gentle in speech, kind in words, and close to God" (Thomson 2009). Prophetic Medicine, grounded on the writings of theologians and religious leaders, was popular among religious Muslims because of its theological basis (although it was weak on scientific medical theory).

Spiritual Medicine

Distinct from Prophetic Medicine (although overlapping with it) was a type of practice called "Spiritual Medicine" or "Spiritual Healing," which emphasized several healing practices that continue to be used by many Muslims today. These include reciting passages from the Qur'an or prayers to Allah either by the sick person or by friends and family to either protect a person from disease or to treat the disease (Nagamia 2003). This might include the ingestion of honey and/or the drinking of water that had been prayed over using verses from the Qur'an (Oyewole 2006). Amulets, while not encouraged by the Prophet, were allowed if used with verses from the Qur'an. Another healing practice of Spiritual Medicine was writing verses from the Qur'an on a piece of paper, dissolving it in water, and then drinking the water, timing the ingestion to specific times during the day such as sunrise (Rahman 1998, p. 89). A text written in the ninth century called *Khawass al-Qur'an* (Properties of the Qu'ran) describes the healing properties of reading passages from the Qur'an, linking specific passages with specific diseases (Al-Tamimi, n.d.). For example, reciting Chapter 38 of the Qur'an over a sleeping person was used to treat breathing problems, whereas writing the verses down on paper and reading them during waking hours was thought to cure illness in general.

Islamic philosopher and theologian Fazlur Rahman[2] describes one example of Spiritual Medicine in a case from the twelfth century. Failing to cure a patient with severe abdominal pain with drugs, the health professional (a pharmacist) recited the opening sura of the Qur'an: "In the name of God, the Lord of Mercy, the Giver of Mercy! Praise belongs to God, Lord of the Worlds, the Lord of Mercy, the Giver of Mercy. Master of the Day of Judgement. It is You we worship; it is You we ask for help. Guide us to the straight path: the path of those You have blessed, those who incur no anger and who have not gone astray" (Qur'an 1:1). Following this, he blew his breath in the direction of the patient. He then prayed "O my Lord, my God, my Master! You have said in your firm, true, and indubitable Book [the Qur'an], 'We send down the Qur'an as a restorer of health and as mercy for the believers' [17,82]" (Rahman 1998, p. 95). He then cleansed himself, stood on his prayer rug, and began to pray. He soon received news that the patient had been cured.

Golden Age of Islam

As a result of Islamic religious teachings, which regulated and stabilized every aspect of daily life, an ethical code developed that balanced the rights of the individual with those of the community. This ethical code brought stability to many regions governed by the Islamic empire. The result was a period of intense learning and scientific progress, which became known as the Islamic Golden Age. This period extended nearly 500 years from the middle of the eighth century, when the Abbasid caliph transferred the Eastern Muslim empire's capital from Damascus to Baghdad, until 1258, when the Mongols conquered Baghdad thus ending the Abbasid dynasty (Gregorian 2003). The supreme religious and political leader of the Islamic state was known as the *caliph* (successor to the Prophet Muhammad). The two most famous caliphs who ruled during the early Golden Age were Al-Mansur (712–775 CE) and Harun al-Rashid (754–809 CE). Al-Rashid was the caliph portrayed in the *Arabian Nights*, a series of stories and folk tales written in

[2] In this chapter we frequently cite the work of Fazlur Rahman (1919–1988), who has been described as "the most learned of the major Muslim thinkers in the second-half of the twentieth century, in terms of both classical Islam and Western philosophical and theological discourse" (http://www.freerepublic.com/focus/fr/531762/posts). In addition to being a highly reputable and exact Islamic scholar, he studied the original sources and translated into English many texts that are now available only in Arabic, Persian, Turkish, or Urdu. Considered a Sunni scholar and philosopher, he was raised in Pakistan and obtained a Ph.D. in Islamic philosophy from Oxford University. He is known widely as a prominent moderate reformer, and served for many years as the leader of the Islamic Research Institute in Pakistan. After leaving that position, he taught at the University of California at Los Angeles and later became the Harold H. Swift Distinguished Service Professor at the University of Chicago and the first Muslim member of the Divinity School faculty at the University of Chicago. He grew up in a Sunni family of the Hanafi school (representing reason). His famous textbook *Islam* (1979, University of Chicago Press) is used as an undergraduate text in many Western universities.

Arabic during this period (although did not receive widespread acclaim until the first English language edition in 1706) (Lyons and Petrucelli 1997).

Early in the ninth century, the House of Wisdom (*bayt al-hikmah*) was established in Baghdad. Here Greek scientific and medical texts brought in from Constantinople and other learning centers were translated into Arabic. The head of this institute was Abu Zakari ya ibn Masawayh, a Nestorian Christian physician from the medical school at Jundishapur. He was the personal physician to four successive caliphs. The House of Wisdom collected, synthesized, and expanded knowledge obtained from ancient Egyptian, Greek, Roman, Chinese, Indian, Persian, and Byzantine scholars. Many original Greek manuscripts on medicine and science by Hippocrates, Aristotle, and Galen were lost due to wars and invasions. However, due to Arabic translations from the House of Wisdom, the knowledge from these manuscripts was preserved for scientists and physicians in both the East and the West.

During the Islamic Golden Age, the Middle East was considered the center of medical and other scientific learning in the world. Only later did such learning spread westward to Europe. Even the *Canterbury Tales* mentions Al-Majusi (Haly), Al-Razi (Razis), and Ibn Sina (Avicenna or Avicen) among the great physicians that fourteenth century readers would be familiar with:

> With us her was a Doctour o Phisyk
> In all this world ne was ther noon him lyk
> To speke of phisik and surgerye,…
> Wel knew he the olde Esculapius,
> And Deiscorides, and eek Rufus,
> Old Ypocras [Hippocrates], Haly [Haly Abbas], and Galien [Galen],
> Serapion, Razis, and Avicen… (Chaucer (1387–1400) 1957)

Islamic Medicine

The advances in science and the arts during the Islamic Golden Age resulted in the emergence of Islamic Medicine. Separate and distinct from pre-Islamic Arabic Medicine, Prophetic Medicine, and Spiritual Medicine (discussed earlier), this form of medicine was more "scientific and analytical" (says Nagamia). Islamic Medicine depended on medical knowledge acquired from translations of Greek, Roman, Indian, Syrian, and Persian writings and from original discoveries made by Islamic physicians themselves.

Islamic Medicine emerged out of interactions between pre-Islamic indigenous local traditions, Greco-Roman influences, and religious beliefs (Nagamia 2003). Initially, there was some debate about whether Islamic physicians should use the medical techniques inherited from Greek, Roman, and Chinese physicians, since these techniques were viewed by some as pagan practices. Eventually, however, Islamic authorities gave Islamic physicians freedom to use whatever medical treatments they wished. As a result, early Islamic Medicine focused on balancing the humors, as Hippocrates had done and Galen in the second century had refined, and incorporated influences from both Indian (Ayurveda) and Iranian Medicine.

The translation of medical knowledge from early scholars (particularly Greeks) into Arabic not only contributed to the development of Islamic Medicine, but later contributed to the development of Western Medicine up through the early Renaissance. Arabic translations occurred primarily between the seventh and tenth centuries, as Islamic physicians examined and compiled the scientific works of Hippocrates and Aristotle, Galen, and Greek scholars from Alexandria (Herophilus, Erasistratus). Eventually translated from Arabic into Latin, this medical knowledge would influence the practice of medicine for nearly 1,000 years (from 600 to 1600 CE) and reach far beyond the Middle East to Western Europe and ultimately to the Americas. For example, the Latin version of *Canon of Medicine*, authored by Islamic physician Ibn Sina, was published more than three dozen times between the fifteenth and sixteenth centuries in Europe.

Surgery in Islamic Medicine. Surgery was not commonly practiced as part of Islamic Medicine (probably due to poor results, says Nagamia). However, a number of surgical procedures were routinely performed in early Islamic societies. These included bloodletting and cauterization. Cauterization involved burning of a wound with a red hot metal rod to slow bleeding or prevent infection. Bloodletting (usually directly from veins) was part of the Galenic tradition of balancing the body's humors. "Cupping" was a form of bloodletting, and could be either wet (incision made and suction provided with a cupping glass) or dry (no incision). To prevent infection after surgery, the wound was often cleansed with wine, oil of roses, salt water, or vinegar (Pormann 2007). In the tenth century, Islamic physicians were not only treating eye diseases with medicines, but were also removing cataracts by a suction technique (see Ali Ibn Isa's "Notebook of the Oculist") (Ayad 2011).

Dissection of the body, however, was generally forbidden—since Muslims believed in the afterlife and that a vital spark (Ruh) was reawakened after death and rewarded in paradise (heaven) (Lyons and Petrucelli 1997). A passage from the early writings of Islamic physician and surgeon Al-Nafis suggests that dissection was not a common practice: "The precepts of Islamic law (shari'ah) have discouraged us from the practice of dissection (tashrih), along with whatever compassion is in our temperaments." Remarking on this passage, Savage-Smith notes that this gives no "clear sense of prohibition or interdiction, but only a general sentiment that the conventions, or perhaps rules, of the shari'ah had discouraged or deterred them (saddana) from the pursuit of dissection (mubsharat al-tashrih)" (Savage-Smith 1995, p. 100). Nevertheless, in a careful review of early Shari'ah laws, she could find nothing about dissection being forbidden.

Pharmacology in Islamic Medicine. Distinctive contributions were also made to the field of pharmacology during the Islamic Medicine period (also, see Al Kindi below). In fact, pharmacy as a distinct discipline separate from medicine was probably established for the first time under Arabic rulers during the Islamic Golden Age. Arabic techniques for identifying and purifying medicines included distillation, crystallization, sublimation, reduction, and calcination—basic processes in chemistry and pharmacy. In the late ninth century, Al-Razi's text *al-Hawi* contained a description of over 800 drugs (Nagamia 2003). In the tenth century, Al-Zahrawi wrote a book titled "Al-Tasrif" that included a section on drug preparations, compounding of drugs, and dosages. This was followed in the eleventh century by Al-Biruni's *Kjtab al-saydalah* (Book of Pharmacology) devoted entirely to drugs and dosages.

Hospitals. Another major contribution of Islamic physicians was the establishment of the hospital (also called the "bimaristan"). In fact, the first Muslim hospital service may have been located in the courtyard of the Prophet Muhammad's mosque in the city of Medina (Alam and Siddiqui 2007). The Prophet had a special tent erected in front of the mosque to provide medical aid to soldiers wounded in battle, and assigned women there to attend the wounded.

Umar ibn Al-Khattāb (634–644 CE), the second caliph after Abu Bakr (632–634 CE), supported the development of public welfare programs that included hospitals. This was paid for by the *zakat* (private contributions by individuals as required by the Qur'an). Not only did these hospitals provide care for sick patients within the building itself, but also sent physicians out into the community to provide care to those living in poorer, remote rural areas. The "ambulant" hospital was carried on camelback in caravan style with food, water, medicine, operating rooms, and a team of physicians, nurses, and other attendants. This was also useful during military campaigns. For example, the caliph sent a company of physicians protected by soldiers to the battlefield during war with Persia. The army of Ghaznavid sultan Mahmud was said to have been accompanied by a medical team carried by 40 camels (Rahman 1998, p. 67). Hospitals were also places where physicians could study and do research.

These were early efforts to provide medical care to the sick and wounded. However, Caliph Al-Walid is said to have built the first "real" hospital in Damascus around 707 CE, which was mainly for the blind who needed help getting about and for lepers to keep them away from healthy people (Miller 2006). Patients were segregated based on their condition, such that lepers had their own separate facilities. Standard hospitals that cared for patients with a range of medical and surgical conditions did not appear until the beginning of the Abbasid Caliphate in 750 CE. These early hospitals were secular, and served all people regardless of race, religion, or financial status (some hospitals even contained a chapel for Christians) (Shanks and Dawshe 1984). Patients could stay in the hospital for as long as necessary for them to get well enough so that they could return to work (Alam and Siddiqui 2007).

In the mid-eighth century, Al-Mansur, the second Abbasid caliph who founded the city of Baghdad, invited Jurjis Bukhtishu, a Christian physician and head of the medical school in Jundishapur, to treat a stomach complaint of the caliph. The treatment was a success, and the Al-Mansur gave Jurjis a position in his court. Although he soon returned to Jundishapur, his grandson Jibril (also Christian) came to Baghdad and established his medical practice there. He rose to prominence after successfully treating Caliph Harun al-Rashid's severe headaches. For his position as physician-in-chief of the main hospital in Baghdad, Jibril was paid 4.9 million dirhams ($1.3 million USD today) per year. In contrast, a doctor working at the hospital for two days and two nights a week was paid 3,600 dirhams ($972 USD) per year (Nagamia 2003). Medical schools and hospitals in Baghdad, and eventually those built by successive caliphs throughout the Muslim world, would be modeled after the medical school in Jundishapur because of Jibril's influence. A Persian Christian, Yuhanna ibn Masawaih (son of a pharmacist brought by Jibril to Baghdad from Jundishapur) eventually took Jibril's place as head of the main hospital in Baghdad. By the early tenth century, many hospitals had been built throughout the Muslim world, including those in Mecca and Medina. These were often headed by Christian physicians (Yuhanna ibn Masawaih, Abu 'Uthman al-Dimashqi, and Sinan ibn Thabit, for example) (Rahman 1998, p. 66). More on this later.

Hospitals were not only built to serve medical and surgical patients, but also to treat psychiatric patients. The first humane psychiatric hospitals (and psychiatric wards in general hospitals) were established during the ninth and tenth centuries, nearly 300 years before such institutions were founded in the West (Mohit 2001). The quality and complexity of hospitals in Jundishapur, Damascus, Baghdad, and Cairo reached their zenith during the Islamic Golden Age, surpassing even Christian hospitals in the East and the West (Lyons and Petrucelli 1997). Besides hospitals, special homes for older women and for orphans were built, and medical teams were even mobilized to visit the sick in jails. Vizier Ali ibn Isa, who served under the 18th Abbasid caliph Al-Muqtadir bi-Allah from 913 to 928 CE, was especially known for establishing hospitals and mobilizing ambulant medical teams (Rahman 1998, pp. 66–67).

The queen of all hospitals, however, was built in Cairo in 1284 CE. The Mansuri Hospital was known as the most luxurious hospital in the entire Middle East and North Africa. The Sultan himself (Mansur Qala'un) participated in its construction by bringing in artists from throughout the East to assist in its design. Patients with conditions such as fever, eye diseases, internal medicine problems, and surgical illnesses were placed on separate wards, as were men and women. The Mansuri Hospital had originally been a palace that could hold more than 8,000 people. There was a chapel for Christians and a mosque for Muslims. According to Rahman (1998, pp. 70–71), the hospital continues to operate today and specilizes in eye diseases. When patients were discharged from the hospital, it was said that they were given five pieces of gold to help them to recuperate (Lyons and Petrucelli 1997).

Islamic Physicians

As noted earlier, Islamic physicians (called *Tabib* or *Hakim*) made many original contributions to medicine, surgery, and pharmacology. This is particularly true in the area of ophthalmology. The writings and research by Ibn al-Haitham remained the most respected work on this subject until modern times (Saunders 1978). Likewise, Hunain ibn Ishaq contributed ten original works on ophthalmology.

Original contributions were also made by Islamic physicians in anatomy and physiology (pulmonary circulation), surgical techniques, infectious diseases (scabies, tuberculosis), psychology, and ethics. Many of these contributions were absorbed into Western Medicine, often without giving credit to the Islamic physicians who discovered them.

Physicians were taught to keep careful records of their treatments in the event that someone accused them of malpractice. In that event, treatment records were reviewed by their peers who would decide on the case. Prior to the existence of medical schools and teaching institutions, most physicians were educated in an apprenticeship system. Those who wanted to become doctors followed experienced physicians around, observing and copying their practices. For many years, it was the physician mentor (not an institution or certifying body) who granted a license (*ijaza*) to practice medicine to new physicians (Rahman 1998, p. 81).

Medicine was practiced primarily by Christian and Jewish physicians during the early years of Islam, a fact that al-Shafi'i (founder of the Shafi'i school of jurisprudence, one of the four Sunni schools of law) lamented in the following quote from the ninth century: "I do not know of any type of knowledge, after the knowledge of what is lawful and what is unlawful, more noble for a Muslim[to acquire] than that of medicine but, alas! They have neglected it—they have neglected one-third of human knowledge—and abandoned it to Jews and Christians" (Al-Dhahabi 1961). Early famous Islamic physicians existed in families, with the Christian Bukhtishu family being the oldest (765–801 CE). Other physician families were the Masawayh family (prolific writers and famous ophthalmologists) and the Ishaq family (first translators of Greek and Syrian medical texts into Arabic). However, Al-Kindi, Al-Tabari, Al-Ruhawi, Al-Razi, Al-Majusi, Al-Zahrawi, Ibn Sina, and Al-Nafis were the physicians who gave Islamic Medicine its reputation during Islamic Golden Age.

One of the first great Islamic physicians was **Al-Kindi** (800–870 CE), who developed a medical formulary (*Aqrabadhin*), which described the preparation of medicines from herbs and plants, animals (musk), and minerals. Besides drugs that had been used by Greek and Roman physicians, he also included medicines from Persia, Egypt, and India. Muslim physicians used an assortment of natural substances to treat patients, including sedatives and pain killers derived from the opium poppy and hemp plant (cannabis).

The first true Arabic encyclopedia of medicine (*Firdous al-Himah* or Paradise of Wisdom) was a seven-volume treatise written by **Al-Tabari** in 860 CE (Meyerhoff 1931). Al-Tabari pointed out the close relationship between psychology and medicine, making original contributions to mental healthcare in the areas of child development, psychotherapy, and counseling (Amber 2004). He also warned that while opium from poppy leaves was useful to treat pain and induce sleep, it could also kill.

One of the earliest surviving Arabic manuscripts on medical ethics is *Adab al-Tabib* (Ethics of the Physician) written in the ninth century by **Al-Ruhawi** and based on the works of Hippocrates and Galen. Interestingly, Al-Ruhawi was a Christian from the Nestorian sect and was still Christian when he wrote *Adab al-Tabib*, which was based on Muslim beliefs and principles (Levey 1967).

According to Nagamia, Al-Ruhawi "examined not only the relationships between a patient and a physician, but also a physician's personal standards of behavior, conduct of daily activities, morality and even his relationship with God" (Nagamia 2003). In *Adab al-Tabib*, Al-Ruhawi stated that it was a physician's duty to integrate spirituality into the care of the patient: "The philosopher can only improve the soul, but the virtuous physician can improve both body and soul. The physician deserves the claim that he is imitating the acts of God the Exalted as much as he can" (Levey 1967). Al-Ruhawi also recommended how a physician should start out the day (before seeing patients): "He should wash his mouth, clean and polish his teeth. Then it is necessary to examine the order of his bodily organs…His clothes should be useful and attractive. Following all this is prayer. Then he should read the book of his religion, then books of the ancients on medicine" (Rahman 1982).

Like Al-Ruhawi, many Islamic physicians viewed the practice of medicine as a holy vocation. Rahman (1998, p. 94) notes that *hakim*, the word for physician in Arabic (meaning full of knowledge and wisdom), is also one of the names of God in Islam. Ishaq the Isra'ilite, a physician who wrote a book of 50 aphorisms in the tenth century said, "Visiting and healing the poor and needy patients is your special duty because a more meritorious work you cannot perform" (Ullman 1970). According to Rahman (1998), "It is clear, then, that theologians and traditionists who wrote Prophetic Medicine works, on the one hand, and the writers of scientific medicine, on the other, valued medicine as a religious vocation of the first order because it helps men and women to help others preserve and restore health" (p. 39).

Indeed, **Al-Razi** (Rhazes in Latin) (865–925 CE) exemplified this tradition, although his approach was more broadly "spiritual" than religious. Al-Razi has been variously called the "father of Islamic Medicine" (Shuttleworth 2010), "the Galen of Arabs," and "the greatest physician of the Muslim World" (Karaman 2011). His name is probably the most recognized of all Islamic physicians. Rahman (1998, p. 94) says that Al-Razi had so many students that patients were seen first by students of his students. Failing a successful diagnosis by the secondary student, the primary student saw the patient next. If the primary student failed to make a diagnosis, the patient was finally seen by Al-Razi himself, who conducted an exhaustive examination. Born in Persia, near present-day Tehran, Iran, Al-Razi studied language and literature, philosophy, mathematics, astronomy, and medicine. He wrote over 200 books, including a 23-volume treatise, *Kitab al-Hawi fi al-tibb* (*al-Hawi*) (Comprehensive Book of Medicine) that brought together all the Islamic medical knowledge of his time. This text would become a primary source for Western Medicine up through the seventeenth century. In fact, a copy of *al-Hawi* resides in the U.S. National Library of Medicine and is considered one of the oldest medical manuscripts in the world in existence today. This book contains a summary of Greek, Syrian, Hindu, Persian, and early Arabic Medicine, all of which Al-Razi was trained in. He was also a scientist who conducted medical research that involved observation and experimentation. Nearly 1,000 years before the germ theory of disease, Al-Razi was convinced that such diseases as smallpox and measles resulted from something in the blood (infection).

Not only a rigorous scientist, Al-Razi was a true clinician, emphasizing the important role that the psychological state of the patient played in their health. In *al-Hawi*, he wrote: "The physician, even though he has his doubts, must always make the patient believe that he will recover, for the state of the body is linked to the state of the mind" (Tibi 2006). His approach to treating patients underscored the importance of trust between physician and patient. The physician was obligated to care for the patient, but the patient was also obligated to comply with the treatments prescribed by the physician. Included in his medical evaluation were questions about the patient's background and any illnesses suffered by family members. Al-Razi's book on medical ethics (*Ahlaq al-Tabeeb* or "Ethics of a Doctor") is a classic. He discussed here how the physician should behave toward patients, presenting a model for ethical behavior by Islamic physicians. Because all religions respect physicians, Al-Razi emphasized that doctors should take pride in their profession and practice it in a way that deserved this high calling.

Al-Razi also wrote a book titled *Al-Tibb al Rawhani* (Spiritual Medicine). Because both medicine and philosophy are closely related to Islamic values, he believed the physician has several responsibilities to the patient. First, the doctor should treat the patient with kindness patience, concern, and professional confidence. Second, physicians should be themselves good and ethical people, otherwise their treatments will not be effective. Third, unless a patient has good morals, he or she cannot be physically healthy either. Thus, Al-Razi believed that good moral health in both the physician and the patient was essential for successful treatment (Rahman 1998, p. 96).

Despite his sensitivity to physician ethics and emphasis on providing free care to the poor, Al-Razi distanced himself to some degree from religion. Although he believed in God, it is said that he rejected formal religion and many of the core teachings of Islam. In an article published on *Muslim Philosophy Online*, Goodman describes a debate in which "Al-Razi answers that God has provided what we need to know, not in the arbitrary and divisive gift of special revelation, which only foments bloodshed and contention, but in reason, which belongs equally to all. Prophets are impostors, at best misled by the demonic shades of restless and envious spirits. But ordinary men are fully capable of thinking for themselves and need no guidance from another" (Goodman 1999).

Fazlur Rahman (1998) challenges critics of Al-Razi who claim that he was not a religious man, that he denied the Prophet Muhammad, and that he did not believe in revelation. Rahman points out (pp. 99–100) that some of what Al-Razi said came out in the heat of debate while defending himself. In fact, the statements by Al-Razi quoted above were made during a famous debate with a conservative Ismaili religious leader, and he was responding to that person's esoteric doctrine involving Al-Talim and electionism. There is no doubt that Al-Razi believed that in order to fully understand a patient, the physician needs to understand both the physical and the spiritual aspects of the person (Karaman 2011). He said that the physical nature involved physical disorders, whereas the spiritual nature involved issues related to the spiritual self, i.e., moral diseases. In Spiritual Medicine, Al-Razi advocated caring for the whole patient and even includes a section on meditation. While he focuses primarily on morality, ethics, and reason in this book, and largely avoids religion, Al-Razi does say that those who live according to their religion have nothing to fear in death. He emphasized that if persons should have doubts about their religion and are unable to establish its truth for themselves, then God is merciful and will forgive them. He notes that God never burdens someone beyond their capacity, and in fact, demands much less of humans than they can usually do (citing 2:286; 6:152, and 7:42 in the Qur'an, which all say that God does not burden people with more than what they can bear) (Rahman 1998, p. 99).

The next great Islamic physician, born in the famous medical city of Jundishapur and of Zoroastrianism faith, was **Al-Majusi** (Haly Abbas in Latin) (930–994 CE). He authored the *Kitab al-Malaki* (The Royal Book), which was one of the earliest illustrations of surgical approaches to skull fractures and other disorders. The text also discussed many internal diseases, their causes and treatments. Al-Majusi was a Persian physician and psychologist whose *Kitab al-Malaki* was considered superior in some respects to Al-Razi's Comprehensive Book of Medicine that preceded it and Ibn Sina's Canon of Medicine that followed. Al-Majusi was probably one of the three greatest physicians of the Islamic empire during this period. *Kitab al-Malaki* was used as a basic text at the medical school in Salerno, the center of medical training in Europe between the tenth and thirteenth centuries. Al-Majusi served as a royal physician during the Buwayhid dynasty in Baghdad. His frequent references to Allah in his writings suggest that he was a deeply religious man (Amber 2004).

A contemporary of Al-Majusi's was **Al-Zahrawi** (Albucasis in Latin) (930–1013 CE). Born in Cordoba, Spain, he was an Islamic physician known for his *al-Tasrif*, a 30-volume medical and surgical text. Considered by many to be the "father of modern surgery," Al-Zahrawi's text is one of the oldest books with illustrations of surgical instruments. In it he described many different operations, including those for varicose veins, skull fractures, removing teeth, forceps deliveries, and a host of others. *Al-Tasrif* was considered more systematic and practical than any other medical text of the time. Serving as a court physician to Al-Hakam II (the Adnalusian caliph of the Western Islamic empire), he is listed as one of the greatest physicians in Moorish Spain. His influence was felt throughout the East and the West, and his writings continue to influence the practice of surgery even today (Belen and Aciduman 2006). Al-Zahrawi discovered the hereditary nature of hemophilia and was the first to accurately describe ectopic pregnancy.

Ibn Sina (Avicenna in Latin) (980–1037 CE) was a great Islamic scholar who was a physician and teacher. According to Nagamia, Ibn Sina was the greatest physician of the Islamic era and possibly the greatest physician of all time, greater even than Al-Razi (Nagamia 2003). This claim is based on Ibn Sina's well-rounded education in many areas of science as well as religion, philosophy, metaphysics, and logic. He is said to have memorized the entire Qur'an by the age of 10 years. Born in Bokhara (present-day Uzbekistan in central Asia), he wrote over 100 books almost all in Arabic and nearly 450 treatises, of which 40 were on medicine. His most famous work was the five-volume *Kitab al-Qanun fi al-Tibb* (Canon of Medicine), which would later be translated into Latin and serve (along with Al-Razi's *al-Hawi*) as the basis for European Medicine. The Canon was a primary textbook taught in European medical schools up through the seventeenth century. Nagamia (2003) quotes a professor of history at the U.S. National Library of Medicine as saying: "The medicine of the day was so brilliantly clarified by these compendia (especially those of Ibn Sina and Al-Majusi) and such order and consistency was brought to it that a sense of perfection and hence stultifying authority resulted" (p. 27).

The Cannon presented basic medical principles, discussed medicines used to treat illnesses, described organ-specific diseases and more general systemic illnesses, and addressed the prevention of illness. Ibn Sina emphasized checking the pulse and the color, cloudiness, and smell of a patient's urine. He also stressed the need to give pure water to infants, and described the diseases that could result from failing to do. He, like Al-Razi, hypothesized that many diseases might be transmitted through the air. Ibn Sina carefully described common diseases of his day such as guinea worm infection, trigeminal neuralgia, and different types of facial paralysis.

Ibn Sina also addressed the area of the mind, and described a number of psychiatric illnesses. However, his perspective was different from Al-Razi's when it came to religion. In his *Kitab al-shifa'* (Book of Healing), he discusses logic, the natural sciences, mathematics, and metaphysics. A deeply religious man, the first problem Ibn Sina tackles in this book is the existence of God based on intuition and reason, presenting both ontological and cosmological arguments to prove the existence of God. While describing a scientific and mathematical theory of the world, he attributed ultimate causation of everything to God (the "first cause"). Ibn Sina argued that that since the soul is incorporeal, it must be immortal and that the decay and destruction of the body did not affect the soul. When his works were translated into Latin, they were said to influence many Christian philosophers including Thomas Aquinas (Kemal 2001).

Ibn Sina's approach is illustrated in the concluding paragraph of his four-volume text titled *Remarks and Admonitions*: "O Brother. In these remarks I have brought forth to you the cream of truth and, bit by bit, I have fed you in sensitive words the best pieces of wisdom (p. 904). Therefore, protect this truth from ignorance, the vulgar, those who are not endowed with sharpness of mind, with skill and experience, those who lend an ear to the crowds, and who have gone astray from philosophy and fallen behind. Thus, if you find a person whose purity of heart and goodness of conduct you can trust, as well as his suspending judgement on that to which doubt hastens (p. 905) and his viewing the truth with the eye of satisfaction and honesty, then gradually, and in bits and pieces, give him the truth he requests, carefully observing what you get from what you have already given (p. 906). Ask him to heed God and the inescapable faith, following your manner in what you give him and taking you as an example. If you divulge or lose this knowledge, God will be the arbitrator between you and me. God is sufficient as a trustee" (Inati 1996, pp. 107–108).

In summarizing the contributions of Islamic physicians, well-known Islamic scholar A.S.B. Ansari notes, "The art of healing was dead, Galen revived it; it was scattered and dis-arrayed, Razi re-arranged and re-aligned it; it was incomplete, Ibn Sina perfected it" (Ansari 1976).

Among the last great Islamic physicians of this period was **Al-Nafis** (1213–1288 CE), who was born in Syria, and studied medicine, law, philosophy, and theology at the medical school in Damascus (Shuttleworth 2010). He focused on the respiratory and cardiovascular systems, particularly the route that blood took from the heart to the lungs. Al-Nafis discovered that blood flowed from the heart to the lungs via the pulmonary circulation, where it was then "purified." This idea challenged Galen's notion that the blood flowed directly from the right side to the left side of the heart through invisible pores in the septum. Al-Nafis' observations came from detailed dissection, although not of the human body (to avoid conflict with his own religious beliefs). He also tried to integrate theology with anatomy, believing that the heart was the place where "spirit" was put into the blood, and that the pumping of the blood was necessary to disperse the invisible spirit throughout the body. His ideas about the heart and lungs could have greatly advanced Western Medicine had scientists been aware of his teachings, which were not widely disseminated. It was not until William Harvey's discoveries in 1628 CE that the work of Al-Nafis was brought to the attention of others. It was not until the microscope was used by Antonie van Leeuwenhoek to study the lungs in 1676 CE that Al-Nafis' observations were confirmed by directly viewing the pulmonary capillaries.

Unlike in the West, a more holistic view of the person and their medical or psychiatric illnesses developed among Islamic physicians, who were influenced by Indian philosophy and Muslim mystical thinkers (Mohit 2001). More and more, the human body and mind became viewed as a product of interactions between body, emotions, diet, soul, society, and behavior, all of which had to be evaluated in order to determine how to treat an illness. As noted earlier in this chapter, many Islamic physicians of this period believed that the person was not just made up of the physical body alone, but contained a life force—the Ruh (spirit or soul)—which enabled the body to function (Nagamia 2003). They believed that the Ruh came from the Almighty (God) to make the human person complete. Thus, Islamic physicians insisted that the Ruh had to be taken into account when treating a patient. The Ruh is mentioned in the Qur'an (17:85): "And they ask you (O Muhammad) concerning the Ruh (the Spirit); Say: 'The Ruh (the Spirit) is one of the things, the knowledge, you (mankind) have been given only a little'" (Al-Hilali and Khan 1996).

Period of Decline

Many factors, both political and environmental, led to a decline in Islamic Medicine and the Islamic Golden Age more generally, beginning in the thirteenth century. One factor was the corruption of rulers who had absolute power, which weakened the empire and made it more vulnerable to enemy invasions. Starting in the Central Asian steppes, Mongols led by the notorious leader Genghis Khan combined forces with the Turks in historical Mongolia, forming the Mongol empire in 1206. Mongol forces spread rapidly to Eastern Europe, covering large parts of Siberia to the north, Southeast Asia to the south, the Indian subcontinent, and penetrating deep into the Middle East.

This culminated in the invasion of the Eastern Islamic empire and in 1258, the takeover of Baghdad, the Abbasid capital and intellectual center. Mongols decimated the region, destroying universities, hospitals, and libraries, reversing many of the scientific and cultural achievements of the Islamic Golden Age. These events were understood by traditionalist Muslims as God's retribution against the people and their leaders for straying from the Sunnah (a view even maintained by the prominent physician and anatomist Al-Nafis) (Beg 2006). Interestingly, within 50 years of their invasion of Baghdad the Mongol conquerors had adopted Islam as their religion.

Many prominent scholars and doctors fled to India at this time, shifting the center of medical learning from the Middle East to this region of the world. According to Rahman (1998, p. 73), the Muslim Turkish Sultans of India—Muhammad ibn Tughlaq (1325–1351) and his successor Firuz Shah Tughlaq (1351–1388)—were physicians who built a broad complex of hospitals and medical clinics in Delhi. However, the quality of medicine declined substantially in Muslim regions after the Mongol invasions. Under the Mongol rulers, medicine was taught largely in religious schools (*madrasas*), which may have discouraged scientific research and progress, while favoring the integration of religion into medical care.

Although the Persian and Turkish Ottoman empires were able to largely hold their own against the Mongolians during this period, other regions of the Middle East were not so fortunate. Mongol rulers blocked the Industrialization and rapid technological advances in Islamic areas that were then taking place in the West. Mohit (2001) notes "no account of any meaningful system of care of ordinary people exists from this area… For example, in Iran during the Qajar dynasty between the seventeenth and late nineteenth centuries, there was an era of unprecedented decline and ignorance. Magic, superstition and fatalistic, rather hopeless attitude replaced the scientific approach to health and disease. The condition in Egypt was more or less the same" (p. 343).

The rise of the second Persian empire also contributed to the decline of the Golden Age. Beginning in 633 CE, the Islamic Arab armies began raiding the Persian Sassanid empire, and by 644, under the direction of Caliph Umar, they had completely conquered the Sassanids and soon the Persian lands were under firm Muslim control. With decline of the Islamic empire, however, Persia began to reassert itself as an independent state, and fought vigorously to maintain control and expand its influence in the region. From 1501 to 1979 (the year of the Iranian revolution), Persia was ruled by a succession of kingdoms including the Safavid, Afsharid, Zand, Qajar, and Pahlavi dynasties. From 1514 to 1823 CE, a series of 12 wars occurred between the Persian and Ottoman empires, but Persia (present-day Iran) remained under its own rulers. These wars, however, decimated many centers of learning and brought scientific progress in medicine to a standstill.

There were perhaps others reasons as well for the decline of the Islamic sciences. Admittedly, the 13 crusades led by European Christian powers against the "infidel" Muslims between 1095 and 1295 CE did not help. Another factor was the rising conflict between Sunni and Shia Muslims. Although many claim that the rise of the West led to a decline in the Islamic Golden Age of scientific and medical achievements, the reverse was more likely. In other words, it was the decline of the Islamic empire that allowed the West to rise. With the fall of the Western Islamic empire in Spain (1492 CE) came the takeover by the West of much of the scientific and medical information accumulated by Muslims. This literature would serve as the foundation for the Renaissance in Europe and the Scientific Revolution in the eighteenth and nineteenth centuries.

The Eastern Islamic empire (which was the center of the Golden Islamic Age) was followed by the Ottoman empire, which lasted for over 600 years from 1299 to 1922 CE and did not value scientific progress and achievement as did its predecessors. A major turning point in the spread of the Ottoman empire was in 1453 CE with the conquering of Constantinople, the capital of the Byzantine Christian Roman empire. Although virtually destroyed during the war, the city was rebuilt and renamed Istanbul (city of Islam). The religion of the Ottoman empire had long been Islam (since 751 CE) and the rule was by Shari'ah law. The sultan was the highest position in the government, and also claimed the position of caliphate, the highest position in Islam. The Ottomans would expand until it peaked in 1520–1566 CE, when the empire controlled large parts of Western Asia, Southeastern Europe, Northern Africa, and much of the Middle East. While the primary religion of the empire was Muslim, the Ottomans were "uniquely" tolerant of people from other religions including the Orthodox Christians and Jews (many non-Muslims continued to be governed by the Greek Orthodox millet system). Unfortunately, there was a relative neglect of science, technology, and medicine in the lands that the Ottoman Turks controlled.

In 1838, the Ottoman sultan established the first Western-style medical school in Istanbul, staffed by Europeans. These westerners argued that the Islamic medical tradition had become outdated. Other Muslims countries soon followed the lead of the Turks. Only in India and Pakistan did the traditions of Islamic and Hindu Medicine survive (Rahman 1998, pp. 131–132).

During the decline and eventual end of the Ottoman empire between 1828 and 1922 CE, European Christian missionary doctors (and colonial armies) began to slowly bring modern scientific medicine into the region. With the growing influence of Western colonialism, the Islamic world was divided into a number of separate independent countries (see below). For some countries, this resulted in European influences on government styles, including the adoption of constitutional models and social changes that included a growing acceptance of Western medical treatments. This was followed by the establishment of public outpatient clinics and hospitals, and a decline in traditional or local forms of treatment. Leaders from Egypt and Iran began a constructive dialogue with Western countries, helping to develop science and technology in their regions. Modern hospitals began to be established, modeled after European hospitals. Islamic Medicine was affected by the rapid spread of Western conventional medicine, which eventually replaced it in most Muslim countries. The practice of traditional Islamic Medicine is now limited to India, Pakistan, and Bangladesh, which continue to have medical schools that teach it, known as "Unani" or "Tibi" medicine (Nagamia 2003).

At the end of World War I in 1922, the Ottoman monarchy was abolished with the signing of the Treaty of Lausanne between Turkey and the allied powers.

With this treaty (and other treaties during the 10 years that preceded it), the lands controlled by the Ottoman empire became independent countries. These include Cyprus, Greece, Romania, Bulgaria, Hungary, Egypt, Palestine, Jordan, Lebanon, Sudan, Syria, Lybia, Iraq, Yemen, and Saudi Arabia (Asir and Hejaz). Since the 1940s, Muslim countries have gradually established their independence from Western colonialism, although according to Rahman, they are *culturally* still under the domination of the West (Rahman 1998, p. 133). Nagamia (n.d.) says that Islamic nations are now in the "dark ages" (p. 7) from which they need to emerge (but on their own terms).

Today, most Muslims see physicians for modern treatments, although continue to rely on their religious beliefs to meet social, cultural, and spiritual needs. Religious beliefs continue to have a strong influence on personal hygiene, diet, alcohol use, tobacco use, and eating, as well as on a variety of health practices across the life span from conception to death (see Chap. 3).

Summary and Conclusions

Religion, medicine, and healthcare have been closely linked throughout the 1400-year history of Islam. Islamic physicians made seminal contributions to the field of medicine through accumulation, preservation, and translation of earlier Greek, Roman, Indian, Syrian, Chinese, Persian, and Byzantine medical texts into Arabic, as well as by their seminal original contributions in many areas of medicine, surgery, and pharmacology. The translation of Arabic texts into Latin and English would later serve as the basis for Western Medicine and for the scientific discoveries that followed and led to a renaissance of learning and discovery in Europe. Many of the first and best hospitals, including those for patients with psychiatric illness, were built during the Islamic Golden Age, and the patients in those facilities were treated in ways that modern hospitals today can only envy. Wars and invasions over the last 700 years have led to the decline of the Islamic Golden Age and Islamic Medicine, resulting in stagnation of science and technology. For over 1,400 years, Islam was a dominant force that directed the evolution of medicine and healthcare in the East and the West, and while its influence has waned some during the past few centuries, its recent growth and spread suggests a bright future ahead—if it can advance in science, medicine, and healthcare on its own cultural and religious terms.

References

Abdullah, A. R. (Trans.) (2003). *Healing with the medicine of the Prophet* (by Imam Ibn Quayyim Al-Jauziyah, written in the 14th century). Houston, TX: Dar-us-Salam Publications.

Alam, M. S., & Siddiqui, M. K. (2007). Development of health sciences and related institutions during the first six centuries of Islam. *The CDR Journal, 3*, 51–63.

Al-Dhahabi, M. I. (1961). *Al-Tibb al-Nabawi (prophetic medicine)* (pp. 107–108). Cairo, Egypt: Mutafā al-Halabī.

Al-Hilali, M. T., & Khan, M. M. (Trans.) (1996). *The Noble Qur'an*. Riyadh, Saudi Arabia: Darussalam.

Al-Tamimi, A.-H. (n.d.). *Khawass al-Qur'an* [Properties of the Qur'an]. Referred to by Fazlur Rahman (1998). Health and Medicine in the Islamic Tradition (p. 89). Chicago, IL: ABC International Group (Kazi Publications).

Amber, H. (2004). Psychology from Islamic perspective: Contributions of early Muslim scholars and challenges to contempoary Muslim psychologists. *Journal of Religion and Health, 43*(4), 357–377.

Ansari, A. S. B. (1976). Abu Bakr Muhammad Ibn Yahya: Universal scholar and scientist. *Islamic Studies, 15*(3), 155–156.

Armstrong, K. (2002). *Islam: A short history*. New York: Random House.

Avalos, H. (1995). *Illness and health care in the ancient near east: The role of the temple in greece, mesopotamia, and israel (harvard semitic monographs)*. Atlanta, GA: Scholars Press.

Ayad, A. (2008). *Healing body & soul*. Riyadh, Saudi Arabia: International Islamic Publishing House.

Ayad, A. (2011). *History of medicine in Islamic civilization*. Retrieved October 3, 2013, from http://www.onislam.net/english/health-and-science/faith-and-the-sciences/454994-history-of-medicine-in-the-islamic-civilization.html?the_Sciences=

Beg, M. A. (2006). *Decline of Islamic civilizations—causes—time for a new paradigm*. Countercurrents.org. Retrieved October 3, 2013, from http://www.countercurrents.org/beg-250706.htm

Belen, D., & Aciduman, A. (2006). A pioneer from the Islamic gold age: Haly Abbas and spinal traumas in his principal work, the royal book. *Journal of Neurosurgery: Spine, 5*, 381–383.

Chaucer, G. (1387–1400) (1957). The Canterbury Tales. In *The works of Geoffrey Chaucer*. Boston, MA: Houghton Mifflin. Retrieved from October 3, 2013, from http://www.nlm.nih.gov/exhibition/islamic_medical/islamic_02.html

Foltz, R. (2011). Zoroastrians in Iran: What future in the homeland? *Middle East Journal, 65*(1), 73–84. (See also BBC Religions). Retrieved October 3, 2013, from http://www.bbc.co.uk/religion/religions/zoroastrian/history/zoroaster_1.shtml.

Goodman, L. E. (1999). *Al-Razi (Rhazes)*. Retrieved October 3, 2013, from http://www.muslimphilosophy.com/ei2/razi.htm (original source: Encyclopedia of Islam. Leiden, The Netherlands: Koninklijke Brill NV, 1999).

Gregorian, V. (2003). *Islam: A mosaic, not a monolith* (pp. 26–38). Washington, DC: Brookings Institution Press.

Heidel, A. (1963). *The Gilgamesh epic and old testament parallels*. Chicago: University of Chicago Press.

Inati, S. (Trans.) (1996). A closing comment and a wish (chapter 32, closing chapter). In *Ibn Sina and mysticism: Remarks and admonitions: Part Four*. London: Kegan Paul International. Retrieved October 3, 2013, from http://www.muslimphilosophy.com/books/inati2.pdf

Karaman, H. (2011). Abu Bakr al-Razi (Rhazes) and medical ethics. *OMUIFD: Ondokuz Mayis University Review of the Faculty of Divini, 30*, 77–87.

Kemal, S. (2001). *Ibn Sina—Abu Ali al-Husayn (980-1037)*. Islamic Philosophy Online. Retrieved October 3, 2013, from http://www.muslimphilosophy.com/sina/art/ibn Sina-REP.htm

Levey, M. (1967). Medical ethics of medieval Islam with special reference to Al-Ruhawi's 'practical ethics of the physician'. *Transactions of the American Philosophical Society, 57*, 1–100.

Lyons, A. S., & Petrucelli, R. J. (1997). *Medicine: An illustrated history*. New York: Harry N. Abrams. (Also see: Medicine under Islam: Arabic Medicine). Retrieved October 3, 2013, from http://www.healthguidance.org/entry/6344/1/Medicine-under-Islam-Arabic-Medicine.html

Meyerhoff, M. (1931). Alî at-Tabarî's "paradise of wisdom", one of the oldest Arabic compendiums of medicine. *ISIS: Journal of the History of Science Society, 16*, 6–54.

Miller, A. C. (2006). Jundi-Shapur, bimaristans, and the rise of academic medical centres. *Journal of the Royal Society of Medicine, 99*(12), 615–617.

Mohit, A. (2001). Mental health and psychiatry in the Middle East: Historical development. *Eastern Mediterranean Health Journal, 7*(3), 336–347.
Nagamia, H. F. (2003). Islamic medicine history and current practice. *Journal of the International Society of Islamic Medicine, 2*, 19–30.
Nagamia, H. F. (n.d.). *A museum and library of Islamic Medical History: A new perspective*. Retrieved October 3, 2013, from http://www.iiim.org/Files/Museum and Library/Museum_and_Library.pdf
Oyewole, Y. (2006). Healing in Islam. Cited in Rodlach A, Dilly B (2011). Religion, health, and healing: An interdisciplinary inquiry. *Journal of Religion & Society*, (Suppl. 7), 150–168.
Paulissian, R. (1991). Medicine in ancient Assyrian and Babylonia. *Journal of Assyrian and Academic Studies, 5*(1), 3–51.
Pormann, P. (2007). *Medieval Islamic medicine* (pp. 115–138). Washington, DC: Georgetown University Press.
Rahman, F. (1982, Winter). Islam and health. *Hamdard Islamicus, 5*, 81.
Rahman, F. (1998). *Health and medicine in the Islamic tradition*. Chicago, IL: ABC International Group (Kazi Publications).
Saunders, J. J. (1978). *A history of medieval Islam* (p. 193). London: Routledge.
Savage-Smith, E. (1995). Attitudes toward dissection in medieval Islam. *Journal of the History of Medicine and Allied Sciences, 50*, 67–110.
Shanks, N. J., & Dawshe, A. K. (1984). Arabian medicine in the middle ages. *Journal of the Royal Society of Medicine, 77*(1), 60–65.
Shuttleworth, M. (2010). *Islamic medicine. Explorable*. Retrieved October 3, 2013, from http://explorable.com/islamic-medicine.html
Taylor, G. M. (2010). *The physicians of Judishapur*. Irvine, CA: University of California.
Thompson, T. L. (2002). *The historicity of the patriarchal narratives* (p. 15). Harrisburg, PA: Trinity Press.
Thomson, A. (Trans.) (2009). *Medicine of the Prophet* (by Jalal As-Suyuti, written in the 15th century). London: TA-HA Publications.
Tibi, S. (2006). Al-Razi and Islamic medicine in the 9th century. *Journal of the Royal Society of Medicine, 99*(4), 206–207.
Ullman, M. (1970). *Die Medizin im Islam: Handbuch der Orientalistik* (p. 224). Leiden, The Netherlands: E.J. Brill. (Referred to by Fazlur Rahman (1998). Health and Medicine in the Islamic Tradition, Chicago, IL: ABC International Group, Inc. (Kazi Publications), p. 93).
Van Der Toorn, K., Becking, B., & Van Der Horst, P. W. (1999). *Dictionary of deities and demons in the Bible* (2nd ed.). Grand Rapids, MI: Wm. B. Eerdmans Publishing Company.
Wisseman, S. U. (2003). *The virtual mummy* (p. 5). Champaigne, IL: University of Illinois Press.

Chapter 2
Muslim Beliefs, Practices, and Values

In order to understand how and why religiosity (degree of and commitment to religious faith) in Islam might influence health, we need to examine the beliefs, practices, and values of those who call themselves Muslims.

Islam is the religion of an estimated 1.6 billion persons worldwide, including the majority of the population in at least 57 countries (Miller 2009). In 2010, countries with the most Muslims were Indonesia (205 million or 13 % of all Muslims), Pakistan (178 million), India (177 million), Bangladesh (148 million), Egypt (80 million), Turkey (75 million), and Iran (75 million). This means that only 20 % of the world's Muslim population lives in the Middle East proper. For comparison, there are only 2.6 million Muslims in the USA and 2.9 million in the UK (Pew Forum 2011).

The word "islam" in a religious context means voluntary submission to God. Islam is divided into two major branches, Sunni (80–90 %) and Shia (10–15 %). A third branch, Sufism (5 % of Muslims today) arose in the twelfth–thirteenth centuries. Sufis may be either Sunni or Shia. Sufism represents the mystical arm of Islam, and emphasizes reliance on the will of God and focusing attention on the inner self. It is known as one of the Islamic groups most tolerant to other religions (Rahman 1998, p. 31). The Sunni branch of Islam has four major schools of religious jurisprudence or law: Hanafi, Maliki, Shafii, and Hanbali. The Hanafi school (representing reason) is the largest, and most adherents live in southern Asia. Hanbali represents the most conservative school, whose adherents live primarily in Saudi Arabia and Qatar. Wahhabi, considered the most conservative Muslims, is a small branch of the Hanbali school. The more moderate Maliki school is widespread in northern and western Africa, while the Shafii school is more dominant in Malaysia and East Africa.

The word Sunni refers to those who follow and maintain the teachings and actions (*Sunnah*) of the Prophet Muhammad. Sunni Muslims revere Abu Bakr as the closest companion of the Prophet and consider him the first caliph (successor) after the Prophet Muhammad. Selected by a group of the Prophet's companions, Abu Bakr was the father-in-law of the Prophet and one of his closest friends.

H.G. Koenig and S. Al Shohaib, *Health and Well-Being in Islamic Societies: Background, Research, and Applications*, DOI 10.1007/978-3-319-05873-3_2,

He was followed as caliph by Ibn al-Khattāb, Ibn Affan, and Ibn Abu Talib, who together make up the four "rightly guided caliphs" in the Sunni tradition.

Belief in the above successorship is one factor that distinguishes Sunni from Shia Muslims, who believe that Ali, the Prophet's son-in-law and cousin, was his rightful successor and first caliph. Shia believe that only God has the right to choose a successor to the Prophet, since the successor is responsible for safeguarding Islam, the Qur'an, and shari'ah law. The origin of the split between Sunni and Shia is a complex one, based in part on this line of succession and who should be revered (Armstrong 2002). The Shia branch consists of three major schools of jurisprudence: Twelver, Zaidi, and Ismaili. The Twelver school originated from the 12 imams or supreme religious–political leaders in early Islam who are believed by adherents to be infallible (Rahman 1998, p. 3). This school has the most adherents (85 % of Shia Muslims) and makes up the majority of the population in Iran (90 %), Iraq, Azerbaijan, and Bahrain. The Twelvers believe that the descendants of the Prophet through his daughter Fatima and son-in-law Ali are the best source of knowledge about the Qur'an and shari'ah and are those who are most worthy of respect and honor.

Although the differences that separate the two largest branches of Islam, i.e., Sunni and Shia, are numerous and complicated, many of the beliefs and traditions of Sunni and Shia Muslims are similar. Therefore, we make no effort to further distinguish Sunni from Shia beliefs and practices in our descriptions. However, given that the overwhelming majority of Muslims are Sunni, the beliefs and traditions discussed below lean more toward this branch of Islam.

Islamic beliefs and practices are based on the Qur'an, the Hadith (sayings of the Prophet reported by others), Sunnah (doings of the Prophet reported by others), and the opinions of early jurists based on their interpretation of the Qur'an, Hadith, and Sunnah (Alsharif et al. 2011). Islamic beliefs and practices are strongly related since devout Muslims do what they think is right and seek to avoid what is wrong in terms of behavior. The five core beliefs (pillars) of Islam are (1) the creed of belief (*shahada*), (2) daily prayers (*salah*), (3) giving to the poor (*zakat*), (4) fasting during Ramadan (*sawm*), and (5) pilgrimage to Mecca (*hajj*). These are required for all believers and are the basis for Muslim life. The deeper the belief, the stronger the practice. Devoutness of belief can grow stronger or weaker with time depending on circumstances, and this may both influence health and be influenced by health.

Islamic Beliefs

The Islamic creed of belief (confession of faith) in Arabic is *lā ilāha illā l-Lāh, Muhammad rasūlu l-Lāh*. Translating, this means "There is no god but God, Muhammad is the messenger of God." This statement emphasizes belief in the oneness (*tawhid*) of God and the acceptance of Muhammad as God's messenger and final prophet. A sincere declaration of this statement is required for anyone to be considered a Muslim. There are six articles of faith in Islam: (1) belief in God,

(2) belief in the Prophets, (3) belief in Divine Books, (4) belief in the Day of Judgement, (5) belief in Angels, and (6) belief in Destiny or fate (*qadr*). Besides these core beliefs, other important beliefs include those regarding life after death, intercession, and the role of the individual. We now describe each of these beliefs in greater depth.

Belief in God. Allah is Arabic for God (literally "the God"). While the Qur'an does not discuss the nature of God per se, He is the basis for all of the teachings in the Qur'an that guide human conduct. Without God, nothing can exist or operate in the universe. Rahman (1998) notes that the relationship qualities of God with respect to humans are "creation, sustenance [love], guidance, and judgement" (p. 11). God is the creator, the infinitely merciful who knows everything. He is the first and the last, the Alpha and the Omega. He does everything for the good of people and nothing in the world is due to chance. God is wise and merciful, but also judges and His punishment can be severe. God sees everything humans do, hears everything, controls everything, and nothing happens against His will. At the same time, people have free choice to do things either according to God's will or against it, and are responsible for those choices. God is merciful to all people, both good and bad, but does not like what bad people do. God created both good and bad people for a purpose. Life is viewed as a kind of test. It is not easy for believers to do their duty and there are many challenges to overcome. One of those challenges is dealing with the actions of those who have gone astray, who need to be shown the right way.

God wants the best for all people, and so the true believer in God will be supported by their belief, which may relieve stress as the person accepts those aspects of life that he or she cannot control. If people choose to follow the will of God and surrender their lives to Him, then it is believed that they will find favor with others as well. Each person carries a great responsibility—the responsibility of being the best person he or she can be. This is dependent, however, on the person's choices (see The Individual below).

Beliefs about God may have psychological consequences. When people feel that they are connected to God, whom they believe has unlimited power and is infinitely merciful, this helps them to relax and makes them more optimistic. This may help them feel that the unfairness they see in the world will not continue forever and that distressing and apparently bad events also have a purpose. While those events may seem terrible and hurt on first glance, they may not turn out to be so bad if people are patient and examine the events more deeply. Knowing God in Islam is considered a gift by itself that will help the individual to have patience and understanding. Muslims believe that God cares for people and will help them, but they must work hard to do right and be optimistic. God is most able to help those who work hard and expect the best. This belief helps create motivation to overcome obstacles and endure bad times based on the faith that good will result because God is in control.

Belief in the Prophets. The Prophet Muhammad (literally "praiseworthy") was born in approximately 570 CE in Mecca. He had no formal education. While meditating in a cave, the angel Gabriel appeared to the Prophet and gave him revelations (*Wahy*).

According to Islamic expert Seyyed Hossein Nasr, "revelation" is a direct conveying of a message from Heaven that comes to prophets alone, and is distinguished from a similar concept, "inspiration," which is available to everyone (Nasr 2002). The angel Gabriel commanded the Prophet to let others know about the revelations, and so he shared them with others who wrote down what the angel said to him, resulting in the Holy Qur'an. When the Prophet first began receiving revelations in 610 CE, most of Arabia was polytheistic and worshiped many different gods (idols, angels, the sun, moon, and other lesser gods). The angel told him that there was only one God. Throughout his life the Prophet would proclaim and insist that there was only one God and that people were to surrender their lives to Him (*islam*). Muslims consider the Prophet Muhammad an exemplar and seek to emulate his life and deeds. This means following the Holy Qur'an, and adhering to the Prophet's sayings as reported by others in the Hadith and his actions in the Sunnah.

The prophets in Islam (the Prophet Muhammad and other prophets) are considered perfect human models (although are not necessarily sinless) (Omar 1993). They worship God and live in the best way. Muslims believe that a prophet is a special creation by God, but would never ask people to worship anyone except God. The fact that prophets are human beings means it is possible for people to follow their guidance and live the way they do. Although regular people cannot be as perfect as prophets, everyone can learn from them and seek to follow their teachings. A prophet demonstrates how people should live at home and treat their families, how to help other people at work, and even how to run a country. Muslims believe that if prophets were not human beings (i.e., were angels or other supernatural beings), then it would not be possible for regular people to do what the prophets have done. Because prophets are humans, this means that people have the ability to live like them. Muslims believe that the Prophet Muhammad was the last and final prophet in a long line of messengers from God that started with Adam (including Noah, Abraham, Ishmael, Jacob, Moses, David, Elijah, and John the Baptist, among others). Also on this list of prophets is Jesus the Christ or Messiah (*Isa al-Mesiah*), who is considered to be the only prophet to have been raised up to heaven by God (3:55). He is believed to be the last prophet before the appearance of the Prophet Muhammad.

Divine Books. In Islam, the Holy Qur'an is the infallible Word of God. Muslims believe that it was dictated directly to the Prophet Muhammad by the angel Gabriel reading from the original "mother book" that resides in Heaven inscribed in Arabic on stone tablets. The Qur'an is believed to have come directly from God, and it is considered blasphemous to attribute the Qur'an to the Prophet Muhammad. The Qur'an is arranged into 114 numbered *suras* (chapters) that contain numbered verses (*ayas*).

A second source of Islamic teaching is the Hadith and Sunnah recorded after the Prophet's death. As noted above, the Hadith involve reports about the sayings and approvals of the Prophet Muhammad. The Sunnah (distinguished from the Hadith, although sometimes described as a type of Hadith) are descriptions of the Prophet's life itself, e.g., how he lived. While very important as a guide for living, the Hadith and Sunnah are not infallible like the Qur'an. There are six primary collections of Sunni Hadith: Sahih Bukhari, Sahih Muslim, Sunan Abu Dawood, Sunan al-Sughra, Jami al-Tirmidhi, and Sunan ibn Majah. Those Hadith with "sahih" in their name are thought to be the most reliable and authentic (i.e., Bukhari and Muslim). There are also other collections of Sunni Hadith that contain authentic hadith but are used less frequently by Islamic scholars. These include the Musannaf of Abd al-Razzaq, Musnad, Mustadrak, Muwatta (Malik), Sahih Ibn Hibbaan, Sahih Ibn Khuzaymah, and Sunan al-Darimi.

Shia Muslims do not follow the six Sunni Hadith, but instead have their own. The four major Shia Hadith collections (associated with the Twelvers school of jurisprudence) are Kitab al-Kafi, Man la yahduruhu al-Fqih, Tahdhib al-Ahkam, and Al-Istibsar. These primary Hadith collections are written by three authors known as the "Three Muhammads": Muhammad ibn Ya'qub al-Kulayni al Razi, Muhammad ibn Babuy, and Shaykh Muhammad Tusi. The differences between Sunni and Shia Hadith are based on their respective scholars' belief in the reliability of the narrators (i.e., early companions reporting the sayings of the Prophet) and transmitters (those who collected these reports). In the Sunni tradition, Muhammad al-Bukhari is considered by far the most reliable of the transmitters. Because of this, and because 85–90 % of Muslims are Sunni, we frequently cite the Hadith collected by al-Bukhari.

Other divine books recognized in Islam are the Torah (*Tawrat*), the Psalms (*Zabur*), and the Gospel (*Injil*). Muslims believe that the Qur'an is the final divine book that has corrected all the previous divine books that contained errors, were corrupted, or were lost. Muslims believe in all of these divine books (Torah, Psalms, and Gospel) as revealed by God in their original form. Muslim scholars believe that the Injil refers to an original Gospel that was revealed by God to Jesus, but does not refer to the current Gospels of the New Testament, which are thought to contain some of Jesus' teachings but are not the original Gospel, which was corrupted or lost (New World Encyclopedia 2008).

The Day of Judgement. Both the Qur'an and Hadith refer to the Day of Judgement (the day of resurrection, the "day after" the end of the world). We will refer to it here as the Day. The Qur'an notes that (1) the Day is known only to God (33:63), (2) the Prophet Muhammad cannot make it happen (6:57), (3) on the Day it will seem to people that they were on earth only a very short time and everyone will recognize one another (10:45), (4) God will resurrect everyone, even those who have turned to dust or stone (17:49), and (5) those who deny God's truth will suffer in the fire of hell (11:17). Before the Day comes, there are three periods of time with some overlap between periods. The first period began when the Prophet Muhammad died and lasted until the death of his companions; the second period lasted 1,000 years; and the third period is the one we are in now and will end with the appearance of the Mahdi. The Mahdi, or guided one, is a leader who will usher in a period of about 7–9 years of justice, equality, and restore true religion, and then the world will end. Jesus the Christ (Isa) is foretold in the Qur'an to appear at this time: "And he [Isa] shall be a known sign for (the coming of) the Hour (Day of Resurrection)" (43:61).[1]

[1] The English translation of the Qu'ran used in this book is that of M.A.S. Abdel Haleem in the Oxford University World's Classics series, *The Qur'an* (Oxford, UK: Oxford University Press, 2005; reissued 2008). Occasionally, to enhance clarity, the translation by Muhammad Asad is used (*The Message of the Quran*), although this will be noted.

Table 2.1 Examples of God's compassion, mercy, and forgiveness in the Qur'an

"But there is also a kind of man who gives his life away to please God, and God is most compassionate to His servants" (2:207)
"...God would never let your faith go to waste [believers], for God is most compassionate and most merciful towards people" (2:143)
"On the day when every soul finds all the good it has done present before it, it will wish all the bad it had done to be far, far away. God warns you to beware of Him, but God is compassionate towards His servants" (3:30)
"Say, 'If you love God, follow me, and God will love you and forgive you your sins; God is most forgiving, most merciful'" (3:31)
"Hurry towards your Lord's forgiveness and a Garden as wide as the heavens and earth prepared for the righteous, who give, both in prosperity and adversity, who restrain their anger and pardon people—God loves those who do good" (3:133-134)
"But if you avoid the great sins you have been forbidden, We shall wipe out your minor misdeeds and let you in through the entrance of honour" (4:31)
"Whoever has done a good deed will have it ten times to his credit, but whoever has done a bad deed will be repaid only with its equivalent—they will not be wronged" (6:160)
"Ask your Lord for forgiveness, then turn back to Him. He will grant you wholesome enjoyment until an appointed time, and give His grace to everyone who has merit" (11:3)
"As for those who who avoid grave sins and foul acts, though they may commit small sins, your Lord is ample in forgiveness" (53:32)

Although the Qur'an emphasizes that the punishments for evil behavior and lack of belief will be severe on the Day of Judgement, it moderates the severity by stressing in many places that there is hope in God's compassion, infinite mercy, and forgiveness (see Table 2.1).

Angels. Muslims believe in angels, i.e., supernatural beings who act under the direction of God. They are not humans and never have been humans. In fact, they were asked by God to bow down to Adam (2:34). The Qur'an identifies Gabriel as the angel who appeared to the Prophet Muhammad, both to deliver the message of the Qur'an (2:97) and to miraculously transport the Prophet to Jerusalem (the Night Journey and ascension, 17:1, 17:60, 53:13–18). Both the angel Gabriel and the angel Michael are described in the Qur'an as message bearers from God (2:97–98; 66:4).

Destiny. Muslims believe in destiny, which means that everything—all events and happenings in life—have a purpose and there are no random occurrences: "It was not without purpose that We created the heavens and the earth and everything in between" (38:27). God has decided everything beforehand and His will is supreme, above even human will (57:22; 81:29). However, Muslims also believe that God gives people free choice in many things, especially the choice to be a good person (to do good things in life) or the choice to be a bad person. This freedom of choice means taking responsibility: "BEHOLD, from on high have We bestowed upon thee this divine writ, setting forth the truth for [the benefit of all] mankind. And whoever chooses to be guided [thereby], does so for his own good, and whoever chooses to go astray, goes but astray to his own hurt; and thou hast not the power to determine their fate" (39:41).[2]

This means that Muslims have no excuse for not working or failing to be productive, since all are accountable for everything they do or not do. On the other hand, there are many things that people do not choose—such as the country or time in which they are born or their race or skin color. People may also receive unpleasant things in life such as diseases or loss of loved ones. In those situations, Muslims believe that they must accept what has happened and be patient, which God will reward (Bukhari 7/70/544–545).[3] This belief helps people to accept disease and other stressful events, and in this way helps them to cope with them. Muslims are taught never to ask the question "why me" when they get a disease or have bad things happen to them. Belief in destiny helps people to accept disease and give support to others who are also afflicted with illness.

Other important beliefs, considered less central than the six beliefs above, include beliefs about life after death, intercession, and the individual (vs. the group).

Life After Death. As death nears, it is the responsibility of the dying person to recite the confession of faith (*shahadah*) and to seek the forgiveness of others whom he or she has wronged. After death, loud wailing by friends and family is forbidden, as is observance of the death beyond 3 days (Rahman 1998, p. 129). The Qur'an makes it clear that death is not the end. Rahman says, "For the Qur'an, the after-death life is as concrete and palpable as the 'life in this world'; there is a natural continuity between the two, and death is the passage between them" (p. 126). The quality of life after death—either heaven or hell—is determined by an individual's performance during this life. For the Muslim, death bed repentence is not allowed, since there is no more opportunity to work and do good. Says the Qur'an, "God is always ready to accept repentance, He is full of mercy. But God only undertakes to accept repentence from those who do evil out of ignorance and soon afterwards repent: these are the ones God will forgive, he is all knowing, all wise. It is not true repentance when people continue to do evil until death confronts them and then say, 'Now I repent'…" (4:16–18).

Intercession. There are two types of intercession. One type involves *praying to God for someone* for the benefit of that person (e.g., for a sick loved one). The other type involves *praying to an intermediary so that the intermediary will pray to God.* With regard to the second type of intercession, the Qur'an emphasizes that there are no intermediaries between a person and God, and that intercession of this type is not allowed, at least not on the Day of Judgement (2:48, 2:254) and perhaps not otherwise

[2] Qur'an translation by Muhammad Asad in *The Message of the Quran* (http://www.usc.edu/schools/college/crcc/private/cmje/religious_text/The_Message_of_The_Quran__by_Muhammad_Asad.pdf) (last accessed April 22, 2014).

[3] Citations to *Sahih Bukhari* (the most respected of all Sunni Hadiths) is based on a 2009 translation M. Muhain Khan (2009). We list the reference by volume, book, and number (vol/book/no). See http://d1.islamhouse.com/data/en/ih_books/single/en_Sahih_Al-Bukhari.pdf (last accessed April 22, 2014).

either (6:51, 6:70, 32:4; 39:43–44). In Islam, people are to pray directly to God and only to God. Less clear, however, is the Qur'anic view toward praying for others (the first type of intercession described above). Several Qur'anic verses indicate that prophets prayed to God for others. Moses prayed to God for the people when they were hungry (2:61) and when there was a plague (7:134–135). The Prophet was also told by God to intercede for the people on several occasions (3:159, 4:64, 63:5). Some suras suggest that God only permits certain people to intercede ("no one will have power to intercede except for those who have permission from the Lord of Mercy" 19:87), and only those with whom God is well pleased (53:26). Several Hadith have also been more tolerant with regard to the first type of intercession, emphasizing that the Prophet himself prayed for the well-being of others (Bukhari 1/12/768).

The Individual. Islam is a religion that systematically directs a person's entire life. Islam regulates an individual's daily activities and relationships with others in a way that builds a more homogenous society. This creates harmony between people, which influences their sense of value as an individual who has rights but also obligations to others that must be fulfilled. Individual identity and boundaries are clear and unambiguous, as are boundaries between individual rights and group rights. As a result, people feel equal to each other with clear individual roles, duties, and obligations to the community. While individual freedom is respected and honored, it cannot be at the expense of the community. Every person in the community is important regardless of role since Muslims believe that they will receive praise for their work from God, not other people. The value of a person is based on how closely their life conforms to these beliefs and practices, not by the material possessions they own or their job status.

The individual, then, plays an important role in Islam. People have the responsibility to make life better for themselves and for others. At the same time, Muslims believe that the individual is still a human being and will continue to make mistakes in life. This should not cause a person to feel frustrated or affect their self-esteem since that is the nature of being human. But, Islam stresses that a person should learn from mistakes and try to avoid them in the future. There is an understanding in Islam that people possess a range of weaknesses and strengths, but the goal is for each person to live the best life possible. Islamic beliefs (customs and societal rules) help to make a person feel more responsible, clear on his or her role, and valued as part of the community.

Islamic Practices

Islamic practices center around (1) daily prayers, (2) giving to the poor (zakat), (3) fasting during the month of Ramadan, and (4) participating in the Hajj at least once during one's lifetime. These practices could influence health by helping people to relax and by decreasing materialistic thinking.

Prayer. Muslims say prayers five times a day. The first prayer is said at dawn, the second at midday around noon, the third around 4:00 PM, the fourth at sunset, and the last prayer 90 min after sunset. In Muslim areas, the call to prayer (*azan*) is announced from the minaret of the mosque by a loudspeaker that can be heard throughout the community. The preparation, dress, and physical activity during prayer are important. Muslims must first wash (feet, hands, forearms, and sometimes head), put on a long white robe (when able), take off their shoes, and prepare their prayer rug. They must bow during prayer so that their foreheads contact the ground. Every mosque around the world has a marker that indicates the direction to Mecca, toward which Muslims must face and bow.

Prayer involves a direct relationship between God and the individual. Prayer is relaxing and controls and organizes time and sleep. All Muslims pray at the same time, and when possible, in the same place. They believe that all are equal before God in prayer. This belief helps to equalize the value placed on the poor and makes the rich more humble. The prayer at dawn is the most important one, since this helps to set the tone for the day. Saying the prayers together in a group helps people to meet and talk with each other and enhances social relationships. Men are required to say their prayers at the mosque on Fridays (weekly), although this is optional for women. Saying prayer at the mosque is believed to be 27 times more beneficial (in reward) than saying the prayer at home (Bukhari 1/8/466). For women, however, praying at home is believed to be better, although women are permitted to go to mosque to seek knowledge and socialize with Muslim sisters (Ansari 2013).

Zakat. Giving to the poor is an important religious practice in Islam. Honor and courage are highly valued by Muslims, and are expressed in part by compassion for those in need. More than 30 verses in the Qur'an refer to *zakat*, which serves to redistribute wealth from the rich to the poor and other dispossessed Muslims. As one of the five pillars of Islam, giving is part of the covenant made between God and humans (see Table 2.2). Rahman (1998) notes that the Qur'an is so intent on emphasizing good works and giving of one's wealth to support the poor (i.e., active rather than passive acts of worship) that in two places it even promises God's favor and salvation to whoever "believe in God and the Last Day and do good" (Muslims, Christians, and Jews) (2:62; see also 5:69) "without mentioning belief in the messengership of the Prophet Muhammad" (p. 24). Although the latter part of that statement by Rahman is controversial, it underscores the importance that the Qur'an places on good actions, especially caring for those in need, perhaps even at the expense of good belief [he is trying to make a point here about the general passivity found in the Hadith compared to the action orientation that pervades the Qur'an].

Zakat involves paying 2.5 % per year of all capital assets (savings of cash) and agricultural goods, gold, silver, stocks, and livestock (all assets owned continuously through the lunar year). Islamic scholars differ in what assets are included in the calculation of the zakat and how the calculation is performed. A person's home, clothing, and household furniture are excluded. Zakat is paid through a voluntary not compulsory system, except in countries such as Saudi Arabia and Pakistan where zakat is obligatory and is collected by the state. The Qur'an specifies who is

Table 2.2 Emphasis on giving to the poor in the Qur'an

"Remember when we took a pledge from the Children of Israel: 'Worship none but God; be good to your parents and kinfolk, to orphans and the poor; speak good words to all people; keep up the prayer and pay the prescribed alms'" (2:83)
"They ask you [Prophet] what they should give. Say, 'Whatever you give should be for parents, close relatives, orphans, the needy, and travellers. God is well aware of whatever good you do'" (2:215)
"Those who spend their wealth in God's cause are like grains of corn that produce seven ears, each bearing a hundred grains. God gives multiple increase to whoever He wishes: He is limitless and all knowing"(2:261)
"None of you [believers] will attain true piety unless you give out of what you cherish" (3:92)
"But those of them who are well grounded in knowledge and have faith do believe in what has been revealed to you [Muhammad], and in what was revealed before you—those who perform the prayers, pay the prescribed alms, and believe in God and the Last Day—to them We shall give a great reward" (4:162)
"Alms are meant only for the poor, the needy, those who administer them, those whose hearts need winning over, to free slaves and help those in debt, for God's cause and for travellers in need" (9:60)
"Give relatives their due, and the needy, and travellers—do not squander your wealth wastefully; those who squander are the brothers of Satan, and Satan is most ungrateful to his Lord" (17:26-27)
"Believe in God and His messenger, and give out of what He has made pass down to you: those of you who believe and give will have a great reward" (57:7)
"[Prophet], have you considered the person who denies the Judgement? Is is he who pushes aside the orphan, and does not urge others to feed the needy. So woe to those who pray but are heedless of their prayer; those who are all show and forbid common kindnesses" (107:1–7)

eligible to receive the zakat that is given. There are eight categories of individuals eligible to receive zakat: (1) those in abject poverty (living on less than $1.25 per day), (2) those who cannot meet their basic needs, (3) those who collect the zakat (the civil service), (4) non-Muslims sympathetic to Islam or those who wish to convert, (5) those who are trying to free themselves from slavery or war (for payment of ransoms or blood money), (6) those whose debts make it unable for them to meet their basic needs, (7) those working for an Islamic cause, i.e., "purely for the sake of Allah" (*Fī Sabīlillā*), which includes defense, religious education, and health, and (8) children living on the street, or to provide facilities for travelers (Table 2.2).

Fasting. Regulation of food intake is important in Islam. Muslims are encouraged not to eat more than what their body requires. They are also responsible for feeding hungry relatives or neighbors if they cannot afford food (see Table 2.2). Muslims are also required to fast. The reason is "so that you may be mindful of God" (2:183). Muslims are obligated (*fard*) to fast during the month of Ramadan from dawn till sunset (2:183–185). Fasting during the day as a community during the month of Ramadan, and doing so in the same way and at the same time, influences feelings of unity and helps to bond people together. Fasting helps people to remember that there are poor people who cannot afford food. Both the rich and poor cannot eat anything during the daytime in the month of Ramadan. When there is no food consumption or tobacco use, and the focus is on prayer and worship, this will impact a person's mood and mental state. There may also be physical health benefits to fasting. These include lowering the risk of degenerative brain diseases, improving the aging brain's resistance to toxins, reducing the damage following stroke, slowing the motor deficits in Parkinson's disease, and lessening the rate of cognitive decline in Alzheimer's disease. These and other benefits of intermittent fasting were described in the January 2013 issue of *Scientific American*, which suggested that fasting breakfast and lunch each day over the long term may produce substantial health benefits (and increase productivity) (Stipp 2013).

Muslims are encouraged to fast at other times during the year besides Ramadan, but this is not obligatory. Some devout Muslims fast 3 days each month and may even fast 2 days a week. Excessive fasting, however, is discouraged (Ali 1990). Besides emphasizing fasting, Islam also encourages people not to overeat: "eat and drink [as We have permitted] but do not be extravagant: God does not like extravagant people" (7:31).[4]

Hajj. The Hajj (pilgrimage) to the Kaaba in Mecca is one of the five pillars of Islam. Approximately three million people make this pilgrimage each year (United Press International 2010). Only Muslims can enter the city of Mecca and go into the mosque (*Masjid al-Haram*) that houses the Kaaba ("The Cube" or "Sacred House"). The Hajj is required at least once in a lifetime for those who can afford to go and are physically able. By "afford," this means having extra finances beyond that needed to support one's family. The Hajj is the largest annual religious pilgrimage in the world. People come from many different countries to the high plains of Arafat outside Mecca in the 12th month of the Islamic calendar (*Dhu al-Hijjah*). The Islamic calendar is a lunar calendar and is 11–12 days shorter per year than the solar calendar, the one followed by those in the Western world. Each month is 29–30 days depending on when the crescent moon appears. For example, Dhu al-Hijjah in 2014 is September 26 through October 24, and in 2015, will be September 15 to October 14. The Islamic calendar is also dated differently than the Gregorian (Western) calendar, and starts in the year 622, when the Prophet Muhammad emigrated from Mecca to Medina. Dhu al-Hijjah is different from the month of Ramadan, which is the ninth month of the Islamic calendar (in 2014, Ramadan will occur from June 29 to July 27).

During the Hajj, men must wear the same dress (long white robes), which is another symbol of equality. Worshiping God together makes Muslims feel that they are not alone but part of something greater than themselves. Pilgrims are asked to leave everything behind them. Individuals must concentrate on their relationship with God and forget everything else that may be stressful in their lives (work, family problems, etc.). Being in an isolated place with a feeling of oneness and a chance to rethink issues provides an opportunity for self-examination and restructuring of attitudes and goals. Pilgrims are forbidden to argue during this time or make any bad remarks about other people. Only healthy discussions and pleasant words are allowed. The Hajj also involves physical exercise with much walking (and some running).

---

[4] Muhammad Asad's translation of 7:31 says: "O CHILDREN of Adam! Beautify yourselves for every act of worship, and eat and drink [freely], but do not waste: verily, He does not love the wasteful!"

Islamic Values and Attitudes

Ethical Values. As noted above, individuals in Islam are valued by their ethical behaviors in preference to what they produce. People are judged by their relationships to those who are close to them. It does not matter how much a person owns or who their father's tribe, language, or country is. Islam teaches that people are judged only on things they have control over. In Islam there are no second class people except those who intend to deviate from Islamic values and persist in doing so. These values, if applied, will influence people's feelings about themselves that could affect their mental health and may stimulate efforts toward self-improvement that could dispel feelings of emptiness or worthlessness.

Islam encourages "downward" comparisons with regard to possessions, but "upward" comparisons with regard to values. In other words, Muslims are taught to compare themselves to those who are less fortunate in terms of material possessions, but to look up to and try to emulate those who live virtuous lives. Great importance, then, is placed on a person's principles and faith. This minimizes a sense of inferiority that Muslims might otherwise feel to those who are rich or better off than they are. Feelings of equality with others and a sense of fairness can help to combat feelings of low self-esteem, thereby enhancing the health of the individual and the community more generally.

Positive Attitudes. Muslims believe in having a positive attitude, and are encouraged by their faith to be optimistic even in their darkest moments: "Who is it that answers the distressed when they call upon Him? Who removes their suffering? Who makes you successors in the earth? Is it another god beside God?" (27:62). The Qur'an in many places discourages sadness, since this life on earth is only a test period and not long enough to feel sad about small things. Feelings of desperation or powerless are also discouraged. One of the greatest sins in Islam is to give up and feel that God doesn't listen or care. Muslims believe that God does listen and may forgive anyone as long as they try their best, even if they make mistakes: "[Prophet] if My servants ask you about Me, I am near. I respond to those who call Me, so let them respond to Me, and believe in Me, so that they may be guided" (2:186). Islam emphasizes that strong believers are better off than weak believers, and so people are encouraged to increase their beliefs, talents, and abilities in every respect and use them to help society. This increases motivation for individuals to help themselves and provides a self-image that may influence mental health, as well as affect apathy and feelings of emptiness. Thus, frustration, dissatisfaction, hopelessness, sadness, and feelings of shame run counter to what Muslims believe.

Importance of Family. Family and kinship are the cornerstones of Muslim life. Islam stresses that caring for family members is a primary responsibility of both the individual and the community (2:83, 2:215, 4:36, 6:151). Marriage is strongly encouraged, as is the raising of children in the proper way. Muslims believe that God will reward individuals who do this. In Islam, there is no excuse for men not to marry, even if they want to have more time to engage in religious activities (the Qur'an does not explicitly forbid celibacy and some Sufis in Islamic history have been celebate, although it certainly does not encourage it—see Rahman 1998, p. 103). Marriage *is considered a religious practice* and taking good care of family members is a priority: "Husbands should take good care of their wives, with [the bounties] God has given to some more than others and with what they spend out of their own money. Righteous wives are devout and guard what God would have them guard in their husbands' absence" (4:34). The individual is responsible for supporting their first-degree relatives if those relatives cannot support themselves (spouse, children, and parents). Taking care of aging parents is especially important, which means supporting them morally, psychologically, and financially (17:23–24, 31:14, 46:15). Islam emphasizes that children should avoid upsetting aging parents about anything either major or minor. On many occasions, the Qur'an stresses respect for parents, particularly when they are old. Extramarital relationships are considered major sins and never allowed in Islam. Supporting women before and after marriage is required of all men. A man must support his wife even if she is rich and owns more than he does.

Adultery. The Qur'an forbids adultery: "And do not go anywhere near adultery: it is an outrage, and an evil path" (17:32). This passage is sandwiched between admonitions not to kill children and not to take a life, and so the prohibition concerning adultery is one about which there is little debate among Islamic scholars. Under Islamic law, the punishment for adultery is 100 lashes of moderate intensity (seldom carried out in most Islamic countries today): "Strike the adulteress and the adulterer one hundred times. Do not let compassion for them keep you from carrying out God's law—if you believe in God and the Last Day—and ensure that a group of believers witnesses the punishment" (24:2). Although the Qur'an does not say the punishment is stoning to death, this is sometimes carried out in countries where a very strict form of shari'ah law is practiced (this is opposed, however, by the Islamic Human Rights Commission).

Polygamy. Muslim men are allowed to have up to four wives, although they must treat each wife equally. This is based on the Qur'an: "you may marry whichever women seem good to you, two, three, or four. If you fear that you cannot be equitable [to them], then marry only one" (4:3). The difficulty of treating each wife equitably is also underscored in the Qur'an: "You will never be able to treat your wives with equal fairness, however much you may desire to do so…" (4:129). In reality, few Muslim men have more than one wife. There are practical reasons for this besides the issue of fairness. In some countries the custom is to ask the approval of the first wife before the husband can take on a second wife. Furthermore, women may specify in a prenuptual agreement that her husband can have only one wife. Despite this, however, systematic research indicates that in Turkey (where the practice has been illegal since 1926) about 2 % of men have more than one wife and in the Arab world the percentage ranges from 2 to 10 %. Researchers have found that the mental health of women in polygamous families is worse than that of women in non-polygamous marriages (Ozkan et al. 2006).

Importance of Work. Islam encourages Muslims to work and makes it clear that people who work and produce are better than those who spend their time doing nothing or even spend it at the mosque in worshiping only. Strong believers work harder than weak believers. People who work (if they are able) are more respected than those who do not. People who work and produce have more self-esteem and respect for themselves and therefore experience better mental health. Work may also have a positive impact on physical health. Supporting one's family or a relative is an activity that is rewarded by God (as reflected by verses cited from the Qur'an in Table 2.2). Islam also teaches people how to spend the money they earn, and this may influence feelings of guilt associated with wrong spending. Those who spend their money according to Qur'anic guideliness may feel better about themselves. Regardless of the type of work a person does, he or she is rewarded by God as long as the work is something useful to the community. This makes Muslims feel proud of their profession regardless of what other people think.

Summary and Conclusions

There are many potential links between Islamic beliefs and practices and mental, social, and physical health. These beliefs and practices have the potential to promote self-esteem and provide rest and peace, even though some beliefs could cause guilt and fear. Muslims believe that surrendering one's life to God and doing good deeds will result in health and happiness on this earth and eternal life and happiness in the world to come (*jannah*). This is promised in the Qur'an, the highest authority and source of truth in Islam (2:25, 3:15, 5:19, 9:72). Muslims also believe that failure to surrender to God and perform good deeds result in the opposite, misery on earth and the tortures of hell (*jahannam*) in the hereafter (4:56, 5:37, 8:40, 9:35). They believe that God will weigh the good deeds against the bad deeds on the Day of Judgement (7:7–8), and this will determine a person's fate after death. Muslims also believe that good deeds cancel out bad deeds (11:111–115) and that a person's ultimate fate rests in the hands of God, who is just but also merciful. Three fundamental terms are emphasized in the Qur'an: *iman* (from the word "faith" whose root "a m n" means to be at peace or to be safe), *islam* (from the root "s l m" which means to be whole and safe, since surrendering to the law of God brings safety and peace), and *taqwa* (from the root "w q y" which means to be protected and guarded against peril through piety or fear of God) (Rahman 1998, pp. 13–14). These beliefs and behaviors, particularly in a religion such as Islam with many devout adherents, ought to have consequences for health and well-being.

References

Ali, M. M. (1990). *The religion of Islam* (6th ed., pp. 358–365). Columbus, OH: The Ahmadiyya Anjuman Isha'at Islam.

Alsharif, N. Z., Galt, K. A., & Kasha, T. A. (2011). Health and healing practices for the Muslim community in Omaha, Nebraska. *Journal of Religion & Society,* (Suppl. 7), 150–168.

Ansari, U. Z. (2013). Why is it better to pray at home for women? *Quibla*. Retrieved April 10, 2013, from http://spa.qibla.com/issue_view.asp?HD=1&ID=8740&CATE=4

Armstrong, K. (2002). *Islam: A short history*. New York: Random House.

Miller, T. (2009). *Mapping the global Muslim population: A report on the size and distribution of the world's Muslim population*. Pew Research Center. Retrieved March 10, 2013, from http://www.pewforum.org/Muslim/Mapping-the-Global-Muslim-Population.aspx

Nasr, S. H. (2002). *The heart of Islam* (p. 17). New York: HarperCollins.

New World Encyclopedia. (2008). *Injil*. Retrieved March 10, 2013, from http://www.newworldencyclopedia.org/entry/Injil

Omar, I. (1993). Khidr in the Islamic tradition. *The Muslim World, 83*(3–4), 279–294.

Ozkan, M., Altindag, A., Oto, R., & Sentunali, E. (2006). Mental health aspects of Turkish women from polygamous versus monogamous families. *International Journal of Social Psychiatry, 52*(3), 214–220.

Pew Forum. (2011, January). *The future of the global Muslim population. Pew Forum on religion and the public life*. Washington, DC: Pew Research Center. Retrieved March 10, 2013, from http://features.pewforum.org/muslim-population/

Rahman, F. (1998). *Health and medicine in the Islamic tradition*. Chicago: ABC International Group (Kazi Publications).

Stipp, D. (2013). Is fasting good for you? *Scientific American, 308*(1), 23–24.

United Press International. (2010, November 16). *Hajj attracts 3 million pilgrims*. Retrieved March 10, 2013, from http://www.upi.com/Top_News/World-News/2010/11/16/Hajj-attracts-some-3-million-pilgrims/UPI-21981289926713/

Chapter 3
Beliefs About Health, Healing, and Healthcare

Islamic beliefs and practices regarding health and healing are based on the Qur'an, the Hadith, and on Arabic folklore that preceded Islam. These religious and cultural traditions have greatly influenced the attitudes and practices of Muslims toward birth, illness, death, and dying, as well as the social, legal, and political regulations that influence health and healthcare. Certain aspects of health, such as diet and personal hygiene, are addressed specifically in Islamic law. We start out by examining what the Qur'an and Hadith say about health and healing, and then address more specifically what Muslims believe and practice regarding healing and healthcare.

Sayings on Health and Healing in the Qur'an and Hadith

While the *Qur'an* is not a medical book and does not specifically focus on health and healing, it contains a number of suras that directly or indirectly address issues of health, medicine, healthcare, and attitudes toward those who are sick. We present these in chronological order in Table 3.1. These verses are believed to be the direct words of God to Muslim believers.

More sayings on health and healthcare are found in the Hadith. Muhammad al-Bukhari was a Persian Islamic scholar and the author of *Sahih al-Bukhari*, one of the six major hadiths in Islam. Sunni Muslims consider this Hadith (which contains over 2,600 sayings of the Prophet) to be one of the three most trusted collections of Hadith in existence. Some Muslim scholars believe that *Sahih al-Bukhari* is second only to the Qur'an in authenticity. According to this Hadith, the Prophet Muhammad encouraged Muslims to seek treatment for illness, just as he sought treatment for himself. Table 3.2 presents examples of Hadith on health and healing from a book in *Sahih al-Bukhari* that is titled *Medicine* (Bukhari 7/71).[1]

[1] Citations to *Sahih Bukhari* are based on a 2009 translation M. Muhain Khan (2009). We list the reference by volume, book, and number (vol/book/no). See http://d1.islamhouse.com/data/en/ih_books/single/en_Sahih_Al-Bukhari.pdf (last accessed April 22, 2014).

H.G. Koenig and S. Al Shohaib, *Health and Well-Being in Islamic Societies: Background, Research, and Applications*, DOI 10.1007/978-3-319-05873-3_3,

Table 3.1 Verses on health and healing in the Qur'an

"People, eat what is good and lawful from the earth…" (2:168)
"You who believe, fasting is prescribed for you, as it was prescribed for those before you, so that you may be mindful of God" (2:183)
"Spend in God's cause: do not contribute to your destruction with your own hands, but do good, for God loves those who do good" (2:195)
"They ask you [Prophet] about intoxicants and gambling: say, 'There is great sin in both, and some benefit for people: the sin is greater than the benefit'" (2:219)
"No soul may die except with God's permission at a predestined time" (3:45)
"You are forbiden to eat carrion[a]; blood; pig's meat; any animal over which any name other than God's has been invoked;…"(5:3)
"You who believe, when you are about to pray, wash your faces and your hands up to the elbows, wipe your heads, washing your feet up to the ankles…" (5:6)[b]
"… if any saves a life it is as if he saves the lives of all mankind…" (5:32)
"You who believe, intoxicants and gambling, idolatrous practices, and [diving with] arrows are repugnant acts—Satan's doing—shun them so that you may prosper. With intoxicants and gambling, Satan seeks only to incite enmity and hatred among you, and to stop you remembering God and prayer" (5:90–91)
"If God touches you [Prophet] with affliction, no one can remove it except Him, and if He touches you with good, He has power over all things: He is the Supreme Master over His creatures, the All Wise, the All Aware" (6:17–18)[c]
"People, a teaching from your Lord has come to you, a healing for what is in [your] hearts, and guidance and mercy for the believers. Say [Prophet], 'In God's grace and mercy let them rejoice: these are better than all they accumulate'" (10:57–58)
"From the fruits of date palms and grapes you take sweet juice and wholesome provisions. There truly is a sign in this for people who use their reason" (16:67)[d]
"And your Lord inspired the bee, saying, 'Build yourselves houses in the mountains and trees and what people construct. Then feed on all kinds of fruit and follow the ways made easy for you by your Lord.' From their bellies comes a drink of different colours in which there is healing for people. There truly is a sign in this for those who think" (16:68–69)
"Do not kill your children for fear of poverty—We shall provide for them and for you—killing them is a great sin" (17:31)
"We send down the Qur'an as healing and mercy to those who believe…" (17:82)
"Eat from the good things We have provided for you, but do not overstep the bound, or My wrath will descend on you" (20:81)[e]
"No blame will be attached to the blind, the lame, the sick" (24:61)
"Prophet, when believing women come and pledge to you that they will not ascribe any partner to God, nor steal, nor commit adultery, nor kill their children, nor lie about who has fathered their children, nor disobey you in any righteous thing, then you should accept their pledge of allegiance and pray to God to forgive them: God is most forgiving and merciful" (60:12)[f]

[a]Carrion is dead and decaying flesh of an animal

[b]*Wudu*, an aspect of Salat, involves washing all the exposed areas of the hands, arms, face, and feet 5 times a day prior to prayer; this encouragement of hand washing likely prevented disease in Muslim areas fourteen centuries before the germ theory of disease was discovered

[c]In other words, accept disease as *Kaffara* (a way of making amends for bad deeds or wrong actions), and ask God to remove the disease

[d]In other words, eat healthy foods such as fruits, dates, and grapes

[e]Muhammad Asad translates 20:81 as: 'Partake of the good things which We have provided for you as sustenance, but do not transgress therein the bounds of equity lest My condemnation fall upon you'

[f]This verse applies to mental health (feeling forgiven)

Table 3.2 Health and healing in *Sahih al-Bukhari* (vol 7, book 71, titled *Medicine*)

"The Prophet said, 'There is no disease that Allah has created, except that He also has created its treatment'" (582)
"The Prophet said, 'Healing is in three things: cupping, a gulp of honey or cauterization (branding with fire) but I forbid my followers to use cauterization (branding with fire)'" (585)[a]
"I heard Allah's Apostle saying, 'There is healing in black cumin for all diseases except death'" (592)
"Aisha used to recommend At-Talbina for the sick and for such a person as grieved over a dead person. She used to say, 'I heard Allah's Apostle saying, 'At-Talbina gives rest to the heart of the patient and makes it active and relieves some of his sorrow and grief''" (593)[b]
"I heard the Prophet saying, 'Treat with the Indian incense, for it has healing for seven diseases; it is to be sniffed by one having throat trouble, and to be put into one side of the mouth of one suffering from pleurisy'" (596)
"that she (the wife of the Prophet) asked Allah's Apostle about plague, and Allah's Apostle informed her saying, 'Plague was punishment which Allah used to send on whom He wished, but Allah made it a blessing for the believers. None (among the believers) remains patient in a land in which plague has broken out and considers that nothing will befall him except what Allah has ordained for him, but that Allah will grant him a reward similar to that of a martyr'" (630)
"The Prophet ordered me or somebody else to do Ruqya (if there was danger) from an evil eye" (634)[c]
"Allah's Apostle used to treat with a Ruqya saying, 'O the Lord of the people! Remove the trouble. The cure is in Your Hands, and there is none except You who can remove it (the disease)'" (640)
"Whenever Allah's Apostle went to bed, he used to recite Surat-al-Ikhlas, Surat-al-Falaq and Surat-an-Nas and then blow on his palms and pass them over his face and those parts of his body that his hands could reach. And when he fell ill, he used to order me to do like that for him" (644)[d]
"The prophet used to treat some of his wives by passing his right hand over the place of ailment and used to say, 'O Lord of the people! Remove the difficulty and bring about healing as You are the Healer. There is no healing but Your Healing, a healing that will leave no ailment'" (646)
"Allah's Apostle said, 'Avoid the Mubiqat, i.e., shirk and witchcraft'" (659)[e]
"I heard Allah's Apostle saying, 'If somebody takes seven 'Ajwa dates in the morning, neither magic nor poison will hurt him that day'" (664)
"Allah's Apostle said: 'The cattle (sheep, cows, camels, etc.) suffering from a disease should not be mixed up with healthy cattle' (or said: 'Do not put a patient with a healthy person')" (665e)
"The Prophet said, 'Whoever purposely throws himself from a mountain and kills himself, will be in the (Hell) Fire falling down into it and abiding therein perpetually forever; and whoever drinks poison and kills himself with it, he will be carrying his poison in his hand and drinking it in the (Hell) Fire wherein he will abide eternally forever; and whoever kills himself with an iron weapon, will be carrying that weapon in his hand and stabbing his abdomen with it in the (Hell) Fire wherein he will abide eternally forever'" (670)

[a]*Cupping* involves applying local suction to the skin (using hand or electrical pumps), which mobilizes blood flow in order to promote healing

[b]*At-Talbina* is a meal made from barley flour, formed by adding milk and honey to the dried barley powder

[c]*Ruqya* involves reciting words from the Holy Qur'an to cure an illness or disease; also used to treat poisonous sting or snake bite (633, 637)

[d]*Surat-al-Ikhlas* (112:1–4): "Say, 'He is Allah, [who is] One, Allah, the Eternal Refuge. He neither begets nor is born, Nor is there to Him any equivalent'"; *Surat-al-Falaq* (113:1–5): "Say, 'I seek refuge in the Lord of daybreak From the evil of that which He created And from the evil of darkness when it settles And from the evil of the blowers in knots And from the evil of an envier when he envies'"; *Surat-an-Nas* (114:1–6) [last sura or chapter of the Qur'an]: "Say, 'I seek refuge in the Lord of mankind, The Sovereign of mankind. The God of mankind, From the evil of the retreating whisperer—Who whispers [evil] into the breasts of mankind—From among the jinn and mankind'"

[e]*Mubiqat* involves destructive sins, including magic; *shirk* is polytheism or worshiping others besides Allah

There are sayings on health and healing contained in other Hadith as well. For example, Usamah ibn Sharik said, "I came to the Prophet and his Companions were sitting as if they had birds on their heads. I saluted and sat down. The desert Arabs then came from here and there. They asked: 'Apostle of Allah, should we make use of medical treatment?' He replied: 'Make use of medical treatment, for Allah has not made a disease without appointing a remedy for it, with the exception of one disease, namely old age'" (Hasan, n.d.).

Thus, there is much within the core religious writings of Islam that guide people on how to stay physically well and encourage them to seek medical care when they are sick. Based on these sacred sayings and others noted below, we now review what most Muslims believe and practice today regarding the body, sickness, and healing.

The Body

Muslims believe that they are accountable to God for taking care of their body and for living healthy lives. There is a Hadith that says, "A person's body has a due right over him" (Al-Dhahabi 1961, p. 6). This applies to living a healthy life to preserve health and engaging in daily hygienic practices. Instructions that forbid over-eating, as mentioned earlier, and passages stressing the importance of ritual washing before prayer and careful attention to oral hygiene, are found thoughout the six major Sunni Hadith (Rahman 1998, p. 34). The emphasis on care of the body in the Qur'an and Hadith is thought to be one reason why the practice of medicine was so highly valued in early Islam. This served as powerful motivation for many Islamic physicians to conduct research and discover new medical treatments during the Islamic Golden Age (see Chap. 1) (Rodini 2011, p. 1).

Obeying God and living according to His commandments contained in the Qur'an and Hadith are integral to the spiritual, mental, and physical health of Muslims (Stacey 2009a). In general, Islam focuses on the maintenance of health, rather than on the treatment of disease once a person is sick (Stacey 2009b, c). This is especially true in the Medicine of the Prophet tradition. The Qur'an says, "…eat and drink [as We have permitted] but do not be extravagant: God does not like extravagant people" (7:31), and "Eat of the good things we have provided for your sustenance, but commit no excess therein, lest my wrath should justly descend on you" (20:81). The Prophet is also reported to have encouraged healthy persons to stay away from those with a contagious disease (such as leprosy), and recommended dietary practices (avoidance of meat from dead animals and from eating pork) that are now known to cause disease (Rodini 2011, p. 3). There were practical reasons for maintaining health and vigor during the early Islamic period. Sick people could not fight in the cause of Islam or serve God with all their strength and might.

Sickness

All become sick and eventually die, as did the Prophet and all the prophets before him. Muslims believe that God created illness and like everything else has a purpose for it.

Purpose of Illness. A common belief in Islam is that physical or emotional sickness is a trial allowed by God to help purify the individual, nullify previously committed sins, and provide an opportunity for future rewards, particularly if the sickness and suffering is handled with patience and forebearance. This belief gives the illness meaning and purpose, which by itself helps to relieve much pain and suffering caused by the illness. Rahman notes that a Hadith suggests that God may intentionally inflict disease, poverty, or bereavement on someone who is spiritually weak, and that by enduring these trials, this provides the person an opportunity to enter into the ranks of the truly faithful (which otherwise might not be possible) (Rahman 1998, p. 37).

Visiting the Sick. There are Hadith in Islam that encourage people to visit and support the sick as a religious duty, which produces benefit and reward for the healthy and the sick. According to one of these, the Prophet is reported by a close companion to have said:

> God shall say on the Day of Judgement, 'O son of Adam! I was sick but you did not visit me.' 'My Lord! How could I visit you when you are the Lord of the whole world,' man will reply. God will say, 'Did you not know that so and so from among my servants [that is, human beings] was sick but you never visited him or her? Did you not know that if you had visited, you would have found me there?' (Robson 1975, pp. 320–321).

Another Hadith says, "Allah's Apostle ordered us to do seven things and forbade us from seven. He ordered us to visit the sick…" (Bukhari 7/69/539). Visiting the sick, according to this Hadith, was the very first practice that the Prophet said Muslims should do. This is reinforced repeatedly throughout the Hadith: "The Prophet said, 'Feed the hungry, visit the sick, and set free the captives'" (Bukhari 7/70/552,553).

Special Role for Sick Person. In one Islamic tradition, a time of illness is considered such a pure and holy state that the sick individual has special influence with God: "The Prophet encouraged visitors to request the sick person to pray for them because the state of the sick and the helpless is so pure that God hears their prayers…God also visits the sick and says, 'O my servant! Health unites you with yourself, but sickness unites you to Me'" (Rahman 1998, p. 59). Thus, one way to give the sick person a sense of purpose and meaning in life (which is often threatened during illness) is to ask him or her to pray for others.

Healing

Healing comes from the German word "heilen," which means "to become whole," "to set right," or "to restore." While Muslims believe that sickness can play an important role in a person's life, the Qur'an was given to mankind to restore them to the state that God had intended during the Creation event: "We send down the Qur'an as a restorer of health and as mercy for the believers" (17:82).

Spiritual Healing. Spiritual healing is practiced by many if not most Muslims today (Alsharif et al. 2011). This includes prayer, recitation of the Qur'an ("it is guidance and healing for those who have faith" [41:44; 17:82]), drinking water that has been prayed over by reciting verses from the Qur'an (and sometimes placing pieces of paper with Qur'anic verses written on them in the water), and by eating certain foods, particularly those that contain honey (see Chap. 1). The use of amulets (except if used in accordance with the Qur'an and Qur'anic prayers) and all forms of magic, omens, or star cults, however, are forbidden, particularly those that might invoke spirits or other powers besides God. The Prophet is said to have recommended Zamzam water to treat fever because of its healing properties (Bukhari 4/54/483). This water comes from a natural spring in the Grand Mosque that surrounds the Kaaba in Mecca, and is believed to be the original spring that saved Ishmael from dying of thirst when his mother and he were sent into the wilderness by Abraham (Genesis 21:19).

Source of Healing. Muslims believe that God is the ultimate cause of all healing that takes place, no matter what a person does to obtain that healing: "It is He who guides me; He who gives me food and drink; He who cures me when I am ill; He who will make me die and then give me life again" (26:78–81). Likewise, the Qur'an says, "When I fall sick, God restores me to health" (26:80). As a result, complete trust in God and resignation to His will (*tawakkul*) in health matters has been emphasized. Some conservative Islamic theologians from the ninth century have been quoted as saying "Medical treatment is permissible, but its abandonment is better" (Rahman 1998, p. 48). Rahman illustrates this point by describing the story of a Sufi saint, who when sick was told by her friend, Sufyani, "If you pray to God he will ease your suffering." She replied, "O Sufyani! Do you not know who has willed my suffering? Is it not God?" He replied, "Yes." She said, "If you know this, why do you ask me to pray for what contradicts His will?" (Rahman 1998, p. 49).

Health and Medical Care

Balancing the redemptive view of illness just described above is the belief that good health is also a great blessing. In *Prophetic Medicine*, Al-Dhahabi (1961, p. 3) writes "Health is the most excellent of God's blessings upon man after [the faith] Islam, for without it man can neither carry on his life business well nor can he obey God's commands. There is, in fact, no other good like it, so man must be thankful for it and not ungrateful, for God's Messenger—peace and blessings of God be upon him—said, 'There are two blessings for which so many people are enviable, health and lack of worry.'"

Says Rahman, "…after faith, the art and practice of medicine is the most meritorious service in God's sight." In fact, the art of medicine is thought to have come from the Prophet Idris (Rahman 1998, pp. 38–39). Idris is Arabic for Enoch, the great-grandson of Adam through Seth, and the great-grandfather of Noah. According to a well-known Hadith, the Prophet Muhammad said, "[Valid or beneficial] knowledge is only of two kinds: knowledge of faith and knowledge of the body" (Al-Azraq 2006).

Arriving at a compromise between the fatalistic view of blind acceptance of God's will vs. seeking medical treatment when sick, Al-Dhahabi in *Prophetic Medicine* says, "…an expert doctor first tries his best by way of treatment and then puts his trust in God for his success" (Al-Dhahabi 1961, p. 103). He compares this to a farmer who plants his seed and then trusts in God to make it grow. This view is consistent with the beliefs of many Muslims today, regardless of how conservative their theology is. Rahman notes that the vast majority of Muslims believe that not only should medical treatment be sought, but that it has spiritual value and may even be religiously obligatory (Rahman 1998, p. 50). The Muslim medical historian Husain Nagamia says, "Thus, in Islam disease is not looked upon as a curse from God to be endured and suffered but as an affliction for which a cure has to be sought and administered, with patience and perseverance" (Nagamia, n.d.).

What is the bottom line here? Muslims are expected to see physicians when they become sick (Stacey 2009d), as the Prophet often advised others to do (Farooqi 2010), and almost certainly did himself (Bukhari 7/71/602; Lyons and Petrucelli 1997; Robson 1975, pp. 947, 949–950).

Supernatural Beliefs

Muslims also have a wide range of health beliefs regarding the supernatural, some rooted in Islam and some in pre-Islamic bedouin beliefs and folklore.

Miracles. The occurrence of miracles (beyond the spiritual healing practices discussed above) is not stressed in Islam today, at least not nearly as much as in Christianity. The Qur'an acknowledges the existence of miracles as performed by Biblical prophets (Moses, Jesus, others). However, it stresses that the prophets themselves were not responsible for the healing but rather God performed these miracles through them. The Qur'an also indicates that because supernatural miracles were never very successful in converting nonbelievers who denied them (17:59), there would be no more of them (Rahman 1998, p. 12). The Prophet Muhammad's response to Meccan critics who demanded that he perform a miracle was that the Qur'an itself was miraculous. Lack of emphasis on supernatural miracles, however, does not discount healing that comes about as a natural result of prayer (although the line here between natural and supernatural healing is a fine one).

Demons. The Qur'an and Islamic theology refer to humans, angels, and jinn as the three beings created by God who can feel, perceive, and be conscious. Jinn are thought to inhabit the unseen world, and can be either good, bad, or neutral, and may be associated with mental illness (Islam and Campbell 2012). Bad jinn are probably close to demons as they are understood in Christianity, although demons are not emphasized as much in Islam. Rahman notes that one reason for this is because the Prophet Muhammad was once accused by members of his own tribe that he was possessed by a spirit or jinn (i.e., madness) because of his adament religious stance, and suggested that he undergo exorcism (Hisham, n.d.). This accusation of insanity has been strongly rejected in the Qur'an, and consequently the existence of demons as a cause of mental or physical illness has not been stressed much in Islam. However, possession by spirits and jinn is a belief common among the general public and is a layover from Arabic folklore. In this regard, a Sufi *shaik* (or Sufi master) might be sought by some Muslims to do an exorcism if possession is thought to be the cause of illness. The attention on demon posession and exorcism in Islam, however, never reached the fervor it did in Christianity during the Middle Ages.

Ethical Issues in Medicine

Muslims have religious beliefs relevant to health and medical care that determine what is ethical and what is not.

Suicide. Committing suicide is strictly forbidden in Islam. The Qur'an says, "…do not contribute to your destruction with your own hands, but do good, for God loves those who do good" (2:195). A well-known Hadith notes, "The Prophet said, 'He who commits suicide by throttling shall keep on throttling himself in the Hell Fire (forever) and he who commits suicide by stabbing himself shall keep on stabbing himself in the Hell-Fire'" (Bukhari 2/23/446). In another Hadith: "The Prophet said, 'Whoever purposely throws himself from a mountain and kills himself, will be in the (Hell) Fire falling down into it and abiding therein perpetually forever; and whoever drinks poison and kills himself with it, he will be carrying his poison in his hand and drinking it in the (Hell) Fire wherein he will abide eternally forever; and whoever kills himself with an iron weapon, will be carrying that weapon in his hand and stabbing his abdomen with it in the (Hell) Fire wherein he will abide eternally forever'" (Bukhari 7/71/670). Even desiring death by the sick person is discouraged, no matter how much they are suffering.

The "right to die" is not found in Islamic teachings, and therefore euthanasia or any shortening of life is not allowed. Do-not-resuscitate orders are permitted although complex (Rehman 1993), and withdrawal of life support from someone in a persistent vegetative state is not clear, since Islam does not formally recognize brain death (although equates cardiac and respiratory death to brain death) (Sarhill et al. 2001). Nevertheless, it is acceptable to discontinue life support in cases where only the life support equipment is allowing the person to survive. The latter, however, may be easily confused with euthanasia or assisted suicide, so this needs to be clarified by physicians to the patient's family (Hassaballah 1996). Physician-assisted suicide is clearly *haram* (forbidden) based on the Qur'an: "Do not kill each other, for God is merciful to you" (4:29), and more to the point, "If anyone kills a believer deliberately, the punishment for him is Hell, and there he will remain: God is angry with him, and rejects him, and has prepared a tremendous torment for him" (4:93).

According to Rahman (1998), "Sick people, as indeed healthy ones too, are strongly prohibited from desiring or praying for death, let alone committing suicide; for if a person is good, he may do more good if he lives longer, and if a person is not good, longer life may afford him a chance for conversion" (p. 60). The faithful are told to see the Prophet as their role model in this regard, especially if suffering becomes unbearable. According to a famous Hadith (*Mishat*), the Prophet went through severe suffering prior to his death in the arms of his youngest and favorite wife (Aisha). She said, "After witnessing the Prophet's [painful] death, I do not mind how much suffering anyone endures at death" (Robson 1975, pp. 326–327). Those who are suffering are encouraged to recite the Qur'an and Hadith, pray to God for mercy, and have hope [and seek the best medical care available, we may add].

Abortion. Abortion is not allowed. The Qur'an says, "Do not kill your children for fear of poverty—We shall provide for them and for you—killing them is a great sin" (17:31; see also 6:151). Thus, the Qur'an is clear that abortion is forbidden if pregnancy wasn't planned, if the baby will interfere with the mother's life, or with her education, or with her career, or because it is a result of unforced adultery. The only exception to this rule after 4 months of pregnancy is in case of grave risk to the mother's life (under the principle that abortion is the lesser of two evils) (BBC 2009a). This is true even if there is a confirmed untreatable fetal anomaly identified after 4 months of pregnancy. This is agreed on by all schools of Islamic law.

Schools of Islamic law differ, however, on the other conditions that would allow abortion and at what time during the course of pregnancy this might be allowed. Even liberal Islamic scholars, however, agree that abortion is wrong—although perhaps not "punishable" based on Islamic law. A general principle is that the older the fetus is when abortion takes place, the more wrong it is. If there is a confirmed untreatable fetal anomaly, then some (but not all) Islamic scholars would argue that it is permissible to abort the fetus if less than 4 months old. More liberal Islamic scholars might even allow this if the baby were born with a physical or mental defect that would prevent him or her from living a normal life, although at least two competent medical specialists need to confirm this (see citation above).

In cases of rape, some Islamic scholars say that abortion is permissible if done within the first 4 months of pregnancy, whereas other scholars say that it is not permitted at any time even in case of rape. However, Islamic law does have some flexibility and compassion depending on the circumstances.

Contraception. Regarding contraception within marriage, eight out of nine Islamic schools of law permit it under the principle that it may preserve the health of the mother and the well-being of the family (BBC 2009b). However, some conservative Muslim traditions may not allow temporary contraception such as use of condoms, taking a birth control pill or using a patch, unless there are medical reasons for this and the husband agrees (Ishmail 2010). Sterilization (male or female) is generally not allowed because it permanently prevents the having of children and because the Qur'an forbids male castration (based on 4:118).

Miscellaneous Health Practices

A variety of other health practices are important to Muslims that could potentially affect health and well-being. These include circumcision, oral care, sleep, exercise, intoxicating substance use, spending of resources, and socializing with others.

Circumcision. Circumcision is practiced in Islam. Although the Qur'an does not mention circumcision, most Islamic jurists say that circumcision is obligatory for men (the opinion of the majority of Muslim scholars). The rationale is that the Prophet Abraham would not have undergone circumcision at such a late age if the practice was not important. This is also based on the Hadith: "I heard the Prophet saying, 'Five practices are characteristics of the Fitra: circumcision, shaving the pubic hair, cutting the moustaches short, clipping the nails, and depilating the hair of the armpits'" (Bukhari 7/72/779). Fitra is a natural predisposition in which one is inclined toward right action and submission to God. Circumcision is also known to have health benefits (Rabin 2012).

Oral Care. Cleansing the mouth and teeth with a *miswak* or *siwak* is encouraged before every prayer. Miswak is a teeth cleaning twig (natural toothbrush) from the Salvadora persica tree, and has a long history in Islamic theology. A Hadith states, "I saw the Prophet cleaning his teeth with Siwak while he was fasting so many times as I can't count." And narrated Abu Huraira, "The Prophet said, 'But for my fear that it would be hard for my followers, I would have ordered them to clean their teeth with Siwak on every performance of ablution.'" The Prophet did not differentiate between a fasting and a non-fasting person in this respect (using Siwak). His wife Aisha said, "The Prophet said, 'It (i.e. Siwak) is a purification for the mouth and it is a way of seeking Allah's pleasures'" (Bukhari 3/31/154). Good dental care is known to be associated with a lower risk of coronary artery disease and stroke (DeStefano et al. 1993; Wu et al. 2000).

Sleep. Types of sleep, importance of sleep, and good sleep practices are emphasized in the Qur'an and Hadith (BaHammam 2011). Muslims are encouraged to sleep at a regular time during the night rather than during the day, except for a brief afternoon nap. Studies show that sleep deprivation increases risk of cardiovascular disease (Malhotra and Loscalzo 2009). Staying up late at night has also been shown to increase insulin resistance, thus increasing risk of diabetes mellitus (Broussard et al. 2012).

Exercise. Muslims are encouraged to walk to the place of prayer, rather than going by car to the mosque. References to horseback riding, shooting, swimming, hunting, fencing, running, and wrestling are found throughout the Qur'an and Hadith because these were important to having a healthy, well-trained military (Kahan 2003). The Prophet is reported to have said in a Hadith by Al-Tabarani, "Any action without the remembrance of Allah is either a diversion or heedlessness excepting four acts: Walking from target to target [during archery practice], training a horse, playing with one's family, and learning to swim." Daily exercise of this kind is known to reduce risk for many cardiovascular (Miller et al. 1997) and metabolic diseases (Carroll and Dudfield 2004).

Substance use. Alcohol is forbidden in Islam, and there are reasons for this. There was first concern that intoxication might interfere with prayer (4:43). Then it was noted that alcohol was both good and evil, but that the evil was greater than the good (2:119). Finally, Muslims were commanded to abstain from alcohol: "You who believe, intoxicants and gambling, idolatrous practices, and [divining with] arrows are repugnant acts—Satan's doing—shun them so that you may prosper. With intoxicants and gambling, Satan seeks only to incite enmity and hatred among you, and to stop you remembering God and prayer. Will you not give them up?" (5:90–91). Illicit drug use was not mentioned in the Qur'an because it was not even a consideration, although several Hadith indicate that any intoxicants that fog the mind are not allowed (see Abu Dawood, Book 26, Hadith 3679).

As with drug use, there are no instructions in the Qur'an with regard to cigarette smoking either since it was not done in the seventh century. However, there is a general rule given in the Qur'an that is applicable. God instructs [the Prophet] who "commands them to do right and forbids them to do wrong, who makes good things lawful to them and bad things unlawful, and relieves them of their burdens, and the iron collars that were on them" (7:157). Given the dangers of cigarette smoking (Das 2003), Islamic scholars have unanimously forbidden this practice: "In view of the harm caused by tobacco, growing, trading in and smoking of tobacco are judged to be haram (forbidden). The Prophet, peace be upon him, is reported to have said, 'Do not harm yourselves or others.' Furthermore, tobacco is unwholesome, and God says in the Qur'an that the Prophet, peace be upon him, 'enjoins upon them that which is good and pure, and forbids them that which is unwholesome'" (Fatwas of the Permanent Committee 2013).

Spending. Islam prohibits overspending of money and going into debt. The Qur'an says, "The servants of the Lord of Mercy are…those who are neither wasteful nor niggardly when they spend, but keep to a just balance" (25:63–67). Overspending and acquiring of debt increase guilt and stress. The general philosophy in Islam is that money only makes you happy when you spend it in the right way: "Neither wealth nor children will bring you nearer to Us, but those who believe and do good deeds will have multiple rewards for what they have done, and will live safely in the lofty dwellings of Paradise" (34:37). Overspending implies a greed for material things. According to a Hadith, when the Prophet was asked "O Messenger of Allah! Narrate to me a hadith, and make it short! So he (SAW) replied, 'Pray your prayer as if it is your last, as if you are seeing Him (Allah), for even if you do not see Him then He sees you. And give up hope (of obtaining) what other's possess, then you will live a rich life. And beware of anything that you might (later) have to make an excuse for'" (documented by Bukhari in *Al-Tarīkh al-Awsaṭ* and by Tabarani in *Al-Mu'jam Al-Awsat*).

Social Relationships. Islamic beliefs encourage the building of strong relationships with relatives and friends. According to a Hadith, "The Prophet said, 'None of you will have faith till he wishes for his (Muslim) brother what he likes for himself'" (Bukhari 1/2/12). Friendships, however, should be based on the love of God: "The Prophet said, 'Allah will give shade, to seven, on the Day when there will be no shade but His. (These seven persons are) a just ruler, a youth who has been brought up in the worship of Allah (i.e. worships Allah sincerely from childhood), a man whose heart is attached to the mosques (i.e. to pray the compulsory prayers in the mosque in congregation), two persons who love each other only for Allah's sake and they meet and part in Allah's cause only….'" (Bukhari 1/11/629). Social relationships are known to influence mental health and extend longevity (House et al. 1988; Uchino 2009). As noted earlier, marriage is encouraged in Islam and extramarital affairs are prohibited. We know that married people live longer (Waite and Lehrer 2003), and extramarital affairs often result in sexually transmitted diseases (Widdus et al. 1990), as well as family and social disharmony (Atwood and Seifer 1997).

Summary and Conclusions

God's will and destiny are important to Muslims, and unavoidable sickness can result in purification from sins and coming closer to God. However, the Qur'an, Hadith, and behaviors of the Prophet Muhammad himself all encourage the seeking of medical care, use of medicine for healing, and adoption of a healthy lifestyle to avoid disease and sickness. These beliefs influence Muslims' attitudes and behaviors regarding health, healing, and healthcare, and have the potential to influence psychological, social, and physical health in many ways, particularly among those who are devout in their faith and practice. A core message from the Qur'an and Hadith is that the key to health for the individual and the community is the remembrance of God in every action and activity: "You who believe! Be mindful of God, and let every soul consider carefully what it sends ahead for tomorrow; be mindful of God, for God is aware of everything you do. Do not be like those who forget God, so God causes them to forget their own souls" (59:18–19). Muslim beliefs and practices described in the last chapter, in particular the five daily prayers, are ways to help ensure that forgetting one's soul (or mind) will not happen: "I am God; there is no god but Me. So worship Me and keep up the prayer so that you remember Me" (20:14).

References

Al-Azraq, I. (2006). *Tashil al-Manafi' fi al-Tibb wa-al-Hikma (Tashil)* (p. 3). Beirut, Lebanon: Dar Sader Publications.

Al-Dhahabi, M. I. (1961). *Al-Tibb al-Nabawi (Prophetic Medicine).* Cairo, Egypt: Mutafā al-Halabī.

Alsharif, N. Z., Galt, K. A., & Kasha, T. A. (2011). Health and healing practices for the Muslim community in Omaha, Nebraska. *Journal of Religion & Society,* (Suppl. 7), 150–168.

Atwood, J. D., & Seifer, M. (1997). Extramarital affairs and constructed meanings: A social constructionist therapeutic approach. *American Journal of Family Therapy, 25*(1), 55–75.

BaHammam, A. S. (2011). Sleep from an Islamic perspective. *Annals of Thoracic Medicine, 6*(4), 187–192.

BBC. (2009a). *Sanctity of life: Islamic teachings on abortion*. British Broadcasting Corporation (BBC). Retrieved March 10, 2013, from http://www.bbc.co.uk/religion/religions/islam/islamethics/abortion_1.shtml

BBC. (2009b). *Islamic views on contraception*. British Broadcasting Corporation (BBC). Retrieved March 10, 2013, from http://www.bbc.co.uk/religion/religions/islam/islamethics/contraception.shtml.

Broussard, J. L., Ehrmann, D. A., Cauter, E. V., Tasali, E., & Brady, M. J. (2012). Impaired insulin signaling in human adipocytes after experimental sleep restriction: A randomized, crossover study. *Annals of Internal Medicine, 157*(8), 549–557.

Carroll, S., & Dudfield, M. (2004). What is the relationship between exercise and metabolic abnormalities? A review of the metabolic syndrome. *Sports Medicine, 34*(6), 371–418.

Das, S. K. (2003). Harmful health effects of cigarette smoking. *Molecular and Cellular Biochemistry, 253*, 159–165.

DeStefano, F., Anda, R. F., Kahn, H. S., Williamson, D. F., & Russell, C. M. (1993). Dental disease and risk of coronary heart disease and mortality. *British Medical Journal, 306*, 688–691.

Farooqi, M. I. H. (2010). *Medicine of the Prophet (Tibb al-Nabvi): A message par excellence*. Islamic Research Foundation International. Retrieved March 10, 2013, from http://www.irfi.org/articles/articles_251_300/medicine_of_the_prophet.htm

Fatwas of the Permanent Committee. (2013). Fatwa 16484, Part 22, Page 214; Fatwa 1000, Part 22 (pp. 181–183); and Fatwa 19966, Part 23 (pp. 53–54). Retrieved March 10, 2013, from http://alifta.com/Default.aspx (search for cigarette smoking)

Hasan, A. (Trans.) (n.d.). *Partial translation of Sunan Abu-Dawud*. Book 28: Medicine (Kitab al-Tibb), 3846. Retrieved March 10, 2013, from http://abudawudshareef.blogspot.com/

Hassaballah, A. M. (1996). Definition of death, organ donation and interruption of treatment in Islam. *Nephrology, Dialysis, Transplantation, 11*(6), 964–965.

Hisham, I. (n.d.). *Sira* (a biography of the Prophet Muhammad's life written around 730-733 by Ibn Ishaq and edited by Ibn Hisham, who died in 833) (Vol. 1, p. 358) (cited in Rahman, 1998, p 85).

House, J. S., Landis, K. R., & Umberson, D. (1988). Social relationship and health. *Science, 241*, 540–545.

Ishmail, M. (2010). *Islamic learning materials: Islam birth control*. Retrieved March 10, 2013, from http://islamiclearningmaterials.com/islam-birth-control/

Islam, F., & Campbell, R. A. (2014). "Satan has afflicated me!" Jinn-possession and mental illness in the Qur'an. *Journal of Religion and Health, 53*(1):229–243.

Kahan, D. (2003). Islam and physical activity: Implications for American sport and physical educators. *Journal of Physical Education, Recreation, & Dance, 74*(3), 48–54.

Lyons, A. S., & Petrucelli, R. J. (1997). *Medicine: An illustrated history*. New York: Harry N. Abrams. (Also see: Medicine under Islam: Arabic Medicine). Retrieved March 10, 2013, from http://www.healthguidance.org/entry/6344/1/Medicine-under-Islam-Arabic-Medicine.html

Malhotra, A., & Loscalzo, J. (2009). Sleep and cardiovascular disease: An overview. *Progress in Cardiovascular Diseases, 51*(4), 279–283.

Miller, T. D., Balady, G. J., & Fletcher, G. F. (1997). Exercise and its role in the prevention and rehabilitation of cardiovascular disease. *Annals of Behavioral Medicine, 19*(3), 220–229.

Nagamia, H. F. (n.d.). *A museum and library of Islamic medical history: A new perspective* (p. 1). Retrieved March 10, 2013, from http://www.iiim.org/Files/Museum and Library/Museum_and_Library.pdf

Rabin, R. C. (2012, August 27). Benefits of circumcision are said to outweigh risks. *New York Times (Science)*. Retrieved March 10, 2013, from http://www.nytimes.com/2012/08/27/science/benefits-of-circumcision-outweigh-risks-pediatric-group-says.html?_r=0

Rahman, F. (1998). *Health and medicine in the Islamic tradition*. Chicago: ABC International Group (Kazi Publications).

Rehman, K. L. (1993). Cardio-pulmonary resuscitation and life support: The current laws and the Muslim perspective. *Journal of the Islamic Medical Association, 25*, 20–22.

Robson, J. (1975). *Mishkat Al-Masabih*. New York: Orientalia Art Ltd. (cited in Rahman, 1998).

Rodini, M. A. (2011). An investigation of medicine science and public health in Holy Quran. *WebmedCentral Public Health, 2*(10), WMC002324.

Sarhill, N., LeGrands, S., Islambouli, R., Davis, M. P., & Walsh, D. (2001). The terminally ill Muslim: Death and dying from the Muslim perspective. *American Journal of Hospice and Palliative Care, 18*(4), 251–5.

Stacey, A. (2009a). *Health in Islam (part 2 of 4): Qur'an is a healing*. Retrieved March 10, 2013, from http://www.islamreligion.com/articles/1891

Stacey, A. (2009b). *Health in Islam (part 3 of 4): Diet and nutrition*. Retrieved March 10, 2013, from http://www.islamreligion.com/articles/1892

Stacey, A. (2009c). *Health in Islam (part 4 of 4): Fitness and exercise*. Retrieved March 10, 2013, from http://www.islamreligion.com/articles/1904

Stacey, A. (2009d). *Health in Islam (Part 1 of 4): A holistic approach*. Retrieved March 10, 2013, from http://www.islamreligion.com/articles/1878

Uchino, B. N. (2009). Understanding the links between social support and physical health. *Perspectives on Psychological Science, 4*(3), 236–255.

Waite, L. J., & Lehrer, E. L. (2003). The benefits from marriage and religion in the United States: A comparative analysis. *Population and Development Review, 29*(2), 255–275.

Widdus, R., Meheus, A., & Short, R. (1990). The management of risk in sexually transmitted diseases. *Daedalus, 119*(4), 177–191.

Wu, T., Trevisan, M., Genco, R. J., Dorn, J. P., Falkner, K. L., & Sempos, C. T. (2000). Periodontal disease and risk of cerebrovascular disease: The first national health and nutrition examination survey and its follow-up study. *Archives of Internal Medicine, 160*, 2749–2755.

Chapter 4
Christian Beliefs, Practices, and Values

We now examine what Christians believe (U.S. Christians, in particular), how they practice their faith, and the values that are important to them, including attitudes toward health, healing, and ethical issues related to health. This information is important in understanding how religion affects health in populations where the majority are Christian, and will provide clues on how and why religion likewise influences health in Islam. There is a wide range in belief and practice among Christians. Although also true in Islam, beliefs and practices are even more wide-ranging in Christianity since there is nothing in this faith tradition comparable to shari'ah law that continues to institutionalize the core beliefs in many Muslim countries.

The four major divisions in Christianity are Protestant, Catholic, Eastern Orthodox, and Restorationism. Among Protestants alone there are thousands of different denominations, although the main ones are listed in Table 4.1, along with the denominations that make up the other three major Christian divisions. Beliefs vary within each of the four Christian divisions above, ranging from radically fundamentalist to orthodox to conservative to moderate to liberal to radically liberal. Admittedly, the Christian beliefs, practices, and values we present below lean toward the conservative (perhaps even orthodox) side of the spectrum. We will return to this issue of range of belief at the end of the chapter.

Christian Beliefs

Based on the most recent and comprehensive survey of 232 countries and territories by the Pew Foundation Research Center in 2010, there are 2.2 billion Christians who comprise one-third of the world's population of 6.9 billion (Pew Research Center 2011). Christians make up the majority of the population of 158 countries and territories (i.e., about two-thirds of all countries). The regional distribution is 37 % of all Christians live in the Americas (north, south, and central America), 26 % in Europe, 24 % in Sub-Saharan Africa, 13 % in the Asia-Pacific region, and 0.6 %

H.G. Koenig and S. Al Shohaib, *Health and Well-Being in Islamic Societies: Background, Research, and Applications*, DOI 10.1007/978-3-319-05873-3_4,

Table 4.1 Christian denominations with membership of one million or more[1]

Catholic	
Latin (Roman)	1,166,000,000
Eastern Catholic	17,000,000
Philippine	6,000,000
Chinese Patriotic	5,000,000
Brazilian Catholic Apostolic	5,000,000
Protestant	
Pentecostalism	136,000,000
Baptist	100,000,000
Anglican	85,000,000
Nondenominational evangelical	80,000,000
Lutheran	75,000,000
Methodist	75,000,000
Presbyterian	40,000,000
African	40,000,000
Continental reformed	30,000,000
Seventh Day Adventist	17,000,000
Restoration Movement	7,000,000
Congregationalist	5,000,000
Anabaptist and Free	5,000,000
Eastern Orthodox	
Russian (in and outside Russia)	125,000,000
Oriental Orthodox	82,000,000
Romanian	23,000,000
Serbian	11,500,000
Church of Greece	11,000,000
Bulgarian	10,000,000
Greek Orthodox	7,500,000
Ukraine	7,200,000
Georgian	5,000,000
Moldovan	3,200,000
Orthodox Church in America	1,200,000
Polish	1,000,000
Restorationism	
Mormon (Latter Day Saints)	14,700,000
Iglesia ni Cristo	10,000,000
New Apostolic	10,000,000
Jehovah Witness	7,650,000

[1]Source: Wikipedia: List of Christian denominations by number of members (http://en.wikipedia.org/wiki/List_of_Christian_denominations_by_number_of_members) (last accessed October 8, 2013)

in the Middle East and North Africa. The United States contains more Christians than any other country with 11.3 % of the world's Christian population. Of those with a religious faith in the United States, 94 % are Christian (excluding the 16 % who are not affiliated with any religious group). The Nicene Creed (statement of doctrine arrived at in 325 CE) provides a list of Christian beliefs that Catholic, Eastern Orthodox, and Protestants generally agree upon (see Table 4.2 below).

Table 4.2 The Nicene Creed (325 CE, revised 381 CE)[1]

We believe in one God, the Father, the Almighty, maker of heaven and earth, of all that is seen and unseen
We believe in one Lord, Jesus Christ, the only Son of God, eternally begotten of the Father, God from God, Light from Light, true God from true God, begotten, not made, one in Being with the Father
Through him all things were made. For us men and for our salvation he came down from heaven: by the power of the Holy Spirit he was born of the Virgin Mary, and became man
For our sake he was crucified under Pontius Pilate; he suffered, died, and was buried
On the third day he rose again in fulfillment of the Scriptures; he ascended into heaven and is seated on the right hand of the Father
He will come again in glory to judge the living and the dead, and his kingdom will have no end
We believe in the Holy Spirit, the Lord, the giver of life, who proceeds from the Father and the Son. With the Father and the Son he is worshipped and glorified. He has spoken through the Prophets
We believe in one holy catholic and apostolic Church
We acknowledge one baptism for the forgiveness of sins
We look for the resurrection of the dead, and the life of the world to come. Amen

[1]Nicene Creed. Encyclopedia Britannica, Academic Edition. Retrieved April 22, 2014, from http://www.britannica.com/EBchecked/topic/413955/Nicene-Creed

God. Based on the Pew Foundation's U.S. Religious Landscape Survey conducted in 2007–2008, approximately 92 % of Americans believe in either a personal God (a Deity with whom people can have a relationship) or an impersonal Force, and 71 % said they are absolutely certain that God exists (Pew Research Center 2008). Almost all conservative Protestants[1] believe in God (99 %) and most (71–79 %) believe in a personal God. Among Catholics, 97 % believe in God and 60 % believe in a personal God. Among American Muslims, 92 % believe in God and 41 % believe in a personal God. Of the 5 % of Americans who say they do not believe in God (either personal or impersonal), 24 % are atheist (1 % of all Americans), 15 % are agnostics, 35 % say they are nothing in particular, 14 % identify themselves as Christian (<1 % of the US Christians overall), and 10 % affiliate with other religious groups (Pew Research Center 2009a, b). The finding in 2007–2008 that 92 % of Americans believe in God is not much different than was reported in 1944, when 96 % said they believed in God (Princeton Religion Research Center 1996, p. 20).

Christians believe in only one God and pray to only one God. Christians do not believe in three gods. They believe that three "persons" exist in one God: God the Father, God the Son, and God the Holy Spirit, each being fully God in essence. Strictly speaking, this is hard to understand and does not make logical sense on the surface. For that reason, this concept is sometimes referred to as a "mystery." The belief is taken on faith, faith that goes beyond logic. One way to explain it is that God exists in three *forms*, like water exists in three forms (ice, vapor, and liquid). Ice is water frozen. Vapor (or steam) is water in the gas state. Liquid is water in a

[1]By "conservative Protestants" we mean members of Evangelical Protestant Churches or Historically Black Protestant Churches, a group that makes up 33.2 % of all Americans.

state between vapor and ice. All three forms, though, are water. There is only one thing called water, not three different waters or three separate waters. So, when Christians pray, they pray to God—whether they pray to God the Father, God the Son (Jesus), or God the Holy Spirit—they believe they are praying to the one and only God. This is why Christianity is universally known to be a monotheistic religion, not a polytheistic one.

Part of the confusion about Christians worshiping three gods (polytheism) may have come from the impressions obtained by observers of the Catholic Church, which arose out of the polytheistic culture of Rome during the first few centuries. At that time, Rome had statues of the many gods that they worshiped. This pre-Christian culture gave rise to an early Christian culture where people often prayed to Mary or prayed to saints or their statues. However, even then Catholics did not pray to these entities as God, but rather as *intercessors* between themselves and God. Mary and the saints (often martyred for their beliefs) were thought to be very holy people whom early Christians believed had greater access to God than they did. Protestant Christians disagreed and so did away with praying to intercessors of this type. Instead, Protestants prayed *directly* to God, as God the Father, God the Son, or God the Holy Spirit. The Christian belief in the triune nature of God is very different from the belief of the early Meccans in the three daughters of God, i.e., al-Lat, al-Uzza, and Manat, who had their own separate shrines near Mecca and were worshiped as three separate gods during the Prophet Muhammad's time. The Prophet vigorously opposed worshipping the three daughters of God, arguing that God did not have children and only God should be worshiped.

Christians have specific beliefs about the nature of God. They believe God is merciful and forgiving, and personal. They believe that God loves humans whom God created in his own image. In Christianity, there is particular emphasis on love (although perhaps not always practiced). The Bible uses the word "love" over 500 times (45 times alone in the Gospel of John chapters 13–21). When Jesus was asked to name the two most important commandments, he included love in both of them: "You shall love the Lord your God with all your heart and with all your soul and with all your mind. This is the great and first commandment. And a second is like it: You shall love your neighbor as yourself. On these two commandments depend all the Law and the Prophets" (Matthew 22:37–40[2]). The very nature of God is described as love: "Beloved, let us love one another, for love is from God, and whoever loves has been born of God and knows God. Anyone who does not love does not know God, because God is love" (1 John 4:7–8). Christians believe that God is entirely good (omnibenevolent), all knowing (omniscient), present everywhere (omnipresent), and all powerful (omnipotent). It is out of God's infinite goodness that flows love for humans. Christians believe that God's personal nature is directly reflected in Jesus.

Christians also believe that God is fair and just, and that God hates sin (i.e., attitudes or actions that hurt or destroy humans whom God loves). They believe that all

[2] Scriptures cited here are from the New International Version (NIV) of the Holy Bible, unless otherwise noted.

humans because of their sinful nature (Original Sin, see below) cannot stop from sinning. It is this sin that keeps them from coming close to God, who as noted earlier is absolutely and completely good.

Original Sin. Christians believe that Adam, the first human created by God, sinned in the Garden of Eden by freely choosing to disobey God by eating forbidden fruit from the tree of knowledge of good and evil (the only command that God gave Adam). Before eating the fruit, Adam and Eve only knew good. After eating the fruit, however, they came to know evil also and became subject to all its temptations. Christians believe that this rebellion against God (the tendency to follow human desires that contradict God's will and cause harm) has been passed down to every human since then. As a result, Christians believe that from birth onward, all humans have a tendency toward sin and evil that is part of their nature: they are self-centered, ignore others' needs, easily angered, aggressive toward those who oppose them, desire revenge, and so forth. Humans are basically concerned primarily with their own survival (see *The Selfish Gene* (Dawkins 1990)). This desire to go their own way and make decisions that favor themselves over others has separated humans from a perfect and holy God who loves all equally. However, Christians believe that God devised a plan that would be just and fair, and enable humans to relate to and come close to God once again (as in the Garden of Eden). Because of God's love for humans and desire to be in relationship with them, Christians believe that God came down as God the Son to live a sinless life and die a humiliating painful death on the cross (crucifixion). This action paid the price as required by God's fair and just nature for the original sin committed by Adam and all sins that his descendents continue to commit, thus enabling humans who acknowledge this sacrifice to be reunited with God in this life and after death for all eternity.

Jesus the Christ. Christians believe that Jesus is God the Son (84 % of Americans believe this (Gallup Poll 1993)). Christians believe that the reason Jesus came into this world was to address the problem of Original Sin that separated humans from a pure and holy God, and to provide a more approachable role model whom humans could identify with and follow. God had tried sending many prophets to guide and lead the Children of Israel over the preceding 2,000 years. These prophets, however, did not succeed in persuading most people to live a Godly life. Instead, people's human nature repeatedly drew them toward sin and caused them to depart from the ways of God. The Bible tells story after story of how the Jews, because of this human nature, fell back into their evil ways after reforming for a little while. At that time, God was viewed as great, magnificent and powerful, distant, unknowable, and unapproachable. The people were scared of God. However, because of God's desire to relate intimately with people, Christians believe God took on a human form to personally show them how to relate to him and to pay the price for the Original Sin of Adam. Thus, Christians believe that Jesus was and is both fully God and fully human, but without sin (Hebrews 4:15; 7:26; 2 Corinthians 5:21). To Christians, Jesus represents and symbolizes God. This (and this alone) justifies their praying to and worshiping Jesus since when they do so, they believe they are praying to and worshiping God.

Christians base the claim that Jesus is God on his own words. Speaking on the night before his reported death and crucifixion, Jesus said "'And if I go and prepare a place for you, I will come back and take you to be with me that you also may be where I am. You know the way to the place where I am going.' Thomas said to him, 'Lord, we don't know where you are going, so how can we know the way?' Jesus answered, 'I am the way and the truth and the life. No one comes to the Father except through me. If you really know me, you will know my Father as well. From now on, you do know him and have seen him'" (John 14:3–7). Later, Jesus said, "I and the Father are one" (John 10:30), a seemingly outrageous claim that his Jewish critics confirm by their violent response, "'We are not stoning you for any good work,' they replied, 'but for blasphemy, because you, a mere man, claim to be God'" (John 10:33). Other New Testament scriptures also claim that Jesus is God (John 20:28; Acts 20:28; Hebrews 1:8; 2 Peter 1:1). Christians argue further that Jesus accepted worship from others (Matthew 2:11, 14:33, 28:9, 28:17; Luke 24:52; John 9:38) and forgave people their sins (Matthew 9:2; Mark 2:5). In a monotheistic religion such as Judaism, Jesus would only have accepted such worship and forgiven people's sins if he believed he was God.

Finally, Christians believe—based on the Gospel of John—that Jesus is the Word of God: "In the beginning was the Word, and the Word was with God, and the Word was God" (John 1:1). Likewise, it says, "And the Word became flesh and dwelt among us, and we have seen his glory, glory as of the only Son from the Father, full of grace and truth" (John 1:14). There is a parallel between the description of Jesus as the Word of God and how Muslims view the Qur'an. Muslims believe that the Qur'an is God speaking to them. The Qur'an, then, is best compared to Jesus, whom Christians believe is the Word of God speaking to them (Nasr 2002). The goal of the Christian's life is to emulate the life that Jesus lived (to follow his teachings and behaviors), just as the goal of the Muslim's life is to imitate the life of the Prophet Muhammad. Christians believe that Jesus serves as a model for all that they do and say. This is a high standard, however, one that most Christians fall far short of. This is the main reason why Christians believe that Jesus had to suffer and die to compensate for their failures and sins, and to reunite them to a holy and perfectly good God.

The Gospel. Christians believe that the Gospel (or "Good News") is the following. God sent his Word to become a human, live on this earth like any other human, face the same temptations as humans do, but never sin. This human named Jesus, the Messiah, was then crucified, died, was buried, and arose from the dead, defeating death by his resurrection. Because God is perfectly just and fair, he could not simply forgive humans and allow sinful people into heaven. In being crucified, Jesus took on himself all the sins of humanity that separated humans from God (Isaiah 53:4–5; Hebrews 9:26–28). Christians believe that Jesus as God in human form was the perfect sinless sacrifice who died in place of all humans (past, present, and future) so that anyone who believes in Jesus can enter heaven after death and experience eternal life: "For God so loved the world that he gave his one and only Son, that whoever believes in him shall not perish but have eternal life" (John 3:16).

This is the "good news"—that sinners by believing in Jesus can have their sins forgiven and be allowed into heaven for all eternity—no matter what sins they have committed: "If you confess with your mouth that Jesus is Lord and believe in your heart that God raised him from the dead, you will be saved" (Romans 10:9). After this confession of faith, Christians respond to this gift from God with overwhelming gratitude/relief and are then motivated by love and appreciation to submit their will to God, change the way they have been living, and strive to serve God's purposes in the world: "The Spirit you received does not make you slaves, so that you live in fear again; rather, the Spirit you received brought about your adoption to sonship. And by him we cry, '*Abba*, Father'" (Romans 8:15).

Salvation. Protestant and Catholic Christians differ on their views about salvation, i.e., what it takes for people to get into heaven after death. Protestants—particularly conservative Protestants—believe that after the individual repents, salvation is by God's grace and by faith in Jesus alone, and that humans do not "earn" salvation by good deeds that they can take credit for. This belief is based on the scripture: "'Sirs, what must I do to be saved?' They replied, 'Believe in the Lord Jesus, and you will be saved…'" (Acts 16:30–31). Doing good works, according to Ephesians 2:8–9, is not enough to be saved. This is so that people cannot boast and be prideful about saving themselves [for both Christians and Muslims, pride is the worst of all sins]. Protestants do not entirely discount good works, and believe that doing good deeds is important. If a person does no good deeds, then there is some question about whether that person is "really saved." Says the apostle James, "What good is it, my brothers and sisters, if someone claims to have faith but has no deeds? Can such faith save them? Suppose a brother or a sister is without clothes and daily food. If one of you says to them, 'Go in peace; keep warm and well fed,' but does nothing about their physical needs, what good is it? In the same way, faith by itself, if it is not accompanied by action, is dead" (James 2:14–17). In the King James Version of the Bible, it says "faith without works is dead" (James 2:26).

Catholics believe that salvation is a process by which a person comes closer to God throughout life. This occurs as he or she participates in the sacraments (Baptism and Holy Communion, especially) and experiences God's grace that comes through the sacraments. Catholics believe in seven sacraments: Baptism (at birth), Holy Communion (early grade school), Confirmation (during adolescence), Confession (from early grade school onward), Marriage, Holy Orders (becoming a priest), and Extreme Unction (blessing given to chronically ill or dying), all of which are administered by a priest through the Catholic church. Works and good deeds, particularly the care of the poor and needy, are very important in Catholicism and strongly emphasized in order to maintain righteousness after Baptism. Catholics do not, however, believe that man plays as important a role as God does, since only God can save a person and that salvation has been made possible through the death of Jesus (God the Son) on the cross. If this were not so, say Catholics, then Jesus would have died for nothing.

Thus, there are differences in the ways that Protestants and Catholics emphasize faith (correct belief) and deeds (correct action). However, there is general agreement that both are necessary for salvation. Furthermore, both Protestants and Catholics agree that no matter what people have done—no matter what terrible sins they have committed—there is always a possibility, right up to the very moment of death, of reconciliation with God.

Day of Judgement. Christians believe that Jesus will come again on Judgement Day at the end of the world. They base this belief on several passages in the Bible. First, Jesus promised to his disciples that he would come back a second time: "And if I go and prepare a place for you, I will come back and take you to be with me that you also may be where I am" (John 14:3). Jesus' second coming is also referred to elsewhere in the Bible: "For the Lord himself will come down from heaven, with a loud command, with the voice of the archangel and with the trumpet call of God, and the dead in Christ will rise first. After that, we who are still alive and are left will be caught up together with them in the clouds to meet the Lord in the air. And so we will be with the Lord forever" (1 Thessalonians 4:16–17). In a description of what will happen on the Last Day in the Bible, it says "'Look, he is coming with the clouds,' and 'every eye will see him, even those who pierced him'; and all peoples on earth 'will mourn because of him.' So shall it be! Amen" (Revelation 1:7). On the last day it is believed that Jesus will judge the living and the dead (all those who have ever lived) (Baker 1995). Interestingly, nearly 50 % of American Christians say they believe that Jesus will definitely or probably return to earth within the next 40 years (Pew Research Center 2013).

The Holy Spirit. Christians believe that the Holy Spirit is God's Spirit, the form of God who is active in the world and helps people to do the right thing (variously described as the "Helper," the "Advocate," or the "Comforter," depending on translation from the Greek) (John 14:26). The belief that the Holy Spirit is God's Spirit is based on numerous scriptures in the New Testament. For example, Jesus said, "And everyone who speaks a word against the Son of Man, it will be forgiven him; but he who blasphemes against the Holy Spirit, it will not be forgiven him" (only God can be *blasphemed* against) (Luke 12:10). Jesus also describes the Holy Spirit as the "Spirit of truth" (John 14:16–18). The Book of Acts says that lying to the Holy Spirit is equivalent to lying to God (Acts 5:3–4). Elsewhere, the Bible describes the Holy Spirit as the Spirit of God (1 Corinthians 6:11) and later equates the Spirit (Holy Spirit) with the Spirit of the Lord (Jesus in context) (2 Corinthians 3:17). Christians believe that the Holy Spirit—being God—was active in the world before and during the time that Jesus lived on earth, and continues to be active after Jesus' death and resurrection. For example, the first verse of the Bible says: "In the beginning God created the heavens and the earth. Now the earth was formless and empty, darkness was over the surface of the deep, and the Spirit of God was hovering over the waters" (Genesis 1:1–2). The Bible also says that Jesus was conceived by the Holy Spirit (Matthew 1:18) and that the Holy Spirit descended on Jesus during his baptism (Matthew 3:16–17). Jesus himself promised to send the Holy Spirit to his followers to give them strength and power after he died and to give testimony to Jesus' life and teachings: "But you will receive power when the Holy Spirit comes on you; and you will be my witnesses in Jerusalem, and in all Judea and Samaria, and to the ends of the earth" (Acts 1:8).

Mary. Christians believe that Mary was the mother of Jesus and that she miraculously conceived him by action of the Holy Spirit: "But the angel said to her, 'Do not be afraid, Mary; you have found favor with God. You will conceive and give birth to a son, and you are to call him Jesus'... 'How will this be,' Mary asked the angel, 'since I am a virgin?' The angel answered, 'The Holy Spirit will come on you, and the power of the Most High will overshadow you'" (Luke 1:30–31, 34–35). Jesus had a special relationship with his mother Mary. Indeed, he spent over 90 % of his earthly life with Mary, from his conception to the beginning of his public life. Mary even accompanied Jesus during his public ministry (John 2:12), and Jesus' first miracle was done at Mary's request (John 2:1–11). She was also at the foot of the cross at the time of his death, when Jesus asked one of his closest disciples to take care of her (John 19:25–27). Catholics, especially women Catholics, highly venerate Mary because she was Jesus' mother and pray that she will intercede to Jesus for them. Protestants, however, do not believe that such intercession is necessary since people can pray directly to Jesus, God the Son, without an intercessor.

The Prophets. Christians believe in all the prophets that were mentioned in the Bible. They believe that God spoke through the prophets. This is based on a passage in the Book of Hebrews: "In the past God spoke to our ancestors through the prophets at many times and in various ways..." (Hebrews 1:1). Jesus, however, is considered unique and special among the prophets: "but in these last days he has spoken to us by his Son, whom he appointed heir of all things, and through whom also he made the universe" (Hebrews 1:2).

Divine Book. The Divine book of Christians is the Bible, which many believe contains the very words of God. Christians view the Bible similar to how Muslims view the Qur'an, although not exactly (see section on Jesus the Christ above). Most Christians in the United States believe that the Bible is either the literal word of God (30 %) or the inspired word of God (49 %) (Jones 2011). By inspired, most mean that God spoke into the minds of humans who wrote down what they heard, but this may have been influenced by human life experiences, culture, and biases of the time. The Bible includes both the Old Testament (part of the Bible written before Jesus) and New Testament (part beginning with Jesus and then after his death), and was canonized or finalized in 367–397 CE. Christians believe the New Testament supercedes the Old Testament, and vary in how much they value and read the Bible. While the Bible is important to Catholics and is read during religious services, Catholics do not emphasize personal reading of the Bible as much as Protestants do, particularly conservative Protestants. Catholics also supplement the Bible with church tradition, which Catholics argue is directly or indirectly based on the Bible and the teachings of the early church leaders. Catholics also include additional books in the Bible beyond the original 66 (i.e., seven additional "apocryphal" books were canonized in 1546 CE). In contrast, Protestants exclude the apocryphal books from the Bible and have done away with much of the Catholic church traditions. Instead, Protestants ground their beliefs on the 66 original books, especially those in the New Testament.

Life After Death, Heaven, and Angels. The majority of Americans (74 %) believe in life after death (Pew Research Center 2010). In fact, 62 % of American Protestants and 45 % of Catholics say that they are "absolutely certain" that there is life after death (Pew Research Center 2009a, b). This is especially true for conservative Protestants, 79–86 % of whom say they believe in life after death and 62–71 % say they are absolutely certain about it. Nearly half of religiously unaffiliated Americans (48 %) also believe in life after death, as do four of ten American Jews (39 %) (Pew Research Center 2008, p. 10).

Similarly, 74 % of Americans believe in heaven, a place where people who have lived good lives are eternally rewarded (Pew Research Center 2008). This includes 86–91 % of conservative Protestants, 82 % of Catholics, and 85 % of American Muslims. Americans unaffiliated with any religious group are less likely to believe in heaven (41 %).

The majority of Americans (68 %) also believe that angels are active in the world. This belief is especially common among conservative Protestants (87–89 %) (Pew Research Center 2009a, b). Many Catholics (69 %) also believe in angels. The three highest ranking angels (called archangels) are Gabriel, Michael, and Raphael. The Bible indicates that the angel Gabriel interpreted the vision of Daniel (Daniel 9:21) and announced to Mary that she would give birth to Jesus (Luke 1:11). Gabriel is believed to be an angel whose specific job is to bring messages from God to humans. Michael (the name meaning "who is like God?") is considered a protector and the leader of the army of God against the evil forces of satan. Raphael, as the name implies (meaning "It is God who heals"), is in both Judaism and Christianity considered the angel involved in healing.

Demons, the Devil, and Hell. The majority of Americans (68 %) also believe that demons or evil spirits are active in the world (the same percentage who believe in angels) (Pew Research Center 2009a, b). This includes 87–89 % of conservative Protestants and 69 % of Catholics. Demons are generally believed to work directly in the service of the devil (satan). About the same percentage of Americans believe in the devil (70 %) (Newport 2007), a belief that if anything has increased since 1994 when only 65 % of Americans said they believed in the devil (Princeton Religion Research Center 1996, p. 20). Christians believe the devil is a fallen angel who because of his pride rebelled against God, and has been given the name Lucifer (based on Isaiah 14:12, KJV). He is believed to be entirely evil and dark, and is determined to destroy mankind. One of Jesus' main purposes while on earth was to "destroy the devil's work" (1 John 3:8). In the Gospel of Matthew alone, Jesus refers to hell and/or the devil at least six times (Matthew 5:22, 29; 10:28; 13:40–42; 25:30, 41). Hell is described as a place of weeping and gnashing of teeth (Matthew 25:30), outer darkness (Matthew 22:13), a place of torment (Luke 16:23), unquenchable fire (Mark 9:44), sorrow (2 Samuel 22:6), and without rest (Revelation 14:11).

A clear majority of Christians (59 % of Americans (Pew Research Center 2008)) believe that hell is a real place where bad people who have not repented will spend eternity. Conservative Protestants (82 %) and American Muslims (80 %) are more likely to believe in hell than other religious groups. A significant number of Christians say they don't believe in a place called hell, and there are also many who say they are not sure. Least likely to say that they believe in hell are Jews (22 %), Buddhists (26 %), the unaffiliated (30 %), and Hindus (35 %).

There are also a variety of beliefs about hell and who will go there. Many conservative Protestants (34–36 %) believe that only belief in Jesus will save people from going to hell and that their religion is the one true faith that will prevent them from going there (based on John 14:6, 10:7–9, Act 4:12) (Pew Religious Landscape Survey 2008). This raises the question of what happens to those who have never "heard" the Gospel or, despite honest and sincere attempts, are unable to believe in Jesus' sacrifice for them or acknowledge that Jesus is God? Conservative Christian theologian CS Lewis says this: "But the truth is God has not told us what His arrangements about the other people [non-Christians] are. We do know that no man can be saved except through Christ; we do not know that only those who know Him can be saved through Him" (Lewis 1944). Other Christians believe that while there is a literal place called hell, God's great mercy and understanding of a person's abilities and circumstances will excuse many from going to hell and only a few people will be there in the end. According to CS Lewis, "the doors of hell are locked from the inside," meaning that only those who *choose* to be there will end up in hell (i.e., they won't feel comfortable in heaven with God) (Lewis 1940). Interestingly, only 27 % of American Protestants overall and 12 % of Catholics believe that "My religion is the one true faith leading to eternal life." The majority of American Muslims (56 %) also say that members of other religious faiths (besides Islam) may get into heaven, whereas only one-third (33 %) say that their's is the only faith that leads to eternal life (Pew Religious Landscape Survey 2008).

Christian Practices

There is a wide range of Christian religious practices. Christians pray, read religious scriptures and other inspirational literature, watch religious TV, listen to religious radio, play religious music, and attend religious services, meet in small groups for religious activities (praying, Bible-study, etc.), volunteer, and donate money for humanitarian and religious causes.

Prayer. Most American Christians (>90 %) pray at least occasionally, and 83 % say that they believe in a God who answers prayers (Jones 2010). Daily prayer is encouraged, but is not required by either Protestants or Catholics (as it is for Muslims). Nevertheless, the latest figures indicate that 58 % of Americans pray at least once a day other than at mealtimes (Pew Research Center 2010). Even 22 % of Americans not affiliated with any religious group say they pray at least once daily.

Conservative Protestants are most likely to pray at least once daily (78–80 %), whereas 58 % of Catholics pray daily or more. Americans over age 65 are most likely to pray daily or more (68 %). When Americans in 1994 were asked to whom they prayed, 75 % said to "a supreme being such as God," 16 % to Jesus Christ, and 3 % to the Lord (Princeton Religion Research Center 1996, p. 37).

Fasting. Emphasis on fasting is different depending on Christian denomination. Many Christians fast from eating (or at least from eating certain foods) on religious holidays and during religious seasons (Trepanowski and Bloomer 2010). For example, Catholics may refrain from eating meat on Fridays and on other holy days as well. Greek Orthodox Christians have three fasting periods when they do not eat meat, dairy products, eggs, or olive oil: the Nativity fast (40 days prior to Christmas), Lent (48 days prior to Easter), and the Assumption (15 days prior to anniversary of Mary being told she would give birth to Jesus). Some Protestant Christians participate in the Daniel fast, during which only water and vegetarian foods are consumed (10–40 days).

Reading Scriptures. Reading the Old and New Testaments of the Bible (especially the New Testament) is strongly encouraged by Protestants, moderate or conservative Protestants in particular. Catholics, as noted above, place less emphasis on reading the Bible, although this is certainly not discouraged (as it once was long ago when priests controlled access to the scriptures). Gallup polls and Pew Foundation surveys of the US population indicate that 35–37 % of Americans read the Bible daily or weekly, and 59 % read it at least occasionally (other than during religious services) (Gallup and Simmons 2000; Pew Research Center 2010). Conservative Protestants read the Bible most often (60 % once/week or more), and Catholics read it the least (21 % once/week or more). Adults age 30 or over are more likely to regularly read religious scriptures (as well as pray) compared to younger adults.

Besides the Bible, Protestants and Catholics also read other religious or inspirational literature by popular Christian writers that helps to increase their faith or provide guidance in dealing with life problems (e.g., Rick Warren, Tim LaHaye, Corrie Ten Boom, CS Lewis, Thomas Aquinas, Thomas a Kempis). About one-third (33 %) of Americans say they've read a Christian book other than the Bible in the past month (Barna Research Group 2002). These popular writings are not considered sacred, as the Bible is, and often refer to the Bible for their authority.

Religious Media. Christians may also listen to popular religious music or watch religious programs on television as an expression of their religious interest and devotion. Slightly over one-half of Americans (52 %) report listening to Christian radio in the past month: 38 % listened to preaching, teaching, or talk shows, and 43 % listened to Christian music (Barna Research Group 2002). Christian music has been one of the fastest growing areas of the US music industry in recent years (Gospel Music Association 2008).

Similarly, 43 % of Americans watch Christian programs on TV in an average month, with an aggregate viewing audience of 90 million (about the same number who attend Christian churches during a typical week) (Barna Research Group 2002).

The audience for both Christian radio and TV tends to be largely conservative Protestants (evangelical Christians). Among those who say they have an "active faith" (i.e., those who read the Bible, attended church, and prayed during the past week, i.e., 30 % of Americans), 93 % watched or listened to Christian media in the past month. Even 37 % of atheists and agnostics said they listened to, watched, or read something related to the Christian faith during the past month.

Attending Religious Services. The majority of Americans (43 %) attend religious services weekly or almost every week (2010), although 45 % say they seldom or never attended religious services (Newport 2010). Again, conservative Christians are most likely to attend services weekly or almost every week (55 %), as are adults over age 65 (53 %) and women (47 %). Note, however, that even many younger Americans (age 18–29) attend religious services weekly or almost weekly (35 %). Furthermore, despite the widely claimed "secularization" of America, the frequency of religious attendance hasn't changed since 1939 when the Gallup poll first began recording this information, when 41 % of Americans said they attended religious services in the past week (Princeton Religion Research Center 1996, p. 29).

Religious Pilgrimage. The World Religious Travel Association claims that 300 million people worldwide make a religious pilgrimage each year (Wright 2009). They also report that if Americans were able to do so, 25 % would like to make a religious or faith-based pilgrimage. A religious pilgrimage is not required or particularly encouraged by any Christian religious denomination, although devout Christians sometimes make a pilgrimage to Jerusalem or other religious places on their own initiative. Although we could find no other systematic data on the percentage of Christians who make a religious pilgrimage, we suspect that only a small percentage of American Christians actually do so. The most common place that Christians are likely to visit (especially Catholic Christians) are the Our Lady of Guadalupe Basilica in Mexico City (10 million visitors/year), the Vatican (4.2 million/year), Jerusalem (2 million/year), Bethlehem (birthplace of Jesus), and Lourdes. Lourdes, France, is where Jesus' mother Mary is believed to have appeared to a 14-year-old peasant girl in the year 1858. Since 1860, over 200 million pilgrims have visited the shrine at Lourdes, where miraculous physical healings have been reported (66 "documented" out of thousands reported) (Plunkett 2002).

Donating and Volunteering. Many Christians are taught that they should "tithe." This means giving 10 % of yearly income to one's religious congregation (or to religious causes). Many fundamentalist and conservative Protestant churches encourage giving 10 % of total yearly income (not what is left over after taxes), as well as "gifts" that are on top of the tithe. According to the latest national US data (2007), only 5 % of Americans tithe (Barna Research Group 2008). Members of religious groups most likely to tithe are evangelical Protestants (24 %); those who have prayed, read the Bible, and attended church service in the past week (12 %); and charismatic or Pentecostal Christians (11 %). Tithing is done by 1 % or less of individuals who are under age 25, those who are single or never married, or those who are self-declared liberals or atheists/agnostics. Two percent of Catholics tithe, compared to 8 % of Protestants overall.

When the Gallup Poll surveyed members of religious groups in America on whether they gave money to charity in 2009, the results (% yes) were as follows: Protestants in general (74 %), Catholics (65 %), Mormons (72 %), Jews (78 %), and Muslims (70 %) (Gallup Inc. 2009, pp. 51–52). All religious groups were more likely to give to charity than members of the general US population (64 %). Giving money to charity is even more prevalent in Muslims outside of America. For example, 70–92 % of Muslims in the Middle East and North Africa say they give *zakat*, although Muslims in Southeast Asia (Indonesia, Malaysia, Thailand) are most likely to do so (93–98 %) (Pew Research Center 2012).

In terms of volunteering time to an organization in the past month in the U.S., percentages by religious denomination are: Protestants in general (44 %), Catholics (34 %), Mormons (60 %), Jews (44 %), and Muslims (36 %) (Gallup Inc. 2009, pp. 51–52). Percentages of the population of England and Wales who formally volunteered in the past 12 months are as follows: Christian (39 %), Muslim (30 %), Hindu (39 %), Sikh (35 %), Buddhist (39 %), Jewish (58 %), and no religious affiliation (39 %) (O'Beirne 2004). In that study, Muslim men were more likely to volunteer than Muslim women (34 % vs. 26 %), which is the opposite pattern seen in Christian groups, where women are more likely to volunteer. The gender gap in volunteering is probably due to cultural factors. Muslim women from devout Muslim families may not be encouraged to spend time outside the home in public activities. There is also lower civic engagement among Muslims who pray and attend religious services more frequently (i.e., are devout) (Sarkissian 2012). Finally, higher rates of volunteering by Christians likely reflect the fact that they have more free time to volunteer, given their higher socioeconomic status compared to Muslims (Heaton 2013).

Christian Values

Ethics. In Christianity, people are valued because they have been created in the imagine of God, and because Jesus said "Love your neighbor as yourself," where a neighbor is defined as virtually everyone, based on Matthew 22:39. Christians believe that each person has intrinsic value and worth, no matter what his or her race, religion, job, wealth, gender, or education level is. Like Islam, Christianity teaches that people are judged only by their actions concerning things they have control over. *Intentions* are very important—if good is done with the wrong intention, then it is not considered a good act. Christians believe that they are responsible for their own actions. They also believe they are responsible for taking care of others in need, i.e., being their "brother's keeper" (Genesis 4:9). Showing respect for elders is also highly valued. The New Testament instructs: "Do not rebuke an older man harshly, but exhort him as if he were your father. Treat younger men as brothers, older women as mothers, and younger women as sisters, with absolute purity" (1 Timothy

5:1–2). The belief is that all people have certain rights—the right to life, liberty, and pursuit of happiness. These rights are guaranteed in the U.S. Declaration of Independence (authored by Christian statesmen). Ethical principles like these spill over into medicine, healthcare, and the conducting of research, where every effort is made to ensure that the rights of patients and research subjects are protected.

Emphasis on Love. Consistent with the ethical principles above, the Bible teaches that Christians should love other Christians, their neighbor (who include non-Christians), and even their enemies. This was a consistent theme in Jesus' teachings: "A new command I give you: Love one another. As I have loved you, so you must love one another. By this everyone will know that you are my disciples, if you love one another" (John 13:34–35). He taught that Christians should love their neighbors as themselves (Matthew 22:39), and when Jesus was asked "And who is my neighbor?" (Luke 10:29), he told the story of the good Samaritan, a non-Jew who went out of his way to help an injured Jew (Luke 10:30–37). The point of the story is that everyone, regardless of religion or belief, is a neighbor and deserves love and respect. Jesus reinforces the point in Matthew 5:43–44, 48: "You have heard that it was said, 'Love your neighbor and hate your enemy.' But I tell you, love your enemies and pray for those who persecute you…Be perfect, therefore, as your heavenly Father is perfect."

Individualism. Individualists place high value on independence and self-reliance, and resist influence or control by society or society's institutions (especially the government, but also religious organizations). Individualists are interested in self-creation and experimentation, not tradition or following popular opinion. They tend to value individual rights, sometimes even at the expense of the community good (e.g., rights of the mentally ill, rights of criminals, rights of animals). Christians in the West, especially Protestant Christians, are likely to value individualism. Part of this has to do with the "Protestant work ethic" that emphasizes working hard and being frugal with resources, in order to avoid becoming dependent on others. Individualism was also important to those who founded America in the eighteenth century. People who came here had to struggle to survive on their own in hostile wilderness environments where attacks by Indian tribes were common. They were also often escaping the domination and control (often religious control) placed on them by the countries they were leaving. Thus, being independent became a sacred value.

Importance of Work. Christians emphasize the importance of work. In the United States, over 50 % of weekly religious attendees view their work as a mission from God, and nearly three-quarters (72 %) say that they pursue excellence in work because of their faith (Dougherty et al. 2011). Indeed, both the Old Testament and the New Testament stress the importance of work. Humans were intended to work from the very beginning of creation: "The Lord God took the man and put him in the Garden of Eden to work it and take care of it" (Genesis 2:15). Likewise, the Book of Proverbs is filled with statements related to work: "All hard work brings a profit, but mere talk leads only to poverty" (Proverbs 14:23; also see 6:6, 13:4, 18:9, 19:15, 20:4, 24:30–34). The New Testament continues to emphasize this: "Anyone who does not provide for their relatives, and especially for their own household, has denied the faith and is worse than an unbeliever" (1 Timothy 5:8). More to the point, Christians are told: "The one who is unwilling to work shall not eat" (2 Thessalonians 3:10). The political process in the United States seeks to balance the ethics of hard work and independence (which Republicans tend to favor) with providing for those in need through welfare programs (which Democrats tend to favor).

Importance of Family. Christians place a high value on the family and on monogamy. The Book of Psalm says, "Children are a heritage from the LORD, offspring a reward from him. Like arrows in the hands of a warrior are children born in one's youth. Blessed is the man whose quiver is full of them" (Psalm 127:3–5). Taking care of family is a priority for Christians, as it is for Muslims. The New Testament says, "Give proper recognition to those widows who are really in need. But if a widow has children or grandchildren, these should learn first of all to put their religion into practice by caring for their own family and so repaying their parents and grandparents, for this is pleasing to God" (1 Timothy 5:3–4).

Preserving the family unit is important. Jesus taught that divorce was wrong: "It has been said, 'Anyone who divorces his wife must give her a certificate of divorce.' But I tell you that anyone who divorces his wife, except for sexual immorality, makes her the victim of adultery, and anyone who marries a divorced woman commits adultery" (Matthew 5:31–32). Furthermore, Jesus said that when a man and woman are married, the two become "one" before God: "So they are no longer two, but one flesh. Therefore what God has joined together, let no one separate" (Matthew 19:6). Christians believe that adultery (sex outside of marriage) is contrary to the 7th Commandment (Exodus 20:14). Adultery was a sin so serious that in the Old Testament the punishment was death for both partners (Leviticus 20:10; Deuteronomy 22:22). Jesus expanded the definition of adultery even further saying, "You have heard that it was said, 'You shall not commit adultery.' But I tell you that anyone who looks at a woman lustfully has already committed adultery with her in his heart" (Matthew 5:27–28).

Despite these clear and unambiguous Biblical doctrines, the latest Gallup poll in the U.S. found that 59 % of Americans found "sex between an unmarried man and woman" morally acceptable, only slightly lower than "buying and wearing clothing made of animal fur" (60 % said the latter was morally acceptable) (Jones and Saad 2012). Likewise many Americans feel that "having a baby outside of marriage" (54 %) and even viewing pornography (31 %) are morally acceptable. However, only 7 % indicated that a sexual affair between a married man and married woman was morally acceptable. Only a small percentage (11 %) thought that polygamy was morally acceptable, although over half (54 %) said that having gay or lesbian relations was acceptable. Unfortunately, the percentages above were not broken down by religious group, so they do not necessarily reflect the beliefs of Christians (although, as noted previously, 84 % of the U.S. population is Christian).

Care for the Needy. As noted above, Christians believe that they are their "brother's keeper" (Genesis 4:9) and are responsible for taking care of vulnerable individuals in need. The New Testament emphasizes that Christians and the Christian church are especially responsible for taking care of those who have no family to care for them. The Bible says, "If any woman who is a believer has widows in her care, she should continue to help them and not let the church be burdened with them, so that the church can help those widows who are really in need" (1 Timothy 5:16). In one of the most powerful scriptures in the entire Bible, a scripture that the Prophet Muhammad is said to have referred to (see Sahim Muslim, 32:6232), Jesus said:

> 'For I was hungry and you gave me something to eat, I was thirsty and you gave me something to drink, I was a stranger and you invited me in, I needed clothes and you clothed me, I was sick and you looked after me, I was in prison and you came to visit me.' Then the righteous will answer him, 'Lord, when did we see you hungry and feed you, or thirsty and give you something to drink? When did we see you a stranger and invite you in, or needing clothes and clothe you? When did we see you sick or in prison and go to visit you?' The King will reply, 'Truly I tell you, whatever you did for one of the least of these brothers and sisters of mine, you did for me' (Matthew 25: 35–40).

Attitudes on Health and Healing

Christians have beliefs and attitudes toward the body and healing that will affect their physical health and emotional well-being, and could directly influence the relationship between religious involvement and health.

The Body. The body is viewed with reverence as the "temple of the Holy Spirit" and Christians are told to "honor God" with their bodies (1 Corinthians 6:19–20). Not taking care of the body by excessive eating, drinking too much alcohol, or exposing the body to venereal diseases through extramarital sexual activity, then, is considered a sin. People cannot love and serve God with all their strength (as the Torah emphasized and Jesus commanded) if they are sick (Hartman 2002).

Sickness. Christians have a wide range of views on whether God causes sickness, or whether God helps people to endure sickness and suffers with them. Some believe that because God is all powerful and in complete control, that nothing happens outside of God's will—including physical or mental illness. The Old Testament is clear that God sent disease on those who disobeyed: "However, if you do not obey the Lord your God and do not carefully follow all his commands and decrees I am giving you today… The Lord will plague you with diseases until he has destroyed you from the land you are entering to possess. The Lord will strike you with wasting disease, with fever and inflammation, with scorching heat and drought, with blight and mildew, which will plague you until you perish" (Deuteronomy 28: 15, 21–22; see also Leviticus 26:16).

Some Christians believe, like Muslims, that sickness is a test from God that can lead to purification and refining of the person and make him or her more holy. God in the Old Testament says: "See, I have refined you, though not as silver; I have tested you in the furnace of affliction" (Isaiah 48:10; also see Job 23:10 and Psalm

66:10–12). Likewise, the apostle James in New Testament says, "Consider it pure joy, my brothers and sisters, whenever you face trials of many kinds, because you know that the testing of your faith produces perseverance…Blessed is the one who perseveres under trial because, having stood the test, that person will receive the crown of life that the Lord has promised to those who love him" (James 1:2–3,12; see also 1 Peter 1:7).

Other Christians believe that sickness was not part of God's original plan in creating humans, and came into the world only through the Original Sin committed by Adam who freely disobeyed God. Jesus said sickness was a result of the devil's actions (Luke 13:16; Acts 10:38). Christians also believe that Jesus carried the pain and suffering of illness and disease with him to the cross ("Surely he took up our pain and bore our suffering…"—Isaiah 53:4; see also Matthew 8:17). While Jesus and his disciples acknowledged that some sickness was due to sin, they also made it clear that some sickness was not (John 9:2–3; James 5:14–15). Whether due to sin or not, whether caused by God or not, however, the New Testament indicates that God can use illness (and all traumatic life experiences) to bring out something good from it: "And we know that in all things God works for the good of those who love him, who have been called according to his purpose" (Romans 8:28).

Healing. Spiritual healing is an important part of Christian theology. Specific instructions are provided in the New Testament on what to do in case of physical illness (whether it is due to sin or not): "Is anyone among you sick? Let them call the elders of the church to pray over them and anoint them with oil in the name of the Lord. And the prayer offered in faith will make the sick person well; the Lord will raise them up. If they have sinned, they will be forgiven" (James 5:14–15). From this scripture comes one of the seven major sacraments of the Catholic church, the sacrament of *extreme unction* or "anointing of the sick." Although originally only given to individuals prior to death, this sacrament is now administered to any Catholic "who, having reached the age of reason, begins to be in danger due to sickness or old age" (Code of Canon Law 2007). In Christianity, as in Islam, the source of all healing (whether spiritual, mental, or physical) is God: "Praise the Lord, my soul, and forget not all his benefits—who forgives all your sins and heals all your diseases…" (Psalm 103:2–3; see also Exodus 15:26).

Seeking Medical Care. Most Christians, with some exceptions (Christian Scientists), believe that people should see a doctor when they are sick and utilize whatever medicines or other treatments that are available to manage or cure illness. Jesus acknowledged that the sick needed a doctor (Luke 5:31). Interestingly, the Talmud forbids anyone from even living in a city without a physician (Bokser 1951). Seeking medical care, then, is obligatory for Christians who are told to honor God with their bodies and to preserve the "temple" given to them (1 Corinthians 6:19–20).

Supernatural Beliefs. Belief in miracles, and in the existence of supernatural spirits (demons) that influence health, is widespread among Christians in the United States. The four New Testament Gospels record 37 separate miracles that Jesus performed (Fairchild, n.d.). Nearly four out of five Americans (79 %) agree somewhat or completely that miracles still occur today as they did in ancient times (Pew Research Center 2008, p. 11). Conservative Protestants are most likely to say that they completely agree that miracles still occur today (58–61 %).

Jesus definitely believed in demons and the scriptures are full of accounts of exorcisms that he performed resulting in the person's return to health and sanity (Hollenbach 1981). More than two-thirds of Christians believe that demons are active in the world today (Pew Research Center 2009a, b). Studies of Christians in the West indicate that many believe that mental illness or emotional problems result from demonic activity. In 1994 a study of 343 mainly Protestant psychiatric outpatients in Switzerland found that over one-third (37.6 %) believed that the cause of their mental disorder was possibly evil spirits (calling this "occult bondage" or "possession") (Pfeifer 1994). In that study, many psychiatric patients (30.3 %) sought prayers for deliverance or exorcism. Likewise, in a more recent study of 85 mentally ill Christians in Waco, Texas, over one-third (34.1 %) indicated that someone in their church suggested that their mental illness was a result of demonic involvement (Stanford and McAlister 2008). In a study of 126 healthy Protestant Christians without mental illness in Australia, 38 % endorsed a demonic cause for major depression and 37 % a demonic cause for schizophrenia (Hartog and Gow 2005). These explanations for mental illness are not greatly different from those in the Muslim world. A study of 134 patients in the Muslim country of Malaysia found that 53 % said that a supernatural agent was the cause of their mental illness (i.e., witchcraft or demonic possession) (Razali et al. 2007).

Suicide. Most Christians believe that suicide is a sin. However, the Christian community is divided on whether the person who commits suicide goes to hell, i.e., commits a "mortal" sin. The concept of mortal sin is based on the scripture that says: "If any one sees his brother committing what is *not a mortal sin* [emphasis added], he will ask, and God will give him life for those whose sin is not mortal. There is sin which is mortal; I do not say that one is to pray for that. All wrongdoing is sin, but there is sin which is not mortal" (1 John 5:16–17[3]). Catholic Christians are taught that suicide is a mortal sin, both for the person who commits the act and for whoever helps him or her do it. Committing suicide is equivalent to murdering oneself. For a person to commit a mortal sin, however, he or she must be mentally competent and fully intend to commit the act (Saunders 2003). Fear, ignorance, passion, or psychological problems can interfere with free will and affect a person's culpability for the act. In that case, suicide would not be considered a mortal sin. Furthermore, Catholics believe that Jesus Christ will judge the deceased fairly and justly based on all knowledge about the situation and the person's ability to resist.

Many conservative Protestants, particularly evangelical Christians, believe that a person's sins—past, present, and future—are forgiven the moment that person confesses Jesus as savior (Tubbs 2006). Therefore, if a person who confesses Jesus as savior commits suicide, he or she would still go to heaven. This "once saved always saved" position is based on the scripture "For I am persuaded, that neither death,

---

[3] Revised Standard Version Catholic Edition of the Bible.

nor life, nor angels, nor principalities, nor powers, nor things present, nor things to come, nor height, nor depth, nor any other creature, shall be able to separate us from the love of God, which is in Christ Jesus our Lord" (Romans 8:38–39). The majority of Protestants believe that Jesus with his death on the cross took the punishment for all human sins, including the sin of suicide, so that whoever commits suicide will not be prevented from heaven because of this act (2 Corinthians 5:21).

Many Christians also believe that physician-assisted suicide (PAS) is a sin that is equivalent to murder. A statement from the Massachusetts Council of Churches (MCC), which itself is a relatively liberal Christian body, reinforces this belief: "After careful reflection and prayer, members of the MCC Board of Directors seriously doubt, and some reject categorically, that physician assisted suicide is an ethically responsible option" (Massachusetts Council of Churches 2001). They emphasized compassion, however, and suggested that dialogue continue on this issue. The American Medical Association's position on PAS is firm: "Physician-assisted suicide is fundamentally incompatible with the physician's role as healer, would be difficult or impossible to control, and would pose serious societal risks" (AMA 1993). In a survey of a US national random sample, persons were asked whether a patient with terminal lung cancer should ask for PAS. Conservative Protestant affiliation, greater frequency of religious attendance, and strength of religious affiliation were among the strongest predictors of opposition to this action (Burdette et al. 2005).

Abortion. Christians generally have negative attitudes toward abortion, although again this is dependent on their level of religiosity. Among Americans in general, 50 % are "pro-life" (have a negative attitude toward abortion) and 41 % are "pro-choice" (have a positive attitude toward abortion) (Saad 2012). Those who are not religious are more likely to be pro-choice (68 %), whereas Catholics (38 %) and Protestant Christians (33 %) are less likely. The latest Gallup polls (December 27–30, 2012) indicate that 18 % of Americans believe that abortion should be illegal regardless of circumstances, 52 % believe it should be legal but only under certain circumstances (rape, incest, etc.), and 28 % say it should be legal under all circumstances (Gallup Inc. 2013). However, only 9 % of those who attend religious services weekly believe that abortion should be legal under all circumstances (Newport and Saad 2006).

Contraception. Today most Americans (89 %), including Catholics (82 %), believe that contraception to avoid pregnancy is morally acceptable (Newport 2012). The Catholic church's official position (as of 2008), however, is that it opposes the use of contraception, including female condoms and morning-after pills (Dignitas Personae 2008). The reason given is because methods of contraception "dissociate procreation from the integrally personal context of the conjugal act." Other Christian groups, such as the Amish, also discourage contraception.

Substance Use. Use of elicit drugs is illegal in the U.S. because these substances are known to produce addiction and increase the risk of disease and death. Christians obey the law and so Christianity prohibits the use of elicit drugs. This is true for all mainstream Christian denominations. They do not, however, forbid the consumption of alcohol, although many Baptists, Pentecostals, Methodists, Seventh Day Adventists, Mormons, and evangelical groups, such as the Salvation Army, strongly discourage alcohol use. Although consuming alcohol is not necessarily sinful even in the latter traditions, it is considered an unwise and poor choice. In fact, abstention is often required for clergy in these religious groups. Members of religious denominations in the United States vary on the extent of actual alcohol use. When asked on how many days in the past 7 days they consumed four to five or more drinks that contained alcohol (considered heavy alcohol use), 31 % of men and 18 % of women indicated they did this at least 1 day/week. Broken down by religious group and gender, the percentages were as follows: Protestants (25 % of men vs. 15 % of women), Catholics (37 % vs. 21 %), Mormons (11 % vs. 5 %), Jews (23 % vs. 19 %), and Muslims (20 % vs. 6 %) (Gallup Inc. 2009, p. 61).

Range of Belief and Practice

As we indicated at the start of this chapter, there is a wide range of beliefs and practices within the broad group of people who call themselves Christians. There are Christians who may not believe in the Gospel, or even believe that Jesus was a real person who lived on this earth. Some may not believe in God, whether a personal God or otherwise. For example, in 2011, a Gallup poll found that 7 % of those in the U.S. said they did not believe in God (personal or impersonal); among those who defined themselves as "liberals," 10–15 % did not believe in God. There are Christians who don't believe in the Bible either. Nearly one in five (17 % of those in the U.S.) don't believe that the Bible is the literal or the inspired word of God, but rather that it is simply a book of fables. There is also a range of beliefs about heaven, hell, and the devil in the United States, where 20 % do not believe in heaven, 30 % not in hell, 20 % not in angels, and 30 % not in the devil (Winseman 2004). Finally, at least 15 % of those in the United States do not believe that Jesus is either God or the Son of God (Gallup and Lindsay 1999). Although many of these individuals likely fall in the non-affiliated group, there are at least some who would say they are Christian.

Summary and Conclusions

In this chapter we described the beliefs, practices, and values of the broad group of people who call themselves Christians, particularly those in the United States (on which such information is most readily available). We also examine attitudes toward healing and healthcare, including beliefs regarding ethical issues. In general, the conservative or Orthodox views of Christians based on the Bible are presented here, although we acknowledge both at the beginning and the end of this chapter that more moderate and liberal Christian views exist. The reason for presenting such information on Christian beliefs and practices is because they help to explain the relationship between religion and health in Christian populations. Since the vast majority of research on religion and health has been done in Western samples composed primarily of Christians, such information is vital not only for determining how religion affects health but also for comparing results from these studies with those in Muslim populations. Furthermore, understanding the differences and similarities between Christian and Muslim theology, contrasted in the next chapter, is of critical importance in appreciating the research findings presented later in this book.

References

AMA. (1993). *Opinion 2.211—Physician assisted suicide*. American Medical Association. Retrieved October 4, 2013, from http://www.ama-assn.org/ama/pub/physician-resources/medical-ethics/code-medical-ethics/opinion2211.page

Baker, K. (1995). Jesus will judge the living and the dead. In *Fundamentals of Catholicism* (Vol. 1, chap. 28, pp. 85–87). San Francisco: Ignatius Press.

Barna Research Group. (2002). *Christians mass media reach more adults with the Christian message than do churches*. Retrieved October 4, 2013, from http://www.barna.org/barna-update/article/5-barna-update/77-christian-mass-media-reach-more-adults-with-the-christian-message-than-do-churches

Barna Research Group. (2008). *New study shows trends in tithing and donating*. Ventura, CA: The Barna Group, Ltd. Retrieved October 4, 2013, from http://www.barna.org/congregations-articles/41-new-study-shows-trends-in-tithing-and-donating

Bokser, B. Z. (1951). *The wisdom of the Talmud* (Erubin 65a; Berakot 62b; Abot 3:14; Gittin 70a; Sanhedrin 17b; Yerushalmi Kiddushin 66d) (p. 133). New York: Philosophical Library.

Burdette, A. M., Hill, T. D., & Moulton, B. E. (2005). Religion and attitudes toward physician-assisted suicide and terminal palliative care. *Journal for the Scientific Study of Religion, 44*, 79–93.

Code of Canon Law. (2007). *Book IV: Function of the Church* (Cann. 834-848), Part I: The sacraments (Cann. 998-1007), Chapter III: Those on whom the anointing of the sick is to be conferred, Cann. 1004-1007). Retrieved October 4, 2013, from http://www.intratext.com/IXT/ENG0017/_P2R.HTM

Dawkins, R. (1990). *The selfish gene*. New York: Oxford University Press.

Dignitas Personae. (2008). *On certain bioethical questions. Congregation for the doctrine of the faith*. Retrieved October 4, 2013, from http://www.ewtn.com/library/CURIA/cdfdigpersbio.HTM

Dougherty, K. D., Draper, S., Franzen, A., Froese, P., Martinez, B., Mencken, F. C., Neubert, M. J., Park, J. Z., & Whitehead, A. L. (2011). *The values and beliefs of the American public: Wave III Baylor religion survey* (p. 21). Waco, TX: Baylor University.

Fairchild, M. (n.d.). *The miracles of Jesus*. About.com: Christianity. Retrieved October 4, 2013, from http://christianity.about.com/od/biblefactsandlists/a/Miracles-Of-Jesus.htm

Gallup Inc. (2009). *Muslim Americans: A national portrait*. Retrieved October 4, 2013, from http://www.gallup.com/strategicconsulting/153572/report-muslim-americans-national-portrait.aspx

Gallup Inc. (2013). *Abortion*. The Gallup Poll, Dec 27–30, 2012. Retrieved October 4, 2013, from http://www.gallup.com/poll/1576/abortion.aspx

Gallup Poll. (1993). *The Gallup organization. Reported in Gallup G, Lindsay DM (1999). Survey the Religious Landscape*. Nashville, TN: Morehouse Publishing.

Gallup, G., & Lindsay, D. M. (1999). *Survey the religious landscape*. Nashville, TN: Morehouse Publishing.
Gallup, A., & Simmons, W. W. (2000). *Six in ten Americans read the Bible at least occasionally*. The Gallup Poll. Retrieved October 4, 2013, from http://www.gallup.com/poll/2416/six-ten-americans-read-bible-least-occasionally.aspx
Gospel Music Association. (2008). *Overview*. Retrieved October 4, 2013, from http://www.cmta.com/GMA_Industry_Overview_2008.pdf
Hartman, D. (2002). *Maimonides: Torah and philosophic quest* (p. 87). Philadelphia: Jewish Publication Society.
Hartog, K., & Gow, K. M. (2005). Religious attributions pertaining to the causes and cures of mental illness. *Mental Health, Religion & Culture, 8*(4), 263–276.
Heaton, T. B. (2013). Religion and socioeconomic status in developing nations: A comparative approach. *Social Compass, 60*, 97–114.
Hollenbach, P. W. (1981). Jesus, demoniacs, and public authorities: A socio-historical study. *Journal of the American Academy of Religion, 49*(4), 567–588.
Jones, J. M. (2010). *Few Americans oppose a national day of prayer*. The Gallup Poll, May 1–2 USA Today/Gallup Poll Survey. Retrieved October 4, 2013, from http://www.gallup.com/poll/127721/few-americans-oppose-national-day-prayer.aspx
Jones, J. M. (2011, May 5–8). *In U.S., 3 in 10 say they take the Bible literally*. Gallup Poll. Retrieved October 4, 2013, from http://www.gallup.com/poll/148427/say-bible-literally.aspx
Jones, J., & Saad, L. (2012). *Gallup Poll social series: Values and beliefs*. Princeton, NJ: Gallup News Service. Retrieved October 4, 2013, from http://cnsnews.com/sites/default/files/documents/GALLUP-ECONOMIC-SOCIAL ISSUES.pdf
Lewis, C. S. (1940/2002). *The complete C.S. Lewis signature classics: The problem of pain* (p. 626). New York: HarperOne
Lewis, C. S. (1944/1986). *Mere Christianity* (p. 65). New York: Macmillan Publishing.
Massachusetts Council of Churches. (2001). *Physician-assisted suicide: A Christian perspective from the Massachusetts Council of Churches*. Retrieved April 19, 2013, from http://www.masscouncilofchurches.org/docs/doc_suicide.htm
Nasr, S. H. (2002). *The heart of Islam* (p. 23). New York: HarperCollins.
Newport, F. (2007). *Americans more likely to believe in god than the devil, heaven more than hell*. The Gallup Poll. Retrieved October 4, 2013, from http://www.gallup.com/poll/27877/americans-more-likely-believe-god-than-devil-heaven-more-than-hell.aspx
Newport, F. (2010, May). *Americans' church attendance inches up in 2010*. The Gallup Poll. Retrieved October 4, 2013, from http://www.gallup.com/poll/141044/Americans-Church-Attendance-Inches-2010.aspx
Newport, F. (2012). *Americans, including Catholics, say birth control is morally acceptable*. The Gallup Poll. Retrieved October 4, 2013, from http://www.gallup.com/poll/154799/americans-including-catholics-say-birth-control-morally.aspx
Newport, F., & Saad, L. (2006, April 3). *Religion, politics inform Americans' views on abortion*. The Gallup Poll. Retrieved October 4, 2013, from http://www.gallup.com/poll/22222/Religion-Politics-Inform-Americans-Views-Abortion.aspx
O'Beirne, M. (2004). *Religion in England and Wales: Findings from the 2001 Home Office Citizenship Survey*. London: Home Office Research Study.
Pew Religious Landscape Survey. (2008). *Comparisons: Views of one's religion as the one true faith*. Washington, DC: The Pew Forum on Religion and the Public Life. Retrieved October 4, 2013, from http://religions.pewforum.org/pdf/table-views-of-ones-religion-as-the-one-true-faith-by-religious-tradition.pdf [paste website into browser].
Pew Research Center. (2008). *Religious landscape survey: Summary of key findings*. Washington, DC: The Pew Forum on Religion and the Public Life. Retrieved October 4, 2013, from http://religions.pewforum.org/pdf/report2religious-landscape-study-key-findings.pdf
Pew Research Center. (2009a). *Not all non-believers call themselves atheists*. Washington, DC: The Pew Forum on Religion and the Public Life. Retrieved October 4, 2013, from http://www.pewforum.org/Not-All-Nonbelievers-Call-Themselves-Atheists.aspx

Pew Research Center. (2009b). *A religious portrait of African-Americans* [with data on all Americans]. Washington, DC: The Pew Forum on Religion and the Public Life. Retrieved October 4, 2013, from http://www.pewforum.org/A-Religious-Portrait-of-African-Americans.aspx

Pew Research Center. (2010). *Religion among the millennials*. Retrieved October 4, 2013, from http://www.pewforum.org/Age/Religion-Among-the-Millennials.aspx

Pew Research Center. (2011). *Global Christianity: A report on the size and distribution of the world's Christian population*. Washington, DC: The Pew Forum on Religion and the Public Life. Retrieved October 4, 2013, from http://www.pewforum.org/uploadedFiles/Topics/Religious_Affiliation/Christian/Christianity-fullreport-web.pdf

Pew Research Center. (2012). *The world's Muslims: Unity and diversity* (p. 8). Retrieved October 4, 2013, from http://www.pewforum.org/Muslim/the-worlds-muslims-unity-and-diversity-2-religious-commitment.aspx

Pew Research Center. (2013). *U.S. Christians' view on the return of Jesus*. Washington, DC: The Pew Forum on Religion and the Public Life. Retrieved October 4, 2013, from http://www.pewforum.org/Christian/US-Christians-Views-on-the-Return-of-Christ.aspx

Pfeifer, S. (1994). Belief in demons and exorcism in psychiatric patients in Switzerland. *British Journal of Medical Psychology, 67*, 247–258.

Plunkett, O. (2002, February). The miracles of Lourdes. *British Medical Journal (studentBMJ), 10*, 1–44. Retrieved October 4, 2013, from http://student.bmj.com/student/view-article.html?id=sbmj020233

Princeton Religion Research Center. (1996). *Religion in America, 1996 Report: Will the vitality of the church be the surprise of the 21st century?* Princeton, NJ: The Gallup Poll.

Razali, S. M., Khan, U. A., & Hasanah, C. I. (2007). Belief in supernatural causes of mental illness among Malay patients: Impact on treatment. *Acta Psychiatrica Scandinavica, 94*(4), 229–233.

Saad, L. (2012, May 29). *In U.S., nonreligious, postgrads are highly "pro-choice"*. The Gallup Poll. Retrieved October 4, 2013, from http://www.gallup.com/poll/154946/Non-Christians-Postgrads-Highly-Pro-Choice.aspx

Sarkissian, A. (2012). Religion and civic engagement in Muslim countries. *Journal for the Scientific Study of Religion, 51*(4), 607–622.

Saunders, W. (2003). *The sin of suicide*. The Arlington Catholic Herald (reprinted by the Catholic Education Resource Center). Retrieved October 4, 2013, from http://catholiceducation.org/articles/religion/re0123.html

Stanford, M. S., & McAlister, K. R. (2008). Perceptions of serious mental illness in the local church. *Journal of Religion, Disability & Health, 12*(2), 144–153.

Trepanowski, J. F., & Bloomer, R. J. (2010). The impact of religious fasting on human health. *Nutrition Journal, 9*, 57.

Tubbs, B. (2006). *Do people who commit suicide go to hell?* Suite 101. Retrieved October 4, 2013, from http://suite101.com/article/do-people-who-commit-suicide-go-to-hell-a65637

Winseman, A. L. (2004). *Eternal destinations: Americans believe in heaven, hell*. The Gallup Poll. Retrieved October 4, 2013, from http://www.gallup.com/poll/11770/eternal-destinations-americans-believe-heaven-hell.aspx

Wright, K. (2009). *World Religious Travel Association—An overview*. Retrieved October 4, 2013, from http://www.slideshare.net/WRTA/worldreligioustravelassociationoverview

Chapter 5
Differences and Similarities

In order to understand why research findings on religion and health in Muslims might differ from or parallel those in Christians, it is important first to recognize the differences and similarities in belief, practice, and values between these faith traditions. In some respects, they are vastly different. In other respects, they are remarkably similar.

Differences

Beliefs

Most differences between Muslims and Christians lie in the area of belief (since their religious practices, values, and views toward health and healing are largely the same).

God. Muslims emphasize the greatness, grandeur, power, and wisdom of God. He is the creator, the sustainer, the guide, and the judge. God is all-knowing and in complete control. God is not like people who become tired from work or have children, and instead operates on a vastly different level than humans. Says the great Islamic intellectual Seyyed Hossein Nasr, "Allah is beyond all duality and relationality, beyond the differences of gender and of all qualities that distinguish beings from each other in this world. Yet He is the source of all existence and all cosmic and human qualities as well as the End to Whom all things return" (Nasr 2002, p. 3). God is infinitely merciful and forgiving, but is also just and can be severe to those who disobey. The human's obligation is to obey and submit, or face the consequences of not doing so.

Christians emphasize the relational characteristics of God—that humans are created in God's image (Genesis 1:27) and so can communicate and interact with God as a person. Much of this view comes from believing that Jesus was both completely

H.G. Koenig and S. Al Shohaib, *Health and Well-Being in Islamic Societies: Background, Research, and Applications*, DOI 10.1007/978-3-319-05873-3_5,

God and completely human, and as a human got tired, angry, loved, and suffered just like people do. Christians focus their theology on the kindness and love of God, and on God's desire to communicate with His created beings on an intimate level. Christians believe that God is immediately present, a friend who is closer than a brother (Proverbs 18:24). God listens and responds to prayer, answering both spoken and unspoken requests, but only in a way that leads to a person's eternal good. The Bible says that God loves his followers: "For the Father himself loveth you," said Jesus (John 16:27, KJV). Christians believe that love for humans flows naturally out of God's perfect goodness. Christians respond to God's love and goodness by surrendering their lives to him, serving God out of love and appreciation for what He has done for them ("perfect love casteth out fear"—1 John 4:18 KJV).

The differences between beliefs about God described above are in degree and emphasis only, especially among the devout. Most Muslims and Christians believe that God is unimaginably great, all-powerful, wise, all-knowing, just and fair, perfectly good, merciful, and forgiving, and is available and approachable to humans (see below). They also both believe that God deserves unlimited reverence, honor, and respect. Almost no objective research, however, has yet compared views of God between Muslims and Christians. Some initial qualitative work seems to support the differences described above, although that research was in children and developmental issues may be a factor (Zuberi 1988).

Physical images of God or the Prophet (aniconism) are absolutely forbidden in Islam, as this comes too close to idolatry. In contrast, many Christians—particularly Roman Catholic Christians—have statues, medals, or pictures of Jesus, Mary, or various saints.

Creation Story. The creation story in Islam differs in several respects from that in Christianity. These differences are mostly minor, but there is also one major difference. The Qur'an is not clear on whether God created Adam in heaven or created Adam on earth and then brought him to heaven, later placing him back on earth (2:30). God gave to Adam the names of all the creatures (2:31) (Adam did not name the creatures himself, as the Christian version has it). The angels were instructed to bow down to Adam (2:34), which is not found in the Genesis story. Muslims believe that Adam and Eve sinned and God expelled them from the garden (2:36), the same as Christians do. However, unlike in the Bible, the Qur'an says that Adam repented of his sin and God forgave him (2:37). As a result, there was no Original Sin that needed to be addressed later by Jesus dying on the cross (this is the major difference).

Original Sin. Christians believe in original sin, the result of Adam's actions, and that all humans have inherited this tendency to sin and rebel against God. As noted above, Muslims believe that Adam confessed his sin and God forgave him. Therefore, Muslims believe that all humans are born perfect and only their decisions to disobey God result in separation from God. Each time they ask forgiveness, because of his great mercy, God forgives them. This is one reason for the five daily prayers. Each prayer cleanses the persons from whatever sins they may have committed since the previous prayer. Since there is no original sin and God completely

Table 5.1 Statements in the Qur'an about the identity of Jesus, the Messiah

"and because they[a] disbelieved and uttered a terrible slander against Mary, and said, 'We have killed the Messiah, Jesus, son of Mary, the Messenger of God.' (They did not kill him, nor did they crucify him, though it was made to appear like that to them; those that disagreed about him are full of doubt, with no knowledge to follow, only supposition: they certainly did not kill him—God raised him up to Himself. God is almighty and wise (4:156–158)"
"(...There is not one of the People of the Book who will not believe in [Jesus] before his death, and on the Day of Resurrection he will be a witness against them)" (4:159)
"People of the Book, do not go to excess in your religion, and do not say anything about God except the truth; the Messiah, Jesus, son of Mary was nothing more than a messenger of God, His word, directed to Mary, a spirit from Him. So believe in God and His messengers and do not speak of a 'Trinity'—stop [this], that is better for you—God is only one God, he is far above having a son, everything in the heavens and earth belongs to Him and He is the best one to Trust. The Messiah would never disdain to be a servant of God..." (4:171–172)
"When God says, 'Jesus, son of Mary, did you say to people, "Take me and my mother as two gods alongside God"?' he [Jesus] will say, 'May You be exalted! I would never say what I had no right to say—if I had said such a thing You would have known it: You know all that is within me, though I do not know what is within You, You alone have full knowledge of things unseen—I told them only what You commanded me to: "Worship God, my Lord and your Lord"'" (5:116–117)
"[But] he [Jesus] said: 'I am a servant of God. He has granted me the Scripture; made me a prophet; made me blessed wherever I may be. He commanded me to pray, to give alms as long as I live, to cherish my mother. He did not make me domineering or graceless. Peace was on me the day I was born, and will be on me the day I die and the day I am raised to life again.' Such was Jesus, son of Mary. [This is] a statement of Truth about which they are in doubt: it would not befit God to have a child. He is far above that..." (19:30–35)
"When the son of Mary is cited as an example, your people [Prophet] [Meccans] laugh and jeer, saying 'Are our gods better or him?[b]—they cite him only to challenge you: they are a contentious people—but he is only a servant We favored and made an example for the Children of Israel..." (43:57–59)

[a]People of the Book (Jews, Sabians, Magians, Christians)
[b]By "our gods," the Meccans were referring to the daughters of God (al-Lat, al-Uzza and Manat) whom they worshipped (a pagan female trinity)

forgives all sins committed after confessing them in prayer, there is no need for Jesus as God the Son to die on the cross.

Jesus the Christ. The biggest difference between Muslims and Christians is the identity of Jesus the Christ and the question of his Divine nature. On the one hand, Christians believe that Jesus was God the Son, worship Jesus as God, believe that Jesus died on the cross and rose from the dead, and many conservative Protestants believe that admittance to heaven requires belief in Jesus' death on the cross as payment for their sins. On the other hand, the Qu'ran is clear that while Jesus is one of the most important prophets in Islam and is very close to God, he is not God and should not be prayed to or worshipped as God (Table 5.1). Muslims believe that worshiping anyone but God is *shirk*, the sin of idolatry or polytheism. Shirk in Arabic means to share as an equal partner with God. Muslims believe that this sin is an unforgivable sin unless the person confesses and repents of this sin prior to death. God forgives any sin except the sin of shirk. This is based on the Qur'an 5:48: "God does not forgive the joining of partners with Him: anything less than that He forgives to whoever He will, but anyone who joins partners with God has concocted a tremendous sin." Joining partners to God was a major issue that the Prophet Muhammad faced when he sought to combat the widespread polytheism of his day, especially the controversy over the three daughters of God—goddesses who were worshiped by Meccans at that time (Ahmed 2004).

Muslims also do not believe that Jesus was killed or crucified. Instead, they believe that it only appeared that way (i.e., it was not Jesus on the cross, but someone else). Muslims do believe, however, that God raised Jesus bodily into heaven and that Jesus will come again at the Day of Judgement (which is what Christians believe also). In the Qur'an, God chastises the Jews: "...No! God has sealed them in their disbelief, so they believe only a little—and because they disbelieved and uttered a terrible slander against Mary, and said, 'We have killed the Messiah, Jesus, son of Mary, the Messenger of God.' (they did not kill him, nor did they crucify him, though it was made to appear like that to them... they certainly did not kill him—God raised him up to Himself..." (4:155–158). These verses are followed by a powerful statement that underscores how important Jesus (as a prophet) is in the Muslim faith: "There is not one of the People of the Book who will not believe in [Jesus] before his death, and on the Day of Resurrection he will be a witness against them" (4:159).

Christians believe not only that Jesus was a great prophet but also that he was God Himself and his death on the cross for their sins is central to their faith. They maintain that if Jesus were not God and was not crucified, then much of what is said about him in the Bible could not be true. Only if he were God incarnate (in the flesh) would the Gospels and New Testament scriptures make any sense. If Jesus were not God as Christians believe, then not only would Muslims be right in saying that Christians are polytheists (although unintentionally), but worse than that, Jesus would probably not have been a prophet at all. Instead, Christians believe, he would have been mentally ill or demon possessed to say the things he did about himself (*if recorded accurately in the Gospels by his disciples*) (Lewis 1952). In fact, being demon possessed is exactly what his critics accused Jesus of: "The Jews answered him, 'Aren't we right in saying that you are a Samaritan and demon-possessed?'" (John 8:48; see also Matthew 9:34; Mark 3:22; Luke 11:15; John 7:20; John 10:20). Even Jesus' own family thought he was out of his mind (insane) and came to rescue him by force (Mark 3:21). Interestingly, recall from Chap. 2 that the critics of the Prophet Muhammad accused him of the same thing. Members of his own tribe in Mecca said that he was possessed by a spirit or jinn (i.e., madness), and even suggested that he undergo exorcism (Hisham, n.d.).

The Holy Spirit. Christians believe that the Holy Spirit is God's spirit, the form of God who is active in the world and is fully God in every respect (see Chap. 4). According to Jesus, as noted in the last chapter, the only unforgivable sin is "blaspheming against the Holy Spirit" (Matthew 12:31). In contrast, Muslims believe that the holy spirit is Gabriel, the angel who brought down the Qur'an to the Prophet Muhammad (2:97) and accompanied him when he was transported to Jerusalem during the Night Journey (Asad 2003). The Qu'ran calls Gabriel the "Trustworthy Spirit" (26:193).

Salvation. A majority of Protestant and Catholic Christians believe that a primary criterion for salvation is repentance for sin and belief in Jesus' sacrifice on the cross as payment for their sins. Many Protestants emphasize that this is the only criterion necessary for salvation (i.e., salvation is by grace alone—a free gift from God—not based on works or good deeds, says Ephesans 2:8). Good deeds, however, are expected to follow salvation (James 2:24). Catholics also stress the need to follow the teachings of the Catholic church and take part in the sacraments, especially the sacraments of Baptism and Holy Communion. Catholics believe that God in the end makes the final decision: "God has bound salvation to the sacrament of Baptism, but he himself is not bound by his sacraments" (Catechism of the Catholic Church 2003).

Muslims believe that entrance into paradise is not determined by belief in Jesus' sacrifice, but on whether they (1) believe in the six articles of faith (God, angels, the prophets, the Divine books, the Day of Judgement, and Fate) (Bukhari 1/2/47),[1] (2) do good deeds (which are weighed against bad deeds on Judgement Day, see below), and (3) repent of sins. The Qur'an says, "but those who repent, who believe, who do righteous deeds, will enter Paradise" (19:60). Again, however, it is God who decides. He controls everything and does what he wills (see 67:1–2; 85:16).

Thus, the majority of both Muslims and Christians believe that God will make the final decision regarding salvation and entrance into heaven based on God's infinite wisdom and unlimited knowledge of the strengths, weaknesses, and resources of the person and on the person's decisions to do good or evil.

The Prophet Muhammad. Since the Prophet lived hundreds of years after the Bible was canonized, there are no specific references to him in the Bible, nor do Christian doctrines or teachings refer specifically to the Prophet. However, some Muslims believe that the Prophet was referred to earlier in the Scriptures by the prophet Isaiah (Isaiah 53:3) and by Jesus himself (John 15:26). Most Christians today, however, know very little about the Prophet Muhammad's life or teachings, other than what they've heard from the Western news media (often inaccurate).

Muslims believe that the very words of God were sent through the Prophet Muhammad to all humanity to form the Holy Qur'an. According to the Qur'an, the Prophet is considered "the seal of the prophets" (33:40), the final prophet in a series of over 100,000 prophets dating back to Adam (Nasr 2002, pp. 17–18). Seyyed Nasr says there has been no major prophet besides the Prophet Muhammad in the last 1,400 years of the caliber of Moses, Jesus, the Buddha, or the founder of any other major world religion, which appears to confirm this claim.

To become a Muslim a person must affirm by saying the Shahada: "There is no god but God, Muhammad is the messenger of God." Yale University theologian, Lamin Sanneh, says "Muhammad was called *uswa hasan* (33:21), 'the beautiful

[1] Citations to *Sahih Bukhari* (the most respected of all Sunni Hadiths) is based on a 2009 translation M. Muhain Khan (2009). We list the reference by volume, book, and number (vol/book/no). See http://d1.islamhouse.com/data/en/ih_books/single/en_Sahih_Al-Bukhari.pdf (last accessed April 22, 2014).

model,' his followers believing that God had sent him 'as a mercy for the worlds' (*rahmatan li-l-'alamin*) and that God and his angels pronounce blessings on him (33:56)" (Sanneh 1996). In the Qur'an, God instructs the Prophet: "Say, 'My Lord has guided me to a straight path, an upright religion, the faith of Abraham, a man of pure faith. He was not a polytheist.' Say, 'My prayers and sacrifice, my life and death, are all for God, Lord of all the Worlds'" (6:161–162).

Divine Books. Christians, along with the Jews, are called People of the Book in the Qur'an. Christians believe in both the Old Testament (the Torah, i.e., the first five books, and 34 additional books) and the New Testament (the four Gospels, and the Epistles or teachings of the disciples of Jesus). The New Testament says that Jesus reaffirmed the importance and truth of the Scriptures that preceded him, saying "Do not think that I have come to abolish the Law or the Prophets; I have not come to abolish them but to fulfill them. For truly I tell you, until heaven and earth disappear, not the smallest letter, not the least stroke of a pen, will by any means disappear from the Law until everything is accomplished" (Matthew 5:17–18). Christians believe that the entire Bible (Old and New Testaments) was sent by God and is useful as a guide for living: "All Scripture is God-breathed and is useful for teaching, rebuking, correcting and training in righteousness, so that the servant of God may be thoroughly equipped for every good work" (2 Timothy 3:16–17).

While Muslims believe that the Torah, the Psalms (*Zaboor*), and the Gospel (*Injeel*) were sent by God to the prophets, they believe that these scriptures have been tampered with. Muslims maintain that the scriptures have been changed from the original revelation to the current versions that now contain errors. The Qur'an has corrected those errors and is the final authority, an exact replica of God's instructions contained in a sacred book that resides on tablets in heaven. Thus, anything that the Bible says that conflicts with the Qur'an is believed to be the result of human tampering and is therefore rejected. Likewise, the Christian Bible claims that it is the final authority, sending a stern warning to anyone who adds to or takes away anything that has been said in it (Revelations 22:17–20).

Muslims believe that the Prophet did not have direct access to the Bible (Emerick 2004). The timeline supports this belief. The Old and New Testament books of the Bible were not widely agreed upon until the middle of the third century and were not canonized until the end of the fourth century CE. The complete Bible was probably just beginning to be translated into Arabic between 570 and 632 CE and was certainly not widely available even among Christians whom Muhammad associated with. Most of these Christians were not very knowledgeable about the Bible, including the New Testament, and probably based their beliefs on a variety of different views—some mainstream and some heretical (like worshiping Mary). Muslims believe, however, that this doesn't make any difference since the Prophet learned not from reading the Hebrew and Christian scriptures (since he could not read or write), nor from his interactions with Christians and Jews of his day, but rather by direct revelation from God of what was spoken to earlier prophets.

Practices

Most practices of Christians and Muslims are the same, although some practices are considered more important than others depending on the tradition.

Prayer. Regular prayer is emphasized more strongly in Islam than in Christianity. There is no doctrine requiring Christians to pray, and so prayer is done spontaneously and out of devotion to God. As a result, while prayer is very important to devout Christians, it is usually performed less than the five times per day that is required in Islam. The form of prayer is also different between the two faiths, with Muslims becoming involved with their entire bodies by kneeling, bowing, and touching their foreheads to the ground during prayer, while facing toward Mecca.

Fasting. Muslims stress the importance of fasting (*sawm*) as exemplified in the month-long fast during Ramadan, which is one of the five pillars or core teachings of Islam. During Ramadan, Muslims fast from dawn to dusk every day when no food or drink can be consumed. Many Muslims fast at other times as well to express their devotion. Fasting is also a respected tradition in most branches of Christianity because of its frequent mention throughout the Bible (among the Jews, for example, the practices of fasting, prayer, and repentance were the pillars of Jewish theology). Fasting was something that Jesus probably assumed most people did during his time and, in fact, Jesus described how one should go about fasting (Matthew 6:17–18). Jesus went on a prolonged fast himself for 40 days in the desert before beginning his public ministry (Luke 4:2). Furthermore, when his disciples could not cast out a demon, Jesus said that "This kind can come forth by nothing, but by prayer and fasting" (Mark 9:29 KJV, see also Matthew 21:17). Nevertheless, most Christians today fast much less frequently than do Muslims. Almost all Muslims (85–98 %) in the Middle East and North Africa say they fast during the day every day during the month of Ramadan (as required) (Pew Research Center 2012, p. 8).

Reading Scripture. In the Middle East and North Africa, 96–100 % of Muslims read the Qur'an and 31–52 % read it at least once daily (Pew Research Center 2012, p. 7). Many Muslims have memorized the entire Qur'an (6,236 verses or about 80,000 words), which they may recite regularly either aloud or quietly. Christians read the Bible and often memorize scriptures, although this practice may vary depending on the person's religious denomination (Protestants vs. Catholics) and level of devotion. However, Christians usually do not read the Bible as often as Muslims read the Qur'an. Muslims are less likely to read popular inspirational books other than the Qur'an and Hadith, whereas Christians are more likely to supplement their Bible reading (see Chap. 4) with such material.

Religious Services. There are differences in the layout and structure of religious services. Christians usually pray, listen to sermons, and sing hymns or religious songs during a Sunday or Wednesday night church service. Muslims do not usually sing at the mosque, especially during *Jumah* (Friday) service when singing is prohibited. Chanting Islamic songs at the mosque at other times is not forbidden as long as it is not accompanied by prohibited musical instruments, is done quietly, and does not interfere with those praying at the mosque. Muslims usually pray, recite the Qur'an quietly, and listen to the sermon during a mosque service. Mosques provide an open area where Muslims place their prayer mats, on which they sit, stand, bow, and perform prayers. Christian churches provide pews, chairs, or benches where members sit and stand during the service (some Catholic churches also have benches for kneeling). Catholic, Greek Orthodox, and some Protestant churches will also conduct rites and rituals during religious services (e.g., perform the sacrament of Holy Communion or the Eucharist). Rituals (except prayer and reading the Qur'an) are not usually performed during Muslim services at the mosque. There are also no pictures or statues in mosques, so that there will be no temptation to worship them as idols. In contrast, Catholic and Greek Orthodox churches often have pictures and statues.

Unlike in Christianity, where 61 % of church attendees are women (National Church Life Survey 2001), Muslim women attend religious services less frequently than men. The gender difference depends on the particular country (Gallup Inc. 2009, p. 59). In Saudi Arabia, for example, 42 % of women say they have attended a mosque service in the last 7 days, compared to 92 % of men. There is a similar gender gap among women and men in Egypt (42 % vs. 79 %, respectively). Interestingly, there is little gender gap in mosque attendance for Muslims in America (40 % of women vs. 42 % of men attend weekly or more). Unlike young American Christians, young American Muslims (ages 18–29) are just as likely—if not more likely—to attend mosque at least weekly compared to older American Muslims (ages 45–64) (41 % vs. 38 %, respectively).

Religious Pilgrimage. Although Christians may occasionally go on religious pilgrimage (see Chap. 4), it is not part of their theology and therefore they do this much less often than Muslims. If they are able, Muslims are required to make a religious pilgrimage to Mecca at least once during their lifetimes. In the Middle East and North Africa, 17 % of Muslims say that they have made a pilgrimage to Mecca at some point in their lives (Pew Research Center 2012, p. 9). However, the low socioeconomic status of many Muslims in undeveloped countries often prevents such travel. Otherwise, the percentage would be much higher as evidenced by the fact that the distance from Mecca is inversely associated with the likelihood of having completed the pilgrimage.

Importance of Good Deeds. Muslims believe that God will weigh a person's good deeds and bad deeds on a scale (*mizan*) on Judgement Day, and that if the bad deeds outweigh the good, then the person will be sent to hell. The Qur'an says, "On the Day the weighing of deeds will be true and just: those whose good deeds are heavy on the scales will be the ones to prosper, and those whose good deeds are light will be the ones who have lost their souls through their wrongful rejection of Our messages" (7:8–9). Likewise, "We will set up scales of justice for the Day of Resurrection so that no one can be wronged in the least, and if there should be even the weight of a mustard seed, We shall bring it out—We take excellent account" (21:47). Finally,

"On that Day when the Trumpet is blown, the ties between them will be as nothing and they will not ask about each other: those whose good deeds were heavy will be successful, but those whose balance is light will have lost their souls for ever and will stay in Hell—the fire will scorch their faces and their lips will be twisted in pain" (23:101–104). In Christianity, people are not saved by doing good deeds, but rather by belief in Jesus' sacrifice on the cross (saved by grace, not by works). As noted in Chap. 4, however, Christians also believe that "faith without works is dead" (James 2:20, KJV).

Values

The values of devout Christians and Muslims are more similar than either their beliefs or their religious practices, and those differences are largely culture related.

Individualism. While Western Christians pride themselves in being individualistic, this is not the case among Muslims. Muslims work, play, fight, and love as families or kin networks. Individualism is not valued or encouraged within Islam. Rather, it is the family and community that takes precedence. This does not mean that Christians don't highly value family and community, but they are less likely than Muslims to elevate these areas above the rights of the individual. Again, both Muslims and Christians respect the individual and value the community, and the differences here are only a matter of degree.

Destiny. Muslims believe that all things are predetermined by God. The belief in predestination has a word in Arabic, *muqaddar*, which literally means "It's been decided." Another Arabic word used to describe this belief is *maktub* ("It is written"), which refers to a person's written destiny, i.e., what is fated, decreed, predestined, or determined. This belief in destiny has been compared to fatalism—"what will be, will be." Christians also believe that God has a purpose: "And we know that in all things God works for the good of those who love him, who have been called according to his purpose" (Romans 8:28). There is even belief by some Protestant Christians in what is called the *doctrine of predestination* (followed by many Presbyterrean and Reformed churches that abide by the teachings of theologian John Calvin). The doctrine of predestination says "God from all eternity did by the most wise and holy counsel of his own will, freely and unchangeably ordain whatsoever comes to pass" (Westminster Confession of Faith 1646). However, most Christians do not believe in the doctrine of predestination, but rather that a combination of person's actions (free will or choice) and God's sovereign will, these determine what happens. Muslims also believe in free will, although don't emphasize it as much in their theology. This difference between Muslims and Christians on destiny could influence decisions on whether to seek healthcare when sick or engage in healthy behaviors to prevent disease.

Women's Rights. Men dominated the ancient Christian world (Genesis 3:16; 1 Corinthians 11:3), just as they did in early Islam. All 12 of Jesus' disciples were men. The Catholic church still does not ordain women as priests and there has never been a woman pope. However, Jesus emphasized the importance of men treating wives equally and defended the rights of women (Matthew 19:3–9), even prostitutes and non-Jews (John 8:3–11; 4:7–26). Women also accompanied Jesus during his travels at a time when women were supposed to stay at home (Luke 8:1–3). His followers continued this tradition of respect for women (Ephesians 5:22–33; Galatian 3:28), although there are some exceptions (1 Corinthians 14:34–35). Because of this Biblical attitude toward women, Christian societies have generally upheld and defended the rights of women (at least in modern times) (Hiers 2012).

In some parts of the Islamic world, women continue to have fewer rights than men today. This was common in the patriarchical societies that dominated the Arabic world in the Prophet Muhammad's time. On the one hand, much has been said about the unequal rights that men and women have in Muslim countries. The Qur'an devotes an entire chapter to women (*Al-Nisa'*), where it justifies polytheism (4:3), unequal share of inheritance (4:11–12), and punishment (4:34). Elsewhere, the Qur'an says that husbands have rights over women (2:228) and that one male witness for a debt is equivalent to two female witnesses (2:282). On the other hand, the Qur'an was far ahead of its time in making every effort to establish the rights of women, ensure their fair treatment, and preserve their safety given the male-dominated bedouin pre-Islamic Arabic culture of the seventh century (Watts 1956). There are many places in the Qur'an giving women rights, such as the right of property ownership, a right which women in Europe did not receive until the nineteenth century (Women's Rights 2006). Women in Islamic countries today, even those under strict Sharia law, are having their rights expanded, including the right to vote and serve in public office (Chulov 2011).

Similarities

There are also many similarities between Muslims and Christians (particularly conservative Christians) with regard to beliefs, practices, and values. These are often ignored, underestimated, or misunderstood. We describe these now.

Beliefs

God. The most important belief that Muslims and Christians have in common is the central and core belief in God. Arabic Christians used the word Allah for God during the Prophet Muhammad's time, and even today, Arabic Christians continue to pray to Allah. Whenever the Christian Bible is translated into Arabic by Christians today, the word Allah is used for God. In fact, the word that Jesus used when he cried out in his native language (Aramaic) to God during the crucifixion was *Alahi* or "My God" (even though Eli is used in many translations: *Eli, Eli, lama sabachthani*) (Matthew 27:45–46) (Missick 2006).

Table 5.2 Only one God in the Bible

Old testament
"You shall have no other gods before me" (Exodus 20:3) (the FIRST of the 10 commandments)
"Whoever sacrifices to any god other than the Lord must be destroyed" (Exodus 22:20)
"Do not worship any other god, for the Lord, whose name is Jealous, is a jealous God" (Exodus 34:14)
"You shall have no foreign god among you; you shall not worship any god other than me" (Psalm 81:9).
"I am the Lord; that is my name! I will not yield my glory to another or my praise to idols" (Isaiah 42:8)
"This is what the Lord says— Israel's King and Redeemer, the Lord Almighty: I am the first and I am the last; apart from me there is no God" (Isaiah 44:6)
Do we not all have one Father? Did not one God create us? (Malachi 2:10)
New testament
"So then, about eating food sacrificed to idols: We know that 'An idol is nothing at all in the world' and that 'There is no God but one.'" (1 Corinthians 8:4)
"yet for us there is but one God, the Father, from whom all things came and for whom we live..." (1 Corinthians 8:6)
What agreement is there between the temple of God and idols? For we are the temple of the living God. As God has said: "I will live with them and walk among them, and I will be their God, and they will be my people." (2 Corinthians 6:16)
"Or is God the God of Jews only? Is he not the God of Gentiles too? Yes, of Gentiles too, since there is only one God, who will justify the circumcised by faith and the uncircumcised through that same faith" (Romans 3:29–30)
"Make every effort to keep the unity of the Spirit through the bond of peace. There is one body and one Spirit, just as you were called to one hope when you were called; one Lord, one faith, one baptism; one God and Father of all, who is over all and through all and in all." (Ephesians 4:3–6)
"The Lord's message rang out from you not only in Macedonia and Achaia—your faith in God has become known everywhere. Therefore we do not need to say anything about it, for they themselves report what kind of reception you gave us. They tell how you turned to God from idols to serve the living and true God," (1 Thessalonians 1:8–9)

Says Seyyed Nasr, "At the heart of Islam stands the reality of God, the One, the Absolute and the Infinite, the Infinitely Good and all-Merciful, the One who is at once transcendent and immanent, greater than all we can conceive or imagine, yet, as the Qur'an, the sacred scripture of Islam attests, closer to us than our jugular vein. The One God, known by His Arabic Name, Allah, is the central reality of Islam in all of its facets, and attestation to this oneness, which is called *tawhid*, is the axis around which all that is Islamic revolves...He is far beyond our reach, yet resides at the center of the heart of the faithful. He punishes the wicked, but also loves His creatures and forgives them" (Nasr 2002, pp. 3, 5).

Both Muslims and Christians believe in one God, i.e., monotheism. The proclamation of faith in Islam makes it clear that only God is to be worshiped: "There is no god but God, Muhammad is the messenger of God." Not only is this statement required to become a Muslim, but it is displayed on the national flags of both Saudi Arabia and Afghanistan. Christians believe likewise that there is no god but God, and only God is to be worshiped. In both the Old Testament and the New Testament the worship of anyone but God was forbidden (Table 5.2). Christians believe that

God is uniquely and completely one. There are no other gods that compare to God. God does not have partners that are equal to God.

Muslims and Christians, particularly those on the conservative or orthodox end of the spectrum, believe that the primary goal in life is to submit and surrender to the will of God, whom they are to love and serve with all their strength, might, and abilities. In the Torah, the first commandment of the ten Commandments is "You shall have no other gods before me" (Exodus 20:3). Moses further emphasized this as the central commandment in Judaism: "Love the LORD your God with all your heart and with all your soul and with all your strength" (Deuteronomy 6:5). When a Jewish lawyer asked Jesus to name the greatest commandment in the Law, he said: "'Love the Lord your God with all your heart and with all your soul and with all your mind.' This is the first and greatest commandment" (Matthew 22:37). The same answer is given by Jesus in two of the other three Gospels in the New Testament (Mark 12:30 and Luke 10:27). In the Gospel of Luke, Jesus was asked, "What must I do to inherit eternal life?" (Luke 10:25–27). His response was that loving God and loving neighbor are required to enter heaven and paradise. Likewise, the first sentence of the Nicene Creed, which states the core tenets of Christianity, is "We believe in one God, the Father, the Almighty, maker of heaven and earth, of all that is seen and unseen."

Thus, for both Muslims and Christians, the central belief that supercedes all other beliefs is belief in and submission to God—the one God, the only God. All other beliefs are secondary to this belief. The Qur'an says, "So [you believers], say, 'We believe in God and in what was sent down to us and what was sent down to Abraham, Ishmael, Isaac, Jacob, and the Tribes, and what was given to Moses, Jesus, and all the prophets by their Lord. We make no distinction between any of them, and we devote ourselves to Him'" (2:136; see also 3:84). The relationship with and devotion to God can have no other competitors—not friends, not family, not lovers, not possessions, not work, not dreams, not ideals, not doctrines, not creeds. All other attachments must take their rightful place after this single supreme command. Devout Muslims and Christians believe that it is the goal of life to bring a person's will into alignment with God's will, and it takes all of life to the very end of life to even approach this goal. The beliefs that divide Muslims and Christians are small and petty compared to this seemingly impossible task that most if not all humans fail to achieve. Says the Qur'an, "Say, 'People of the Book, let us arrive at a statement that is common to us all: we worship God alone, we ascribe no partner to Him, and none of us takes others beside God as lords'..." (3:64). Jesus agreed—love God with all your heart, your soul, and your mind.

Both faith traditions believe that being constantly aware and thoughtful of God will assist in progressing toward this goal of surrender and submission. The five daily prayers of Muslims are intended for this purpose. Regular, continuous prayer by Christians seeks a similar goal. The Bible says, "Pray without ceasing" (1 Thessalonians 5:17, KJV) or "pray continually" (NIV translation). Muslims as a group, because the five daily prayers are part of Islamic culture and because reminders are given by loudspeaker from every mosque at the designated time, are more likely to do this than Christians, who have few reminders in their increasingly secular Western societies.

Creation Story. The names of Adam and Eve in Islam are the same as in Christianity. A well-known Hadith from Muhammad ibn Muslim says, "I asked Abu Ja'far, may peace be upon him, concerning that which is narrated, that God created Adam, may peace be upon him, in His form (*surah* literally, form, image). He replied, 'It is a form that was originated and created. He elected it and chose it over all the other different forms and attributed it to Himself, in the same way that He has attributed the Ka'bah and the Spirit (*ruh*) to Himself…'" (Rizvi 2012). While form does not mean God's physical image, it does mean God's names and qualities, which is very close to what the Bible means by "God created mankind in His own image" (Genesis 1:27). Muslims and Christians believe that all humans can be traced to a single being: "He created you all from a single being, from which He made its mate…" (Qur'an 39:6). The Qur'an says that God created man from clay and breathed His Spirit into him: "Your Lord said to the angels, 'I will create a mortal out of dried clay, formed from dark mud. When I have fashioned him and breathed My spirit into him, bow down before him'"… (15:28–29). The Bible also says that "…the LORD God formed man of the dust of the ground, and breathed into his nostrils the breath of life" (where the Hebrew phrase "breath of life" is often translated as "spirit") (Genesis 2:7).

Jesus the Christ. Although Muslims don't believe that Jesus is God incarnate, Muslims and Christians have a lot of beliefs in common about Jesus. Jesus is highly esteemed in Islam, far more than Jesus is honored by any other major world religion. Jesus or Isa is mentioned nearly 100 times in the Qur'an—always with great reverence (see Table 5.3 for examples). The Qur'an teaches that Jesus was born from a virgin (19:20–22), committed no sin (was pure) (19:19), performed miracles (3:49, 5:110) and was given "signs" (2:87, 2:253), and is "one of those brought near to God" (3:45; 3:55). Jesus is also described as "a Word from God" (3:39, 3:45; see also 4:171).[2] Muslims believe that those who help Jesus are helping God: "When Jesus realized they[3] [still] did not believe, he said, 'Who will help me in God's cause?' The disciples said, 'We will be God's helpers; we believe in God—witness our devotion to Him'" (3:52; see also 61:14, which refers again to this passage).

The Qur'an gives Jesus the title of "the Christ" or "the Messiah" (3:45), i.e., the "anointed one" or "savior," who was prophesized about in the Old Testament (Daniel 9:26; Psalm 2:2). The Qur'an indicates that Jesus is favored among God's messengers: "We favoured some of these messengers above others. God spoke to some; others He raised in rank; We gave Jesus, son of Mary, Our clear signs and strengthened him with the holy spirit" (2:253). Finally, the Qur'an indicates that among all the prophets, Jesus is the only prophet to have been raised up by God and to return at the Day of Judgement (3:55; 4:158–159; 43:61; see also Sahih Muslim 41:6931) (Poston 2010). According to Sahih al-Bukhari, Jesus will descend as a just ruler on

[2] This is different from the way Christians describe Jesus ("the Word of God"). By Word, most Muslims believe it refers to God's command to "Be!" in foretelling Mary's miraculous pregnancy (3:47).

[3] "They" refers to the Children of Israel.

Table 5.3 Statements in the Qur'an about Jesus

"We gave Moses the Scripture and We sent messengers after him in succession. We gave Jesus, son of Mary, clear signs and strengthened him with the Holy Spirit. So how is it that, whenever a messenger brings you something you do not like, you[a] become arrogant, calling some impostors and killing others?" (2:87)
"These are the revelations of God which We recite to [Muhammad] with the truth, and you truly are one of the messengers. We favored some of these messengers above others. God spoke to some; others He raised in rank; We gave Jesus, son of Mary, Our clear signs and strengthened him with the holy spirit." (2:253)
"The angels said, 'Mary, God gives you news of a Word from Him,[b] whose name will be the Messiah, Jesus, son of Mary, who will be held in honor in this world and the next, who will be one of those brought near to God. He will speak to people in his infancy and in his adulthood. He will be one of the righteous.'" (3:45–46)
"God said, 'Jesus, I will take you back and raise you up to Me: I will purify you of the disbelievers. To the Day of Resurrection I will make those who follow you superior to those who disbelieved. Then you will all return to Me and I will judge between you regarding your differences.'" (3:55)
"We sent Jesus, son of Mary, in their footsteps, to confirm the Torah that had been sent before him: We gave him the Gospel with guidance, light, and confirmation of the Torah already revealed—a guide and lesson for those who take heed of God. So let the followers of the Gospel judge according to what God has sent down in it…" (5:46–47)
"[But] he said: 'I am a servant of God. He has granted me the Scripture; made me a prophet; made me blessed wherever I may be. He commanded me to pray, to give alms as long as I live, to cherish my mother. He did not make me domineering or graceless. Peace was on me the day I was born, and will be on me the day I die and the day I am raised to life again.' Such was Jesus, son of Mary." (19:30–34)
"We sent Noah and Abraham…We sent other messengers to follow in their footsteps. After those we sent Jesus, son of Mary: We gave him the Gospel and put compassion and mercy into the hearts of his followers…" (57:27)

[a]Children of Israel
[b]Jesus is given the epithet "a Word from God" (word is capitalized in the majority of English translations of the Qur'an)

the Day of Judgement that applies even to Muslims. Narrated Abu Huraira, "Allah's Apostle said, 'By Him in Whose Hands my soul is, son of Mary (Jesus) will shortly descend amongst you people (Muslims) as a just ruler and will break the Cross and kill the pig and abolish the Jizya (a tax taken from the non-Muslims, who are in the protection of the Muslim government). Then there will be abundance of money and no-body will accept charitable gifts'" (Bukhari 3/34/425).[4]

The Qur'an indicates that God has the most beautiful names (7:180), including "perfection" (*Kamal*), "beauty" (*Jamal*), and "majesty" (*Jalal*), as well as "the gentle," "the generous," "the beautiful," and "the most loving" (59:22–24, 85:14). According to Seyyed Nasr, "Striving after the realization of that oneness, or *tawhid*, is the heart of Islamic life; and the measure of successful religious life is the degree

[4]Citations to *Sahih Bukhari* (the most respected of all Sunni Hadiths) is based on a 2009 translation M. Muhain Khan (2009). We list the reference by volume, book, and number (vol/book/no). See http://d1.islamhouse.com/data/en/ih_books/single/en_Sahih_Al-Bukhari.pdf (last accessed April 22, 2014).

to which one is able to realize *tawhid*, which means not only oneness, but also the integration of multiplicity into Unity" (Nasr 2002, p. 6). Christians believe that Jesus is another name for God, and that the multiplicity of God the Father, God the Son, and God the Holy Spirit is integrated into that great Unity.

The Prophets. Muslims and Christians believe in the prophets Noah, Abraham, Moses, David, Joseph, John the Baptist, and others (Qur'an 6:84–87). They believe that people should obey the ten commandments that both faith traditions say God gave to Moses (Qur'an 7:144–145; Exodus 20:1–17).

Mary. Both Christians and Muslims believe that Mary was the mother of Jesus and was a virgin when she conceived Jesus, so that Jesus was miraculously born. Neither faith tradition believes that Mary was Divine or that she should be worshiped as a partner of God (see Chap. 4).

Divine Books. The Qur'an repeatedly says that the revelations to the Prophet were a confirmation of the revelations given previously to the People of the Book (Table 5.4). Muslims believe that the Torah and the Gospel were sent by God, although believe that they were altered by Jews and Christians from the original texts, making the Qur'an necessary to correct those distortions. The Qur'an, however, does not say that the actual texts above have been changed. Rather, it says that the People of the Book have twisted the Scriptures *with their tongues* (i.e., what they say about the Scriptures): "There are some who twist the Scripture with their tongues to make you [people] think that what they say is part of the Scripture when it is not; they say it is from God when it is not; they attribute lies to God and they know it" (3:78). The Qur'an also emphasizes that those who follow the Scriptures are righteous before God: "But as for those who hold fast to the Scripture and keep up the prayer, We do not deny righteous people their rewards" (7:170). Thus, the Divine books of both Christians and Muslims convey a message that is largely the same to the servants of God.

Although there are differences between what the Bible and the Qur'an say about Isaac and Ishmael, the Bible stresses how God blessed Ishmael. "And Abraham said to God, 'If only Ishmael might live under your blessing!' Then God said, 'Yes, … And as for Ishmael, I have heard you: I will surely bless him; I will make him fruitful and will greatly increase his numbers. He will be the father of twelve rulers, and I will make him into a great nation'" (Genesis 17:18–20). The Bible says further: "God was with the boy as he grew up. He lived in the desert and became an archer. While he was living in the Desert of Paran, his mother got a wife for him from Egypt" (Genesis 20:20–21). Arabic and Islamic traditions hold that the wilderness of Paran is broadly speaking the area of Tihamah today, which is located along the Red Sea coastal plain of Arabia.

Arab Muslims believe that they descended directly from Ishmael, and while controversial, there is actually some support for this in the Bible, where the line of Ishmael's kin is referred to: "These are the names of the sons of Ishmael, listed in the order of their birth: Nebaioth the firstborn of Ishmael, Kedar, Adbeel, Mibsam, Mishma, Dumah, Massa, Hadad, Tema, Jetur, Naphish and Kedemah. These were

Table 5.4 Qur'an confirming what is contained in the Torah and Gospel

"When it is said to them, 'Believe in God's revelations,' they [Children of Israel] reply 'We believe in what was revealed to us,' but they do not believe in what came afterwards, though it is the truth confirming what they already have..." (2:91)
"So [you believers] say 'We believe in God and in what was sent down to us and what was sent down to Abraham, Ishamel, Isaac, Jacob, and the Tribes, and what was given to Moses, Jesus, and all the prophets by their Lord. We make no distinction between any of them and we devote ourselves to Him.'" (2:136)
"Step by step, He has sent the Scripture down to you [Prophet] with the Truth, confirming what went before: He sent down the Torah and the Gospel earlier as a guide for people and He has sent down the distinction [between right and wrong]..." (3:3–4)
"He will teach him the Scripture and wisdom, the Torah and the Gospel, He will send him as a messenger to the Children of Israel:.." (3:48–49) (God speaking to Mary about Jesus)
"I have come to confirm the truth of the Torah which preceded me, and to make some things lawful to you which used to be forbidden. I have come to you with a sign from your Lord. Be mindful of God, obey me;" (3:50) (Jesus speaking to the Jews)
"We sent Jesus, son of Mary, in their footsteps, to confirm the Torah that has been sent before him: We gave him the Gospel with guidance, light, and confirmation of the Torah already revealed—a guide and lesson for those who take heed of God. So, let the followers of the Gospel judge according to what God has sent down in it. Those who do not judge according to what God has revealed are lawbreakers." (5:46–47)
"Say 'People of the Book you have no true basis [for your religion] unless you uphold the Torah, the Gospel, and that which has been sent down to you from your Lord,'..." (5:68)
"Then God will say, 'Jesus, son of Mary! Remember My favour to you and to your mother: how I strengthened you with the holy spirit, so that you spoke to people in your infancy and as a grown man; how I taught you the Scripture and wisdom, the Torah and the Gospel...'" (5:110)
"Once again, we gave Moses the Scripture, perfecting [Our favour] for those who do good, explaining everything clearly as guidance and mercy, so that they might believe in the meeting with their Lord. This [the Qur'an], too, is a blessed Scripture which We have sent down—follow it and be conscious of your Lord, so that you may receive mercy—lest you say, 'Scriptures were only sent down to two communities before us: we were not aware of what they studied,' or 'If only the Scripture had been sent down to use, we would have been better guided than them.' Now clear evidence, guidance, and mercy have come to you from your Lord. Who could be more wrong than someone who rejects God's revelations and turns away from them?..." (6:154–157)
"Nor could this Qur'an have been devised by anyone other than God. It is a confirmation of what was revealed before it and an explanation of the Scripture—let there be no doubt about it—it is from the Lord of the Worlds." (10:37)
"So if you [Prophet] are in doubt about what We have revealed to you, ask those who have been reading the scriptures before you. The Truth has come to you from your Lord, so be in no doubt and do not deny God's signs..." (10:94)
"...This revelation [the Qur'an] is no fabrication: it is a confirmation of the truth of what was sent before it; an explanation for everything; a guide and a blessing for those who believe" (12:111)
"[We said] 'John, hold on to the Scripture firmly.' While he was still a boy, We granted him wisdom, tenderness from Us, and purity. He was devout, kind to his parents, not domineering or rebellious. Peace was on him the day he was born, the day he died, and it will be on him the day he is raised to life again." (19:12–15) (referring to John the Baptist)
"The disbelievers say, 'We will believe neither this Qur'an nor the Scriptures that came before it'..." (34:31)
"The Scripture We have revealed to you [Prophet] is the Truth and confirms the scriptures that preceded it. God is well-informed about His servants, He sees everything." (35:31)

(continued)

Table 5.4 (continued)

"[Prophet], do you see how deluded those who dispute God's messages are—those who reject the Scripture and the messages We have sent through Our messengers? They will find out when, with iron collars and chains around their necks, they are dragged into scalding water, and then burned in the Fire..." (40:69–72)
"So [Prophet] call people to that faith and follow the straight path as you have been commanded. Do not go by what they desire, but say, 'I believe in whatever Scripture God has sent down...'" (42:15)
"Yet the scripture of Moses was revealed before it [the Qur'an] as a guide and a mercy, and this [the Qur'an] is a scripture confirming it in the Arabic language to warn those who do evil and bring good news for those who do good" (46:12)

the sons of Ishmael, and these are the names of the twelve tribal rulers according to their settlements and camps. Ishmael lived a hundred and thirty-seven years. He breathed his last and died, and he was gathered to his people. His descendants settled in the area from Havilah to Shur, near the eastern border of Egypt, as you go toward Ashur [Assyria]" (Genesis 25:13–18, NIV). Havilah is a region associated with the northern Arabian peninsula just to the north and east of the region between Mecca and Medina in Saudi Arabia.

The Prophet Muhammad was of the Banu Hashim clan of the Quraysh tribe (which controlled Mecca and the Kaaba during his time). The Quraysh was Nadhr, the 12th tribal generation down from Kedar, the son of Ishmael mentioned in the Bible (McAuliffe 2005). Thus, the Bible and genealogical tracings document the Prophet's direct lineage from Ishmael. This, together with repeated referrals in the Qur'an to the Torah, Psalms, and Gospel, demonstrates common ground between the Divine scriptures and the traditions of Christians and Muslims.

Angels, the Devil, and Demons. Although Muslims tend to be more interested in angels than Christians, the gap in interest is not that large. Consider the hit TV series "Touched by an Angel" that had 211 episodes over nine seasons in America between 1994 and 2003, with over 17 million viewers in its fourth season. No doubt, many Christians believe in angels, especially Raphael, Michael, and Gabriel, who are considered good angels who bring messages from God. The angel Gabriel is mentioned as having appeared to Jesus' mother Mary to foretell his birth (Luke 1:19, 26). The angel Gabriel is also mentioned earlier in the Bible as appearing to Daniel to interpret his vision (Daniel 8:16, 9:21). He is considered an "archangel" (high level angel) by both Christians and Muslims. The Qur'an identifies Gabriel as the angel who appeared to the Prophet Muhammad, both to deliver the message of the Qur'an (2:97) and to miraculously transport the Prophet to Jerusalem (the Night Journey and ascension, 17:1, 17:60, 53:13–18). Both Gabriel and Michael are described in the Qur'an as message bearers from God (2:97–98; 66:4).

Muslims and Christians also believe in the devil (*Iblis* or *Shaytan* in Islam). In the Bible, the devil is believed to be a fallen angel, given the name "Lucifer" by Christians (based on Isaiah 14:12, KJV). The Qur'an says that the devil (Iblis) was a fallen angel (or more accurately, a *jinn* at the level of an angel) whose pride or arrogance caused him to be thrown out of the garden and into hell (2:34; 7:12–18).

The Qur'an says that this is because he did not bow to Adam, as God told him (and all the angels) to do (2:34). Muslims, like many Christians, believe that there are demons active in the world (evil *jinn*) that serve the devil and cause problems in people's lives (the Qur'an devotes an entire chapter to The Jinn or *Al-Jinn*, 72: 1–28). Some of Jesus' most dramatic miracles were casting out demons from the possessed (Matthew 12:22; Matthew 17:14–20; Mark 1:23–24; Mark 3:11; Mark 5:1–20; Mark 9:20–21; Luke 4:33–36).

Day of Judgement. Both Muslims and Christians believe in a Day of Judgement (or Resurrection), when people will need to give an account for their lives here on earth. This is clearly documented in the New Testament (Matthew 10:15,12:36; 1 Corinthian 4:5; Revelations 20:11–15) and in the Qur'an (7:172; 9:18–19; 10:15; 50:21–23).

Hell and Heaven. The majority of Muslims and Christians believe in life after death and that after judgement, people will go either to heaven/paradise or to hell. These are part of the core belief systems of each faith tradition (see Chaps. 2 and 4).

Believers. Muslims and Christians are both "believers." The Qur'an does not place Christians and Jews in the same category as "disbelievers" or "infidels" (people who don't believe in God), a group destined for hell: "[Believers], argue only in the best way with the People of the Book, except with those of them who act unjustly. Say, 'We believe in what was revealed to us and in what was revealed to you; our God and your God are one [and the same]; we are devoted to Him' (29:46). The Qur'an also says: "The [Muslim] believers, the Jews, the Christians, and the Sabians—all those who believe in God and the Last Day and do good—will have their rewards with their Lord. No fear for them, nor will they grieve" (2:62; also see 5:69).

Practices

Prayer. Both Muslims and Christians pray to God. They pray either privately when alone or with family, or corporately as a group at the mosque or church. Although the frequency may be different, prayer is valued as the most important and intimate religious practice in both religions. Five times daily prayer is one of the five pillars of Islam. In the Middle East and North Africa, 60–85 % of Muslims pray several times daily and 53–83 % pray five times per day (as required); adults over age 35 are more likely to pray than younger adults (the same age pattern seen in Christians) (Pew Research Center 2012, pp. 3–4). Frequency of prayer varies by Christian denomination, although 78–80 % of conservative Protestants pray daily or several times daily (Pew Research Center 2010).

Reading Scriptures. Christians read and memorize passages in the Bible, and Muslims read and memorize sections of the Qur'an. In the Middle East and North Africa, 31–52 % of Muslims read the Qur'an daily and most of the remaining Muslims read the Qur'an but less than daily (Pew Research Center 2012, p. 5).

In the United States, 60 % of conservative Protestants read the Bible at least weekly outside of religious services (Pew Research Center 2010). These holy scriptures are used during religious services and for religious education of children and adults. Members of both traditions seek to live their lives based on the principles contained in their holy scriptures.

Attending Religious Services. About one-half of Muslims and Christians attend religious services regularly. The latest figures place weekly or almost weekly attendance at religious services among Christians (those in the United States) at 43 %, with 35 % attending one or more times per week (Newport 2010). In the Middle East and North Africa, depending on country, between 35 and 65 % of Muslims attend services at the mosque at least weekly for *jumah* (Friday) prayer, whereas 15–38 % attend more than once a week (Pew Research Center 2012, p. 5).

Fasting. Although there is nothing comparable to fasting during the month of Ramadan in Christianity, many Christians fast for religious reasons (Oppenheimer 2011). This is done in both Islam and Christianity as an act of devotion to God. Just as the Prophet emphasized fasting, so did Jesus in many Gospel passages (see Chap. 4 on Christian fasting).

Importance of Deeds. Obeying God by doing good works and good deeds is of central importance in Islam. So important, in fact, that it is a primary factor determining whether one goes to heaven or hell. The Qur'an confirms this in many verses (e.g., 2:25; 3:15–17; 7:8–9; 34:37–38). The doing of good deeds is also of central importance in Christianity (Matthew 25:35–40; Hebrews 13:16; James 2:14–17; 1 John 3:17). Jesus stressed that loving and doing good to others was second in importance only to loving and serving God, stressing this in three of four Gospels (Matthew 22:37; Mark 12:30; Luke 10:27). Jesus also said, "Why do you call me, 'Lord, Lord,' and do not do what I say?" (Luke 6:46), implying that good deeds are of crucial importance. According to the famous Baptist theologian of the nineteenth century, Charles Spurgeon, "Faith and obedience are bound up in the same bundle. He that obeys God, trusts God; and he that trusts God, obeys God" (Spurgeon 2007). In Revelation (the final book of the Bible), God says: "Let the one who does wrong continue to do wrong; let the vile person continue to be vile; let the one who does right continue to do right; and let the holy person continue to be holy. Look, I am coming soon! My reward is with me, and I will give to each person *according to what they have done* [authors' italics]. I am the Alpha and the Omega, the First and the Last, the Beginning and the End" (Revelation 22:11–13).

Loving God and Others. As noted in Chap. 4, Christians believe that love of God and others is of central importance to their religion, and without it, their faith is meaningless: "If I speak in the tongues of men or of angels, but do not have love, I am only a resounding gong or a clanging cymbal. If I have the gift of prophecy and can fathom all mysteries and all knowledge, and if I have a faith that can move mountains, but do not have love, I am nothing. If I give all I possess to the poor and give over my body to hardship that I may boast, but do not have love, I gain nothing" (1 Corinthians 13:1–3).

Table 5.5 Love in the Qur'an

Love of God for people[a]
"… God loves those who do good" (2:195; see also 3:134; 3:148; 5:13; 5:93)
"… He loves those who keep themselves clean" (2:222) or "purify themselves" (9:108)
"… God loves those who are mindful of Him" (9:4; see also 3:76; 9:7)
"… God loves those who are steadfast" [or "patient in adversity"[b]] (3:146)
"… God loves those who put their trust in Him" (3:159)
"Ask forgiveness from your Lord and turn to Him in repentance: my Lord is merciful and most loving" (11:90)
"… God loves the just" [or "those who act equitably"[b]] (60:8; see also 49:9)
"…God truly loves those who fight in solid lines for His cause…" (61:4)
"… and He is the Most Forgiving, the Most Loving" [or "And He alone is truly-forgiving, all-embracing in His love"[b]] (85:14)
Love of people for God
"Say, 'If you love God, follow me, and God will love you and forgive you your sins. God is most forgiving, most merciful'" (3:31)
"Hence, when thou art freed [from distress], remain steadfast, and unto thy Sustainer turn with love"[b] (94:7)
Love of people for other people
"The believers, both men and women, support each other… God will give His mercy to such people: God is almighty and wise." (9:71)
"No reward do I ask of you for this [message] other than [that you should] love your fellow-men" (42:23).[b]
"… [those] who love all that come to them in search of refuge… it is they, they that shall attain to a happy state!" (59:9).[b]
"If two groups of the believers fight, you [believers] should try to reconcile them…The believers are brothers, so make peace between your two brothers and be mindful of God so that you may be given mercy" (49:9–10)
"and He does not forbid you to deal kindly and justly with anyone who has not fought you for your faith or driven you out of your homes: God loves the just" (60:8)

[a]All are translations by M.A.S. Abdel Haleem, except where noted
[b]Qur'an translation by Muhammad Asad

Muslims also believe in loving God and showing love and mercy toward others based on many verses in the Qur'an (Table 5.5). For example, seeking love and peace between believers is encouraged by the following: "Hence, if two groups of believers fall to fighting, make peace between them; but then, if one of the two [groups] goes on acting wrongfully towards the other, fight against the one that acts wrongfully until it reverts to God's commandment; and if they revert, make peace between them with justice, and deal equitably [with them]: for verily, God loves those who act equitably!" (49:9–10).[5] Just as Jesus instructs Christians (Matthew 5:43–48), the Qur'an instructs Muslims to show kindness even towards unbelievers (and enemies): "As for such [of the unbelievers] as do not fight against you on account of [your] faith, and neither drive you forth from your homelands, God does not forbid you to show them kindness and to behave towards them with full equity: for, verily, God loves those who act equitably" (60:8) (see footnote 5).

[5]Qur'an translation by Muhammad Asad.

The love of neighbor is also strongly emphasized in the Hadith. According to the *Mishkat*, the Prophet said, "God has no mercy for the one who has no mercy for the people" (Robson 1975, p. 1031). In fact, a hadith indicates that the Prophet said that the Angel of Revelation (Gabriel) was so insistent on emphasizing the good treatment of neighbor that Muhammad thought that the neighbor might become a legal inheritor! (Robson 1975, pp. 1038–39). Another hadith describes a man who came to the Prophet and asked him how he could know if he was a good man or not. The Prophet replied, "Find out from your neighbors what they think of you" (Robson 1975, pp. 1033–39).

Values

Values are important for the health of individuals and nations. People who have solid values and goals usually experience greater emotional balance. They know that even good people experience difficult life events, but that because of their principles and responsibilities, they cope with and endure these troubles. It is in the area of values that similarities between Muslims and Christians are greatest.

Ethics. The rights of people, healthy and sick, are important to both Muslims and Christians. Although Islam may appear to hold the community in greater esteem than the individual, the individual is also important (see Chap. 2). Although Christianity, based in a Western culture, emphasizes the rights of the individual, it also places great value on community and does not condone the sacrifice of community welfare for the rights of the individual (laws in Western societies as in Islamic societies favor the community good). Indeed, the core religious teachings of both faith traditions hold justice and fairness in great esteem. These ethics especially apply to individuals who are vulnerable because of physical or mental illness or because of age or gender.

Importance of Family. Christianity and Islam seek to preserve the traditional family (husband, wife, and children), which is considered the fundamental unit of society. Children are highly valued, as is their training and upbringing, and marriage between a man and a woman is considered sacred (among conservatives in both traditions). Divorce is not morally acceptable, nor is having sexual relations with anyone except one's spouse during marriage. Both religions teach that care for parents and older family members is a responsibility of younger family members (1 Timothy 5:3–8; Qur'an 2:215; 6:151;17:23–24, 26). Viewing pornography is forbidden in both Christianity and Islam, except in the most liberal branches of these traditions. As noted earlier, Jesus said that even looking at a woman with lust is the same as committing adultery (Matthew 5:27–28). The Qur'an says basically the same thing (24:30–31; 41:19–20).

Importance of Social Relationships. Muslims and Christians also place great importance on relationships outside the family (women with women, men with men).

Hebrews 10:24 instructs members of the Christian church to meet often together and gives the reason: "And let us consider how we may spur one another on toward love and good deeds, not giving up meeting together, as some are in the habit of doing, but encouraging one another—and all the more as you see the Day approaching." Likewise, the Qur'an instructs Muslims to form friendships and alliances with believers, not unbelievers: "The believers should not make the disbelievers their allies rather than other believers—anyone who does such a thing will isolate himself completely from God…" (3:28). The Prophet encouraged close friendships between men (Bukhari 1/2/12), but those friendships were to be based on a mutual love for God (Bukhari 1/11/629). Muslim women are also encouraged to go to the mosque to develop friendships with other women (Ansari 2013).

Muslim–Christian Relationships. Although some verses of the Qur'an suggest that Christians and Jews should not be taken as friends, what is actually said is that Muslims should not take them on as guardians or protectors, make alliances with them, or make friendships with them if they are unjust, under the wrath of Allah, or make a mockery of Islam (4:139; 5:51, 5:57; 60:13). In the Prophet Muhammad's time (particularly the Medinan period), there was concern about making political alliances with Jews and Christians, since this could weaken the Prophet's position and made him and his followers vulnerable to attack (Armstrong 2007). On the personal level, however, the Qur'an does not prohibit Muslims from relating with Christians or Jews who are believers, particularly those whom the Qur'an describes as "righteous" (3:113–114; 3:199). In fact, the Qur'an even allows a Muslim man to marry a Christian or Jewish women: "Today all good things have been made lawful for you. The food of the People of the Book is lawful for you as your food is lawful for them. So are chaste, believing women as well as chaste women of the people who were given the Scripture before you, as long as you have given them their bride-gifts and married them, not taking them as lovers or secret mistresses…" (5:5).

Likewise, Jesus said to his followers that they are to love their neighbors as themselves. As noted earlier, when Jesus was asked by an expert in the Jewish law to define what he meant by "neighbor," he told the lawyer a parable about someone with a different belief system (a Samaritan) who helped a Jew in distress, and then Jesus instructed the lawyer to do likewise (Luke 10:29–37). Jesus even healed the child of a Canaanite woman, whose beliefs completely contrasted with those of Jewish believers (Matthew 15:22–28). Based on the Qur'an and the Bible, then, there is no logical reason why Muslims and Christians cannot form personal friendships with each other.

Concern for the Poor. Both Muslims and Christians are instructed in their holy scriptures to have concern for the poor and needy. The *zakat* (one of the five pillars of Islam) is meant for this purpose. In Christianity, individuals and the institutional church are instructed to do likewise. There are more than 300 verses in the Bible that express God's concern for the poor and for issues involving social justice. Jesus, in particular, was clear on the issue of caring for the poor (Matthew 5:42; Matthew 19:21; Matthew 25:35–40; Luke 3:11; Luke 12:33; Luke 14:12–14), as were his followers (James 1:27; 1 Timothy 6:18–19; 1 John 3:17). In fact, when a rich young ruler asked Jesus what he should do to inherit eternal life besides obeying the ten commandments, Jesus told him: "If you wish to be complete, go and sell your possessions and give to the poor, and you will have treasure in heaven; and come, follow Me" (Matthew 19:21).

Likewise, the Qur'an is filled with verses describing God's love and reward for those who care for the poor (2:215; 2:261; 3:92; 17:26–27; 107:1–3) and describes what the attitude should be of those who give: "Those who spend their wealth in God's cause, and do not follow their spending with reminders of their benevolence or hurtful words, will have their rewards with their Lord…You who believe, do not cancel out your charitable deeds with reminders and hurtful words, like someone who spends his wealth only to be seen by people…" (2:262–264). This is similar to what Jesus told his disciples: "Be careful not to practice your righteousness in front of others to be seen by them. If you do, you will have no reward from your Father in heaven. So when you give to the needy, do not announce it with trumpets, as the hypocrites do in the synagogues and on the streets, to be honored by others" (Matthew 6:1–2).

Importance of Work. Working hard, being frugal (although not miserly), and avoiding waste (or extravagant living)—all are highly valued in both Islam and Christianity (see Qur'an 6:141; 7:31; 17:26–27; see Proverbs 18:9; John 6:12; Ephesians 4:28). People with high values understand the need to work hard since this is the nature of life and the greater their goals, the greater the efforts needed to achieve them. Work is considered a right and a duty in Islam. Says the Qur'an, "Has he not been told what was written in the Scriptures of Moses and of Abraham, who fulfilled his duty; that no soul shall bear the burden of another; that man will only have what he has worked towards; that his labour will be seen and that in the end he will be repaid in full for it" (53:39–41). Persons who value work are less likely to remain passive and hope that things will change. Instead, they will make strong efforts toward their goals and remaining optimistic about achieving them even when they encounter resistance. Christianity likewise emphasizes the importance of work: "The one who is unwilling to work shall not eat" (2 Thessalonians 3:10). However, the motivation for work should be to serve God, not men: "Whatever you do, work at it with all your heart, as working for the Lord, not for human masters" (Colossians 3:23).

Care for the Body. As noted in earlier chapters, both Christians and Muslims are instructed by their holy texts to respect, honor, and care for the physical body. In Christianity, the physical body is the "temple of the Holy Spirit" that has been "bought at a price" (1 Corinthians 6:19–20). In Islam, Muslims are told to care for their bodies by not eating excessively (7:31), by engaging in exercise (Kahan 2003), and by going to see a doctor when sick (see Chap. 3).

Pro-life. Abortion, suicide, and assisted suicide are all forbidden in both Christianity and Islam. The majority of both American Muslims (78 %) (Rheault and Mogahed 2008) and American Christians (52–59 %) (Saad 2009) are pro-life and anti-abortion. Suicide (and assisted suicide) is likewise morally unacceptable based on the theological teachings of both faith traditions (see previous chapters), as demonstrated by the fact that level of religiosity is a strong determinant of such attitudes (Pew Research Center 2006; Stack and Kposowa 2011; Boyd and Chung 2012).

Intoxication and Other Behaviors. Although alcohol is not forbidden for Christians as it is for Muslims, Christians are instructed not to drink in excess: "Do not get drunk on wine, which leads to debauchery. Instead, be filled with the Spirit" (Ephesians 5:18). Drunkenness is listed among a long list of behaviors that are forbidden in the Bible: "The acts of the flesh are obvious: sexual immorality, impurity and debauchery; idolatry and witchcraft; hatred, discord, jealousy, fits of rage, selfish ambition, dissensions, factions and envy; drunkenness, orgies, and the like. I warn you, as I did before, that those who live like this will not inherit the kingdom of God" (Galatians 5: 19–21). Most practicing Muslims would agree with Christians that these behaviors are forbidden (*haram*).

Similarities Acknowledged in the Qur'an

The Qur'an states that Christians are closer to Muslims than any other religion that exists: "You [Prophet] are sure to find that…the closest in affection towards the believers are those who say, 'We are Christians,' for there are among them people devoted to learning and ascetics. These people are not given to arrogance, and when they listen to what has been sent down to the Messenger, you will see their eyes overflowing with tears because they recognize the Truth [in it]. They say, 'Our Lord, we believe, so count us amongst the witnesses. Why should we not believe in God and in the Truth that has come down to us, when we long for our Lord to include us in the company of the righteous?' For saying this, God has rewarded them with Gardens graced with flowing streams, and there they will stay: that is the reward of those who do good" (5:82–85).

Differences Acknowledged

Besides having many beliefs, practices, and values in common, we acknowledge that there are serious differences in belief and theology, as discussed earlier in this chapter. We believe that Muslims and Christians must work through these differences so they can have true dialogue with one another, which is paramount not only for individual health but also for the health of our world community. The major stumbling block that stands between Muslims and Christians is the Christian belief that Jesus is God. Christians say that only if they believe in the divinity of Jesus can they call themselves monotheists rather than polytheists. Muslims say that worshiping Jesus as God is polytheism. If Muslims are correct and Jesus is not God, the faith of Christians would not make much sense and they would be guilty of what Muslims call "a tremendous sin" (4:48). If Christians are correct and Jesus is God, then not everything that is said in the Qur'an would be true since it categorically and vehemently denies the divinity of Jesus. Thus, Christians and Muslims stand at an impasse. This is an issue that may not be resolvable between the two faith traditions. Whether Jesus is God, whether the Bible or the Qur'an is the Word of God, or whether God even exists—none can be proven by any objective or scientific method. These beliefs are entirely a matter of faith and cannot be resolved by argument or objective reasoning.

Allahu Akbar! God is great, and fully able to decide and judge all on the Last Day. This is one belief that Muslims and Christians agree on. The Qur'an says, "In fact, any who direct themselves wholly to God and do good will have their reward with their Lord: no fear for them, nor will they grieve…God will judge between them on the Day of Resurrection concerning their differences" (2:112–113). The Bible says, "What business is it of mine to judge those outside the church [i.e., Christian church]? Are you not to judge those inside? God will judge those outside…" (1 Corinthians 5:12–13). The Qur'an repeatedly and relentlessly claims that God is all-knowing and wise (4:92, 104, 110, 148, 170; 5:54,75; 6:12, 83, 95, 112; 7:199, 8:42, 61, 71, etc.) and is infinitely merciful: "…God is limitless in His bounty unto the believers" (3:152). The Qur'an also clearly defines and distinguishes believers from disbelievers: "[The believers are] those who turn to God in repentance; who worship and praise Him; who bow down and prostrate themselves; who order what is good and forbid what is wrong and who observe God's limits. Give glad news to such believers" (9:112). Many Christians and Muslims fit into this category.

The Qur'an also provides some space for differences in belief, saying "Every community is sent a messenger, and when their messenger comes, they will be judged justly; they will not be wronged" (10:47). Referring to Christians and Muslims, it also says, "…We have assigned a law and a path to each of you. If God had so willed, He would have made you one community, but He wanted to test you through that which He has given you, so race to do good: you will all return to God and He will make clear to you the matters you differed about" (5:48).

Thus, it is the believer's duty to be faithful to the revelation, be it the Bible or the Qur'an, that God has revealed to him or her and then live by that truth. We believe that Muslims and Christians can be brothers and sisters under God, and engage in true dialogue. This will be possible, however, only if each can acknowledge and accept the differences in belief, tolerate and respect those differences, and love one another so as to honor the great, magnificent, one and only God whom both Muslims and Christians must worship and surrender their lives to.

Summary and Conclusions

Although Muslims and Christians believe in the same God who created and sustains all that exists, share many of the same practices, and hold almost identical values and ethical principles, there are major differences in belief and minor differences in the way they worship God. Although Muslims highly respect and honor Jesus as one of the holiest prophets, they do not believe that Jesus is God. Islam emphasizes pure monotheism which entails worshipping God alone without any partners (e.g., statues, saints, prophets). Muslims believe that God cannot be given attributes of His creation (such as being tired, being in need of food, suffering, and having sons or daughters). Muslims do not believe in the triune nature of God, which is a core doctrine of Christianity. Christians believe the Bible is the final word of God, whereas Muslims believe that the Qur'an is the final word of God. There is no doubt that these differences in belief separate Muslims and Christians. However, the similarities between the two faiths are also striking. Perhaps no two major world religions have more in common than Muslims and Christians, particularly those who are devout adherents.

In the end, the differences between Christians and Muslims described above, including the true identity of Jesus, have very little to do with what both faith traditions say is their ultimate and final goal. The Qur'an says, "True Religion, in God's eyes, is *islam*: [devotion to Him alone]" (3:19). The same claim is made in Christianity, as Jesus instructed (Matthew 7:21) and demonstrated (Matthew 26:39; Mark 14:36; see also James 4:7). According to Seyyed Hossein Nasr, "Even when the Qur'an states that 'the religion with God is al-islam' (3:19) or similar statements, *al-islam* refers to that universal surrender to the One and that primordial religion contained in the heart of all heavenly inspired religions, not just to Islam in its more particular sense" (Nasr 2002, p. 17). The extent of this devotion to God, in fact, may be the critical factor and key mechanism that explains the relationship between religion and health in both Christianity and Islam.

The methods of science cannot substantiate the truth claims made by either Muslims or Christians. Nevertheless, scientific research can be quite useful in other respects. The scientific method can help to determine—in an objective and systematic manner—the impact that the beliefs, practices, and values of each tradition has on the emotional, social, and physical health of believers. Research can help to determine whether the differences (and similarities) between Christians and Muslims described in this chapter influence the relationships between religiosity and health in each tradition. Nevertheless, we acknowledge that the scientific method, as powerful as it is, does not have the final word nor is it nearly as accurate and objective as most in the secular world would like to believe—especially when examining a relationship as complex as this one (Koenig 2011). The scientific approach to examining the religion–health relationship, however, is at least a place to start. We now examine what that research has found—first in Christians and then in Muslims.

References

Ahmed, S. (2004). Satanic Verses. In J. D. McAuliffe et al. (Eds.), *Encyclopaedia of the Qur'ān*. Brill: Leiden.

Ansari, U. Z. (2013). *Why is it better to pray at home for women*? Quibla. Retrieved October 4, 2013, from http://spa.qibla.com/issue_view.asp?HD=1&ID=8740&CATE=4

Armstrong, K. (2007). *Muhammad: A biography of the Prophet*. New York: HarperOne.

Asad, M. (2003). *Commentary by Muhammad Asad in The Message of the Koran* (p. 845). Retrieved October 4, 2013, from http://www.usc.edu/schools/college/crcc/private/cmje/religious_text/The_Message_of_The_Quran__by_Muhammad_Asad.pdf

Boyd, K. A., & Chung, H. (2012). Opinions toward suicide: Cross-national evaluation of cultural and religious effects on individuals. *Social Science Research, 41*, 1565–1580.

Catechism of the Catholic Church. (2003). Second edition. Part II: Celebration of the Christian Ministry, Section II: The Seven Sacraments of the Church, Chapter One: The Sacraments of Christian Initiation, Article 1: The Sacrament of Baptism. New York: DoubleDay Religion. Retrieved October 4, 2013, from http://www.scborromeo.org/ccc/p2s2c1a1.htm - 1257

Chulov, M. (2011, September 25). *Saudi women given the right to vote and stand for election in four years.* The Guardian. Retrieved October 4, 2013, from http://www.guardian.co.uk/world/2011/sep/25/saudi-women-right-to-vote

Emerick, Y. (2004). *The complete idiot's guide to understanding Islam* (2nd ed., p. 89). New York: Alpha.

Gallup Inc. (2009). *Muslim Americans: A national portrait.* Retrieved April 16, 2013, from http://www.gallup.com/strategicconsulting/153572/report-muslim-americans-national-portrait.aspx

Hiers, R. H. (2012). *Women's rights and the Bible: Implications for Christian ethics and social policy.* Eugene, OR: Wipf and Stock.

Hisham, I. (n.d.). *Sira* (a biography of the Prophet Muhammad's life written around 730-733 by Ibn Ishaq and edited by Ibn Hisham, who died in 833) (Vol. 1, p. 358) (cited in Rahman F (1998). *Health and Medicine in the Islamic Tradition.* Chicago, IL: ABC International Group, Inc., p 85).

Kahan, D. (2003). Islam and physical activity: Implications for American sport and physical educators. *Journal of Physical Education, Recreation, & Dance, 74*(3), 48–54.

Koenig, H. G. (2011). *Spirituality and health research: Methods, measurement, statistics, and resources* (pp. 406–408). Conshohocken, PA: Templeton Foundation Press.

Lewis, C. S. (1952). *Mere Christianity* (Rev. ed., p. 55ff). New York: Macmillan/Collier.

McAuliffe, J. D. (Ed.). (2005). *Encyclopaedia of the Qur'an (5 vols.)* (1st ed.). Leiden: Brill.

Missick, S. (2006). *The words of Jesus in the original Aramaic* (p. 75). Maitland, FL: Xulon Press.

Nasr, S. H. (2002). *The heart of Islam.* San Francisco: HarperCollins.

National Church Life Survey. (2001). *Gender profile of church attendees.* Retrieved October 4, 2013, from http://www.ncls.org.au/default.aspx?sitemapid=137

Newport, F. (2010, May). *Americans' church attendance inches up in 2010.* The Gallup Poll. Retrieved October 4, 2013, from http://www.gallup.com/poll/141044/Americans-Church-Attendance-Inches-2010.aspx

Oppenheimer, M. (2011, January 21). Many choices on the menu of religious fasts. *New York Times.* Retrieved October 4, 2013, from http://www.nytimes.com/2011/01/22/us/22beliefs.html?_r=0

Pew Research Center. (2006). *Strong public support for right to die.* Retrieved October 4, 2013, from http://www.people-press.org/2006/01/05/strong-public-support-for-right-to-die/

Pew Research Center. (2010). *Religion among the Millennials.* Retrieved October 4, 2013, from http://www.pewforum.org/Age/Religion-Among-the-Millennials.aspx

Pew Research Center. (2012). *The world's Muslims: Unity and diversity.* Retrieved October 4, 2013, from http://www.pewforum.org/Muslim/the-worlds-muslims-unity-and-diversity-2-religious-commitment.aspx

Poston, L. (2010). The second coming of 'Isa: an exploration of Islamic premillennialism. *The Muslim World, 100*, 108–109.

Rheault, M., & Mogahed, D. (2008). *Moral issue divide Westerners from Muslims in the West.* Gallup Poll. Retrieved October 4, 2013, from http://www.gallup.com/poll/107512/moral-issues-divide-westerners-from-muslims-west.aspx

Rizvi, E. (2012). *Hadith 39: The meaning of god's Creation of Adam in His image. Authentic Hadith narrated through the Prophet [s] and his Ahl al-Bayt.* Pure Islam. Retrieved October 4, 2013, from http://pureislamofficial.blogspot.com/2012/12/forty-hadith-authentic-ahadith-narrated.html

Robson, J. (1975). *Mishkat Al-Masabih*. New York: Orientalia Art Ltd. (cited in Rahman, 1998).

Saad, L. (2009). *More American "pro-life" than "pro-choice" for first time*. Gallup Poll. Retrieved October 4, 2013, from http://www.gallup.com/poll/118399/more-americans-pro-life-than-pro-choice-first-time.aspx

Sanneh, L. (1996). *Piety and power: Muslims and Christians in West Africa* (p. 46). Maryknoll, NY: Orbis Books.

Spurgeon, C. S. (2007). *Faith in all its splendor* (p. 57). Lexington, KY: Sovereign Grace Publishers, Inc.

Stack, S., & Kposowa, A. J. (2011). Religion and suicide acceptability: A cross-national analysis. *Journal for the Scientific Study of Religion, 50*(2), 289–306.

Watts, W. M. (1956). *Muhammad at Medina*. New York: Oxford University Press.

Westminster Confession of Faith. (1646). *Of god's eternal decree*. Chapter III, verse1. Retrieved October 4, 2013, from http://www.reformed.org/documents/index.html?mainframe=http://www.reformed.org/documents/westminster_conf_of_faith.html

Women's Rights. (2006). *Women's rights in Islam. Islam's women: Jewels of Islam*. Retrieved October 4, 2013, from http://www.islamswomen.com/articles/do_muslim_women_have_rights.php

Zuberi, A. K. (1988). A qualitative study of Muslim children's concepts of god. *Pakistan Journal of Psychological Research, 3*(1–2), 1–22.

Part II
Research

In this section we focus on research that has examined relationships between religiosity and health in Christian and Muslim populations. Although there has been much friction between religion and science over the years, there is a long tradition both within Christianity and Islam that has encouraged scientific research. Guessoum (2010) cites many verses from the Qur'an and Hadith that emphasize the value and importance of seeking knowledge (ilm), and quotes theoretical physicist and Islamic philosopher, Mehdi Golshani, as saying "We believe that the spectrum of knowledge recommended by Islam is very wide. It includes both specifically religious teachings and those branches of knowledge that are beneficial to the welfare of individuals and human societies" (p. 63).

Indeed, the first revelation from the angel Gabriel to the Prophet Muhammad when he was instructed to read was: "Read! In the name of your Lord who created: He created man from a clinging form. Read! Your Lord is the Most Bountiful One who taught by [means of] the pen, who taught man what he did not know. But man exceeds all bounds when he thinks he is self-sufficient: [Prophet], all will return to your Lord" (96:1–8). This scripture underscores the importance that Islam places on knowledge, and why early Islamic scholars made such efforts to translate the earlier writings on science and medicine (Greek, Indian, etc.) into Arabic so that they could be studied. This verse from the Qur'an also ends with the warning that there are limits to what humans can learn and discover on their own.

According to Rahman, modern Muslim reformers have emphasized a number of other passages in the Qur'an stressing that God made the universe and that nature should be subservient to humans, not the other way around (Rahman, 1998, p. 12). Here are a few:

> It was He who created all that is on the earth for you, then turned to the sky and made the seven heavens; it is He who has knowledge of all things (2:29)

> [People], do you not see how God has made what is in the heavens and on the earth useful to you, and has lavished His blessings on you both outwardly and inwardly? (31:20)

> It is God who subjected the sea for you—ships sail on it by His command so that you can seek His bounty and give Him thanks (45:12)

These passages have been used to argue that Muslims need to become more involved in science, after centuries of lapse following the Golden Age of Islam. Reformers maintain that conducting research to better understand nature (including human nature, in our view) will bring glory to God through the discoveries of the incredible intricacies of the universe and of the human person that only the Divine could be responsible for. This approach was also consistent with the motivations of many scientists from Christian backgrounds who believed that science is simply a process of discovering how God made the natural world, and furthermore, that it was the responsibility of humans to learn about these magnificent laws that would prove God's existence. For example, Sir Isaac Newton—one of the most influential scientists of all time and a key figure in the Scientific Revolution—said:

> This most beautiful system of the sun, planets, and comets, could only proceed from the counsel and dominion of an intelligent Being… This Being governs all things, not as the soul of the world, but as Lord over all; and on account of his dominion he is wont to be called "Lord God" παντοκρατωρ [pantokratōr], or "Universal Ruler"… The Supreme God is a Being eternal, infinite, [and] absolutely perfect (Newton, 1687).

Indeed, it is within nature that Christians are told that the proof of God's existence lies. Consider the following verses from the Bible ("the Book," as the Qur'an calls it):

> The heavens declare the glory of God; the skies proclaim the work of his hands. Day after day they pour forth speech; night after night they reveal knowledge (Psalm 19:1–2)

> For since the creation of the world God's invisible qualities—his eternal power and divine nature—have been clearly seen, being understood from what has been made, so that people are without excuse (Romans 1:20).

With this introduction, we now proceed in the next eight chapters to review and discuss the scientific research that has examined relationships between religion and health in Christian and Islamic societies.

Chapter 6
Religion and Health in Christian Populations

This chapter reviews research on religious involvement and health in non-Muslim populations, where the vast majority are Christians (over 90 %). The review is systematic, i.e., including all published quantitative research from the 1950s through the middle of 2010. These studies have been individually described and summarized in the first and second editions of the *Handbook of Religion and Health* (Koenig et al. 2001, 2012). Only quantitative research, studies that objectively measure and quantify religious involvement and correlate it with similarly quantified health outcomes, are included here. We briefly summarize the results of that research, removing studies that focus on Muslim-majority populations, which will be the focus of chapters that follow this one. After defining the terms "religion," "religious coping," and "spirituality," we organize the research into sections on mental health, social health, health behaviors, and physical health. We then briefly examine the psychological, social, behavioral, and genetic mechanisms that may underlie the relationship between religion and physical health in Christian populations.

Definitions

Before discussing the research, we must define what we mean by religion, religious coping, and the increasingly popular term, spirituality.

Religion is in disfavor today because it tends to divide people and cause conflict because of differing beliefs (as discussed in the last chapter). However, religious beliefs and practices can be easily measured and quantified. Most importantly, they are quite distinct from the health outcomes that religion might influence. We define religion as beliefs, practices, and rituals related to the Transcendent, where in monotheistic traditions, the Transcendent is also called God, Allah, or HaShem. Religion may also involve beliefs about spirits, angels, demons, or other supernatural forces. Religions usually have doctrines about life after death and rules to guide behavior during the present life to prepare for the life to come. Religion is often organized as

H.G. Koenig and S. Al Shohaib, *Health and Well-Being in Islamic Societies: Background, Research, and Applications*, DOI 10.1007/978-3-319-05873-3_6,

a community and maintained as an institution. Religion, however, can also exist outside of an institution and may be practiced alone and involve private expressions of devotion to the Transcendent. At its core, religion involves an established tradition that arises out of a group of people with common beliefs about and rituals concerning the Transcendent.

Religious coping involves the use of religious beliefs or practices to cope with and make sense of difficult life experiences that involve loss or change. For example, in monotheistic traditions, religious coping involves behaviors such as praying to God in order to derive comfort and hope during emotionally trying times, reading religious writings for inspiration and guidance, attending religious services to be uplifted by worshiping God together, and seeking support from members of one's congregation or giving support to others for religious reasons. Religious coping may also involve cognitive processes, including beliefs about a better life after death when pain and suffering will be no more or beliefs in a loving, caring God who is in control, has a purpose for the world and individuals in it, and has the power to transform difficult circumstances so that good outcomes are possible. Thus, both behaviors and beliefs are involved in religious coping.

Spirituality, in its original use, was a term describing a subset of deeply religious people who had submitted their lives to God or the Transcendent. Examples of "spiritual" people often included the clergy or the prophets described in the Holy Scriptures. These were persons whose lives centered on their faith. Spiritual individuals were distinguished from the vast majority of other religious people for whom religion was important, but not fully integrated into their lives. The definition of spirituality, however, has changed over the past 25 years. The modern definition of spirituality has become a vague, nebulous concept that people often define for themselves, becoming so broad that it has lost all distinction. The term spirituality has even expanded to include those who are not religious at all and those who have rejected traditional religion (*secular* spirituality). Furthermore, there is now considerable overlap between definitions of spirituality and positive aspects of mental health, such as peacefulness, being connected with others, having meaning and purpose, and experiencing existential well-being, which are used to characterize the spiritual person. Because of its nebulous and vague nature, its definition as a positive state of mental health, and the difficulty involved in measuring it as a distinct and unique construct, the modern definition of spirituality is not useful in research studies whose aim is to determine relationships with mental or physical health. Attempts to do so have resulted in findings that are impossible to interpret given the tautology in the constructs being correlated. Note, however, that the situation is quite different in clinical settings, where the goal is to find common ground with patients, both religious and nonreligious, so that conversation may take place (see Chap. 14). In those circumstances, the term spirituality can be quite useful. Spirituality as defined today, however, is not useful when conducting research.

For the reasons described above, we prefer the traditional definition of spirituality (i.e., referring to a subset of deeply religious persons) when conducting research. Therefore, as we discuss and summarize the research, we will use the term religion (or use the terms religion or religious, and spiritual or spirituality, interchangeably, i.e., R/S). We will now summarize the research on R/S and mental, social, behavioral, and physical health in Christian-majority populations.

Mental Health

R/S beliefs and practices are used by many Christians to cope with psychological stressors, important losses, traumatic events, and changes in physical health. A study of medically ill patients in North Carolina in 1998 found that 90 % said they used religion to cope with health problems (Koenig 1998). Similarly, a national random survey of the U.S. population during the week following the September 11, 2001, terrorist attacks on the World Trade Centers, found that 90 % of Americans turned to religion to cope with the anxiety and stress of that time (Schuster et al. 2001). Literally hundreds of studies (454 in the two editions of the *Handbook*) have examined the role that R/S plays in coping with stress or illness. The vast majority indicate that people turn to religion during these times and often find it beneficial (Koenig 2012). Of the studies on religious coping, more than 93 % ($n=423$) were conducted in Christian-majority samples, 2.4 % ($n=11$) in Muslim-majority samples, 2.0 % ($n=9$) in Chinese or Southeast Buddhist populations, 2.0 % ($n=8$) in Jewish samples (Israel), and 0.6 % ($n=3$) in Hindu populations (India). The ability of religion to provide meaning and purpose to negative life circumstances, guidance on how to deal with negative events, and a community of people for psychosocial, social, and practical support are major pathways by which R/S helps to neutralize negative emotions and increase positive ones.

Negative Mental Health

We now review research that has examined relationships between level of R/S involvement, negative emotions, and mental disorders. Examined in the present section are studies focused on relationships between R/S and depression, suicide, anxiety, psychosis, and alcohol/drug use or abuse in Christian-majority populations.

Depression. Of 444 quantitative studies, 414 (93 %) were in Christian-majority populations. The remaining studies were in Muslim ($n=13$), Buddhist ($n=9$), Jewish ($n=5$), or Hindu ($n=2$) majority samples. Of the 414 studies in Christians, 254 (61 %) reported significant inverse relationships between R/S and depression, including 6 studies at a statistical trend level ($0.05>p<0.10$), whereas 26 studies (6 %) reported a significant positive relationship between R/S and greater depression, including 2 studies at a trend level. There were 28 clinical trials, of which 17 (61 %) reported that R/S interventions for depression were significantly more effective than standard treatments or a control condition, and 2 studies (7 %) found that R/S interventions were less effective.

Suicide. Of 141 studies that examined relationships between R/S and suicidal thoughts, attempts, or completed suicide, 126 (90 %) were in Christian-majority populations, whereas the other reports came from Muslim-majority countries ($n=5$), Israel ($n=4$), China ($n=4$), India ($n=1$), and the USA and Kuwait ($n=1$). Of the studies in Christian populations, 99 (79 %) found inverse relationships between religiosity and attitudes toward suicide, suicidal thoughts, or suicidal behaviors (4 at a trend level). Two found positive relationships (2 %). There were also 30 studies that examined attitudes toward physician-assisted suicide and R/S, and all 30 (100 %) found significant inverse relationships.

Anxiety. Of 299 studies that explored relationships between R/S and anxiety level, 245 (82 %) were conducted in Christian-majority countries. The other 54 studies came from Muslim-majority countries ($n=23$), Buddhist-majority countries ($n=13$), Israel ($n=13$), and India ($n=5$). Of studies in Christian populations, 120 (49 %) reported significant inverse relationships between R/S and anxiety (4 at a trend level), whereas 24 (10 %) found significant positive relationships between R/S and anxiety.

Psychosis. Of 43 studies that examined relationships with R/S, 39 (88 %) were in Christian-majority countries, whereas 1 each came from India, Israel, China, and Egypt (Muslim). Of studies among Christians, 11 (28 %) found significant inverse relationships with R/S (1 at a trend level) and 9 (23 %) reported more psychotic symptoms among those who were more R/S (1 at a trend level). The remaining studies reported no association (29 %) or mixed findings (21 %) depending on the R/S characteristic measured.

Alcohol Use/Abuse. At least 278 studies have examined R/S and alcohol use/abuse, of which 269 (97 %) were conducted in Christian-majority countries. The remaining studies were in Buddhists (Singapore, Thailand, South Korea), Jews (4 studies from Israel), and Muslims (one each in Turkey and Lebanon). Of studies in Christians, 233 (87 %) reported significant inverse relationships (11 at a trend level) with R/S and 4 (1 %) reported positive relationships (1 at a trend level).

Drug Use/Abuse. Of 185 studies that focused on R/S and illicit drug use/abuse, 182 (98 %) were in Christian-majority populations. The other three studies were among Jews in Southeast Asia, Jews in Israel, and Muslims in Bosnia. Of those 182 studies in Christians, 154 (85 %) found significant inverse relationships (3 at a trend level) and 2 studies (1 %) found positive relationships.

Positive Mental Health

Religious involvement not only helps to neutralize negative emotions but may also be associated with positive emotions such as overall happiness, life satisfaction, well-being, hope, optimism, meaning and purpose, self-esteem, sense of control, and a wide range of positive character traits (forgiveness, altruism, etc.).

Well-Being. Of 326 studies that examined R/S and well-being, happiness, or life satisfaction, 301 (92 %) were conducted in Christian-majority countries. The remaining studies were from Muslim-majority countries ($n=8$), Israel ($n=8$), Singapore ($n=3$), India ($n=3$), and from China, South Korea, and East Asia (one study each). Of studies in Christians, 237 (79 %) reported significant positive relationships between R/S and greater well-being (8 at a trend level), whereas 3 (<1 %) reported inverse relationships.

Hope. At least 40 studies have examined R/S and hope, with 39 in Christian-majority populations and 1 among Muslims in Kosovo and Bosnia. Of studies in Christians, 29 (74 %) found significant positive relationships (2 at a trend level) and none reported inverse relationships.

Optimism. Of 32 studies, 30 (94 %) were in Christian populations, whereas the remaining 2 studies were in Muslim (Kuwait) and Buddhist (Singapore) countries. Of those in Christians, 25 (83 %) reported significant positive relationships. No studies found lower optimism among those who were more R/S.

Meaning and Purpose. Of 45 studies that examined R/S and meaning or purpose in life, 44 (98 %) were in Christian-majority populations and 1 was conducted in Israel. Of those in Christians, 41 (93 %) reported significant positive relationships.

Self-Esteem. There have been at least 69 studies on R/S and self-esteem, of which 65 (94 %) were in Christian-majority countries, 3 were in Muslim-majority countries (Iran, Pakistan, Iraq), and 1 was conducted in Singapore (Buddhist). Of studies in Christians, 40 (62 %) found significantly great self-esteem in those who were more R/S and 2 (3 %) found significantly lower self-esteem.

Sense of Control. Sense of control is often categorized as either having an *internal* locus (where persons believe they control their own destiny through personal decisions) or an *external* locus (where persons believe they are helpless to direct their lives and that powerful other people or institutions control the future). Usually, the notion of God being in control is not included in having an external locus of control (although some might interpret it that way). Instead, God locus of control should be assessed using a different measure (e.g., God Health Locus of Control Scale), which measures to what extent a person believes that God is in control of health outcomes or that God empowers the person to take control of their health. For our purpose here, we focus on the relationship between R/S and the more traditional measures of personal control (internal or external locus of control). Internal locus of control has long been associated with better mental health and external locus of control with worse.

At least 22 studies had examined R/S and locus of control, of which 20 (91 %) were in Christian-majority populations, 1 in Iran, and 1 in Israel (examining Arabs and Jews). Of studies in Christians, 12 (60 %) reported a greater sense of personal or internal control among those who were more R/S, whereas 3 studies (15 %) found significantly lower internal or personal control.

Personality Traits

Personality traits are long lasting, enduring ways that people relate to others (often with a strong genetic basis). The most widely used model for understanding personality traits is the "Five-Factor Model." This model examines five aspects of personality called "the Big Five" (extraversion, neuroticism, conscientiousness, agreeableness, openness to experience). These are usually measured using the NEO Personality Inventory. We now summarize research on R/S and these five personality traits in Christians.

Extraversion. Extraverted people tend to be more outgoing, talkative, and energetic in social situations, which contrasts with introverted people who tend to be more reserved, less outgoing, more reflective, inner focused, and tend to avoid social situations. Our systematic review identified 50 studies that examined relationships with R/S, of which 46 (92 %) were in Christian-majority populations, 2 in Muslim countries, and 2 in Israel. Of studies in Christians, 18 (39 %) found that R/S was related to greater extraversion, 3 (7 %) with less extraversion, and the remaining studies reported that there was no association.

Neuroticism. Neurotic people are characterized by a long-standing pattern of anxiety, moodiness, worry, feeling uptight, and jealous. They tend to be self-conscious, shy, and react poorly to stress. Of 54 studies that have examined R/S and neuroticism, 51 (94 %) were from Christian-majority populations, 2 from Israel, and 1 from Malaysia. Of studies in Christians, most studies (61 %) found no relationship with R/S, whereas a small proportion (24 %, $n=12$) reported inverse relationships (less neurotic) and even a smaller percentage (10 %, $n=5$) found a positive relationship (more neurotic).

Conscientiousness. Conscientious individuals tend to be efficient, thorough, well organized, systematic, neat, careful, and self-disciplined, in contrast to those who are more laid back, less goal oriented, and more likely to engage in antisocial or criminal behavior. Of 30 studies, 28 (93 %) were in Christian-majority populations, and 1 each was from Israel and Malaysia. Of studies in Christians, 19 (68 %) reported significant positive relationships with R/S and 1 study (4 %) found a significant negative relationship (using the controversial Quest scale as a measure of R/S and the negative relationship was found only in men).

Agreeableness. Those characterized by this trait tend to be cooperative, kind, sympathetic, warm, and considerate toward others. These people are more likely to be considered trustworthy, honest, and good by other people. We identified 30 studies that examined the relationship with R/S, of which 28 (93 %) were in Christian-majority populations, and 1 each in Israel and Malaysia. Of studies in Christians, 24 (86 %) reported significant positive relationships with R/S and no studies found negative relationships.

Openness to Experience. Those who score high on this trait tend to have active imaginations, prefer variety, and are more intellectually curious. They tend to reject conventional or traditional beliefs or ideas and prefer new experiences to familiar routines. There have been 26 studies examining relationships with R/S, of which 24 were in Christian-majority populations and 1 each in Israel and Malaysia. Of studies in Christians, 10 (42 %) reported significant positive relationships with R/S and 2 (8 %) found negative relationships (both measuring traditional or conservative religious beliefs).

Social Health

Social health involves a number of domains, including social support (number and quality of social connections), marital stability, delinquency or crime (antisocial behaviors), and social capital. Each of these social factors has been associated with mental and physical health in a wide range of studies.

Social Support. Social support includes emotional support and tangible support (physical help) received from others. Components of social support include size of social network, number of contacts per week (by telephone, in person, and, nowadays, via social media), and a person's subjective sense that people are available and willing to provide support when needed. Of 74 studies identified in our systematic review, 70 (95 %) were in Christian-majority populations, 2 were in Muslim countries, and 1 each in Taiwan and Israel. Of studies in Christians, 58 (83 %) reported significant positive relationships with R/S and no studies found negative relationships.

Marital Stability. Marital stability involves maintaining marital ties (vs. divorce), satisfaction with marriage, and absence of spousal abuse. Of 79 studies that have examined the relationship with R/S, 75 (95 %) were in Christian-majority populations, 2 in Israel, and 2 in Muslim countries. Of the studies in Christians, 64 (85 %) reported significant positive relationships with R/S (1 at a trend level) and no studies found negative relationships.

Delinquency and Crime. At least 104 studies have examined relationships between R/S and either youth crime (delinquent acts) or adult criminal behavior, of which 99 (95 %) were in Christian-majority populations, 3 were in Muslim countries, and 1 each in Israel and Taiwan. Of the studies in Christians, 79 (80 %) found significantly less delinquency/crime in those who were more R/S (5 at a trend level), whereas 2 studies (2 %) reported greater delinquency/crime.

Social Capital. Social capital is a measure of community health and is often measured by level of community participation, volunteerism, trust, and membership rates in civic, political, or social justice organizations. Our systematic review uncovered 14 studies that examined relationships with R/S, of which 12 (86 %) were in Christian-majority populations, 1 was in Korea, and 1 was in Turkey. Of the studies in Christians, 10 (83 %) found significant positive relationships with R/S and none found negative relationships.

Health Behaviors

Health behaviors are key to living a healthy disease-free life and avoiding chronic illness. Activities that influence physical health include cigarette smoking, exercise, diet, weight, and sexual behavior.

Cigarette Smoking. At least 137 studies have examined R/S and smoking, of which 125 (91 %) were in Christian-majority populations, 6 in Israel, 5 in Muslim-majority countries, and 1 in Thailand (a country that is 69 % Buddhist). Of the studies in Christians, 114 (91 %) found significant inverse relationships between R/S and cigarette smoking (3 at a trend level) and no studies found higher rates of smoking in those who were more R/S.

Exercise. Of 37 studies that examined relationships with R/S, 34 (92 %) were in Christian-majority populations and 3 were conducted in Israel (including 1 among Muslims). Of those in Christians, 25 (74 %) reported greater exercise or physical activity in those who are more R/S (2 at a trend level), and 4 (12 %) reported significantly less exercise/activity among the more religious.

Diet. At least 22 studies have examined relationships with diet or nutritional status, and all (100 %) were in Christian-majority populations. Of those, 12 (55 %) found better diet among those who were more R/S (1 at a trend level) and 1 found worse diet.

Weight. Of all health characteristics, maintaining an ideal body weight is the one health behavior that religious people have trouble with. In general, those who are more religious weigh more than those who are less religious. Of 36 studies that examined the relationship, 33 (92 %) were in Christian-majority populations and 3 were from Israel (1 that focused on Muslims). Of studies in Christians, 5 (15 %) found lower weight (or less underweight) among the more R/S, whereas 13 (39 %) reported heavier weight or higher body mass index. Christian communities encourage eating together as part of fellowship, and the food that is served is not always low in calories.

Sexual Behavior. We identified 95 studies that examined R/S and risky sexual behavior, of which 93 (98 %) were in Christian-majority populations, 1 was from Israel, and 1 was from Iran. Of the studies in Christians, 80 (86 %) reported inverse relationships between R/S and risky sexual activity (1 at a trend level), and 1 study found more such activity among imprisoned sex offenders in Australia who were more religious.

Physical Health

Areas of physical health in which researchers have examined R/S include coronary heart disease, hypertension, cerebrovascular disease, dementia, immune function, endocrine function, metabolic disorders, cancer, self-rated health, and mortality.

Heart Disease. Our systematic review examining R/S and coronary artery disease (CAD) uncovered 20 studies published through the middle of 2010, of which 13 (68 %) were in Christian-majority populations, 3 were from Israel, 2 from India, and 1 from Muslim countries (Albania and Saudi Arabia). Of studies in Christians, 7 (54 %) found significantly lower rates of CAD in those who were more R/S, whereas 1 study found a higher rate of CAD in the more R/S.

In addition, 16 studies have explored links between R/S and cardiovascular functions (cardiovascular reactivity, heart rate variability), surgical outcomes, or levels of inflammatory markers or coagulation factors that predict higher CAD risk (C-reactive protein, fibrinogen). Most of these studies (75 %) were in Christian-majority populations, 3 were from Turkey, and 1 from India. Of the 12 studies in Christians, 8 (67 %) reported significantly better cardiovascular functioning in the more R/S (3 at a trend level) and 1 study reported worse cardiovascular functions in college students who were more R/S.

Hypertension. At least 63 studies have examined relationships with R/S, of which 53 (84 %) were conducted in Christian-majority populations, 5 in Muslim-majority populations, 3 in Buddhist countries, and 1 each in Jewish (Israel) and Hindu (India) populations. Of studies in Christians, 31 (58 %) reported lower blood pressure (BP) or less hypertension in those who were more R/S (5 at a trend level), whereas 7 studies (13 %) found higher BP among the more R/S (1 at a trend level).

Cerebrovascular Disease. Only a few studies have examined the relationship between R/S and stroke or cerebrovascular disease. Our systematic review identified 9 such studies, of which 7 (78 %) were in Christian-majority populations and 2 in Muslim countries. Of studies in Christians, 4 (57 %) reported inverse relationships with R/S (1 at a trend level), whereas 1 study reported greater carotid artery thickening (known to predict an increased risk of stroke) in those who were more R/S.

Dementia/Alzheimer's Disease. There have also been 21 studies that examined relationships between R/S and presence of dementia, Alzheimer's disease, or the decline in memory associated with increased age. Of those, 17 (81 %) were in Christians and the remaining 2 studies were from Taiwan and Israel. Of studies in Christians, 10 studies (59 %) reported significant positive relationships between R/S and memory, including several prospective studies, whereas 2 studies (20 %) found more rapid memory decline or greater dementia in the more R/S.

Diabetes. The findings are less consistent for metabolic disorders such as diabetes, hypercholesterolemia, and overall allostatic load (not surprising given that those who are more R/S tend to be overweight). Concerning diabetes, we identified 17 studies, of which 11 were in Christian-majority populations, 4 were in Muslim countries, and 1 each in Israel and India. Among Christians, 2 studies (18 %) reported significantly better diabetic control in those who were more R/S, 3 (27 %) reported worse diabetic control, and the remainder found no association.

Cholesterol. With regard to cholesterol levels or allostatic load, our systematic review identified 24 studies, of which 16 (67 %) were in Christian-majority populations, 7 in Muslim-majority countries, and 1 in India. Of the 16 studies in Christian populations, 7 (44 %) reported lower cholesterol or lower allostatic load in those who were more religious and 2 studies (13 %) reported significantly higher cholesterol levels.

Immune Function. We identified 30 studies that examined relationships between R/S, immune function, and pro- or anti-inflammatory cytokine levels (indicators of immune system functioning). Of those, 24 (83 %) were in Christian-majority populations, 2 were in Buddhist countries, 3 in Muslim countries, and 1 in southern India. Of studies in Christians, 16 (67 %) found positive relationships with better immune function or lower levels of pro-inflammatory markers (1 at a trend level). Although no studies in Christians found only worse immune function, one study in breast cancer patients reported mixed findings, three reported positive findings (increased CD4/CD3, natural killer cells, and total lymphocytes), and one found worse immune function (lower cutaneous immune response to antigens).

In addition, two studies examined the effects of R/S interventions on interferon gamma, both finding a significant increase as a result of the intervention. Interferon gamma (produced by natural killer cells) is important to the immune system because it can inhibit viral replication directly and has immunostimulatory and immunomodulatory effects. A third study reported that a R/S intervention decreased levels of anti-inflammatory cytokines IL-4 and IL-10 (which were increased above normal at baseline in patients with recently diagnosed breast cancer, thus indicating a positive effect for the intervention).

Susceptibility to infection and virus concentration in blood (viral load) have also been examined as a proxy for immune function in 12 studies, of which 11 were in Christian-majority populations and 1 was in southern India. Of studies in Christian populations, 7 (64 %) reported significantly less susceptibility to infection or reduced viral load in those who were more R/S (no studies found greater susceptibility or increased viral load).

Endocrine Function. We identified 31 studies that examined relationships with R/S or effects of R/S interventions on endocrine function. These studies focused on the stress hormones cortisol, epinephrine, and norepinephrine. Again, most of these studies (27 or 87 %) were in Christian-majority populations and 4 were in Buddhist-majority countries (China or Thailand). Of studies in Christians, 20 (74 %) found positive relationships with better endocrine function or reported that a R/S intervention (often meditation) improved endocrine function. No studies reported a relationship with worse endocrine function or greater stress hormone levels.

Cancer. Our systematic review identified 29 studies that examined connections between R/S and either susceptibility to cancer or prognosis of cancer after it had developed. Of those studies, 28 (97 %) were in Christians and 1 study was in Buddhists/Taoists (China). About half the studies in Christians (54 %) found lower risk of cancer or a better prognosis (one at a trend level). Two studies (7 %), however, reported that women raised in Protestant homes had higher risk of breast cancer than those with no religious affiliation, and that women involved in religious occupations had a higher death rate from cancer.

Self-Rated Health. Self-rated health is a person's sense of their overall physical health condition and is usually rated from poor to excellent. Such ratings are strongly correlated with actual health and mortality (Idler and Benyamini 1997). Our systematic review uncovered 50 studies that examined relationships with R/S, of which 48 (96 %) were in Christian-majority populations and 1 each was from Taiwan and Israel. Of studies in Christians, 29 (60 %) reported significantly better self-rated health in those who were more R/S, whereas 5 (17 %) reported worse self-rated health.

Mortality. We identified 121 studies that examined prospective relationships between R/S and overall mortality, of which 106 (88 %) were in Christian-majority populations, 9 were from Israel, 5 from Taiwan/China, and 1 from Japan. Of studies in Christians, 72 (68 %) found significantly greater longevity or reduced mortality in those who were more R/S (3 at a trend level), whereas 7 (6 %) reported greater mortality.

Mechanisms and Pathways

Based on the research above, and reports from qualitative studies that have asked Christians to describe the role that religion plays in their health, we present here a theoretical model of how R/S involvement in the Christian tradition might influence physical health and extend longevity. The source of the health benefits of Christian faith in this model is a close personal attachment to God, which has been shown to influence the relationship between religious involvement (such as prayer) and mental health outcomes (Bradshaw et al. 2008). This model is based on the role that religious faith plays in coping with negative life events involving loss, change, or trauma. It hypothesizes that Christian beliefs provide meaning and purpose to traumatic life events, foster positive human traits (such as forgiveness, altruism, gratefulness, etc.), and provide guidance on how to make decisions that enhance individual and community health and well-being. Such influences increase the experience of positive emotions (peace, well-being, happiness) and decrease negative emotions (depression, anxiety, addiction). Christian beliefs and practices may also boost social support, increase social interactions, and encourage the providing of support to others, all of which help to buffer stressful events and negative life circumstances. Finally, religious involvement is thought to reduce negative health behaviors such as alcohol intake, cigarette smoking, a sedentary lifestyle, unhealthy diet, and risky sexual behaviors, thereby improving health. These are the primary pathways by which R/S within the Christian tradition might impact physical health (Fig. 6.1).

Note, however, that the effects of R/S are likely impacted by genetic factors, developmental experiences (both in childhood and adult life), and by personality

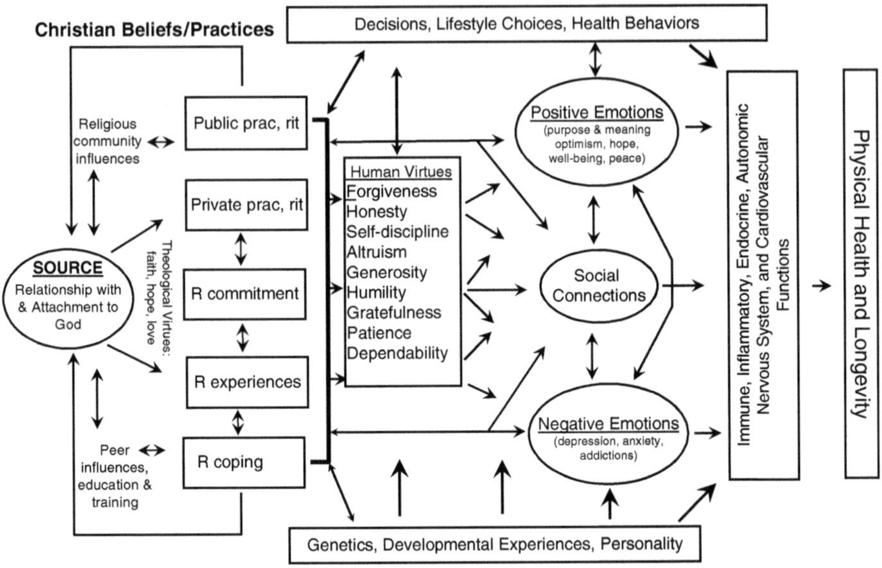

Fig. 6.1 Theoretical pathways by which Christianity is hypothesized to influence mental and physical health. This figure has been adapted from Figure 28.1, p 587, *Handbook of Religion and Health,* 2nd ed. New York, NY: Oxford University Press, 2012. Used with permission

factors (rooted in genetic predispositions and early environmental influences). Thus, the relationship is a complex one that is related to beliefs, behaviors, and decisions made by the individual and by a combination of genetic and environmental factors that are operating independent of the individual.

Summary and Conclusions

Most studies that have examined relationships between R/S and mental, social, behavioral, and physical health have been conducted in populations where the majority of participants are Christian (see Table 6.1 for summary). A majority of these studies report that those who are more religious or spiritual experience fewer negative mental health problems (less depression, suicide, anxiety, alcohol and drug use), more positive emotions (greater well-being, hope, optimism, sense of meaning and purpose, self-esteem, and internal sense of control), and more positive personality traits (greater conscientiousness and agreeableness). Most studies also find that Christian beliefs and behaviors are related to greater social support and marital stability, less delinquency/crime, and overall greater social capital. Negative health behaviors such as cigarette smoking, a sedentary lifestyle, poor diet, and risky sexual behaviors are less frequent among those who are more R/S (although religiosity in Christians is related to being overweight). Physical health also appears better

Table 6.1 Summary of studies and findings in Christian-majority countries through mid-2010 based on systematic review[a]

	Studies in Christians		Findings in Christians	
All studies	Total no.	No. (% of total)	Positive[b] no. (%)	Negative no. (%)
Negative mental health				
Depression	444	414 (93)	254 (61)	26 (6)
Suicide	141	126 (90)	99 (79)	2 (2)
Anxiety	299	245 (82)	120 (49)	24 (10)
Psychosis	43	39 (88)	11 (28)	9 (23)
Alcohol use/abuse	278	269 (97)	233 (87)	4 (1)
Drug use/abuse	185	182 (98)	154 (85)	2 (1)
Negative mental health				
Well-being	326	301 (92)	237 (79)	3 (1)
Hope	40	39 (98)	29 (74)	0 (0)
Optimism	32	30 (94)	25 (83)	0 (0)
Meaning/purpose	45	44 (98)	41 (93)	0 (0)
Self-esteem	69	65 (94)	40 (62)	2 (3)
Sense of control	22	20 (91)	12 (60)	3 (15)
Personality traits				
Extraversion	50	46 (92)	18 (39)	3 (7)
Neuroticism	54	51 (94)	12 (24)	5 (10)
Conscientiousness	30	28 (93)	19 (68)	1 (4)
Agreeableness	30	28 (93)	24 (86)	0 (0)
Openness	26	24 (92)	10 (42)	2 (8)
Social health				
Social support	74	70 (95)	58 (83)	0 (0)
Marital stability	79	75 (95)	64 (85)	0 (0)
Delinquency/crime	104	99 (95)	79 (80)	2 (2)
Social capital	14	12 (86)	10 (83)	0 (0)
Health behaviors				
Cigarette smoking	137	125 (91)	114 (91)	0 (0)
Exercise	37	34 (92)	25 (74)	4 (12)
Diet	22	22 (100)	12 (55)	1 (5)
Weight	36	33 (92)	5 (15)	13 (39)
Sexual behavior	95	93 (98)	80 (86)	1 (1)
Physical health				
Heart disease[c]	35	25 (71)	15 (60)	2 (8)
Hypertension	63	53 (84)	31 (58)	7 (13)
Cerebrovascular disease	9	7 (78)	4 (57)	1 (14)
Dementia/Alzheimer's disease	21	17 (81)	10 (59)	2 (20)
Diabetes	15	11 (73)	2 (18)	3 (27)
Cholesterol/allostatic load	24	16 (67)	7 (44)	2 (13)
Immune function[d]	44	38 (86)	26 (68)	0 (0)
Endocrine function	31	27 (87)	20 (74)	0 (0)
Cancer	29	28 (97)	15 (54)	2 (7)
Self-rated health	50	48 (96)	29 (60)	5 (17)
Mortality	121	106 (88)	72 (68)	7 (6)

[a]*Handbook of Religion and Health*, 1st and 2nd editions (Oxford University Press 2001 and 2012)

[b]"Positive" means *better* health and "negative" means *worse* health

[c]Includes coronary artery disease, cardiovascular functions (i.e., cardiovascular reactivity), surgical outcomes, etc.

[d]Includes 12 studies examining susceptibility to infection or virus concentration in blood, an indirect measure of immune function

among those who are more R/S, including less CAD, better cardiovascular functions, lower blood pressure, less cerebrovascular disease, less dementia and slower decline in memory with age, better immune functions, better endocrine functions (lower stress hormone levels), lower rates of cancer, better self-rated health, and greater overall longevity. There are plausible reasons why R/S involvement in Christians might be related to better health, operating through psychological, social, and behavioral pathways known to influence physiological functions responsible for physical health and vigor. In the following chapters, we examine whether relationships between R/S and health in Muslim populations are similar to or different than those found in Christians, and then try to understand why.

References

Bradshaw, M., Ellison, C. G., & Flannelly, K. J. (2008). Prayer, God imagery, and symptoms of psychopathology. *Journal for the Scientific Study of Religion, 47*, 644–659.

Guessoum, N. (2010). Science, religion, and the quest for knowledge and truth: An Islamic perspective. *Cultural Studies of Science Education, 5*, 55–69.

Idler, E. L., & Benyamini, Y. (1997). Self-rated health and mortality: A review of twenty-seven community studies. *Journal of Health and Social Behavior, 38*(1), 21–37.

Koenig, H. G. (1998). Religious beliefs and practices of hospitalized medically ill older adults. *International Journal of Geriatric Psychiatry, 13*, 213–224.

Koenig, H. G. (2012). Religion, spirituality and health: The research and clinical implications. *ISRN Psychiatry, 2012*, 1–33. Article ID 278730.

Koenig, H. G., McCullough, M. E., & Larson, D. B. (2001). *Handbook of religion and health.* New York: Oxford University Press.

Koenig, H. G., King, D. E., & Carson, V. B. (2012). *Handbook of religion and health* (2nd ed.). New York: Oxford University Press.

Newton I (1687). Principia, Book III; cited in. In H. S. Thayer (Ed.), Newton's philosophy of nature: Selections from his writings (p. 42). New York: Hafner Library of Classics, 1953.

Rahman, F. (1998). *Health and medicine in the Islamic tradition.* Chicago: ABC International Group, Inc./Kazi Publications.

Schuster, M. A., Stein, B. D., Jaycox, L., Collins, R. L., Marshall, G. N., Elliott, M. N., et al. (2001). A national survey of stress reactions after the September 11, 2001, terrorist attacks. *New England Journal of Medicine, 345*(20), 1507–1512.

Chapter 7
Religion and Negative Emotions in Muslims

Introduction to Review

In the next five chapters we describe quantitative research examining relationships between religion and health in Muslims. Studies identified through our exhaustive review of the published literature are described in detail. Although our description of study after study may bore some readers, there is a reason for providing an in-depth account of individual studies and citations for each study. First, this is the first comprehensive review of research on religion and health in Islamic societies. Therefore, providing details on the populations studied, methods used, and findings reported will give the reader a sense of what exactly has been done so far. This will facilitate the design of future research that will extend our knowledge, rather than simply repeat what has already been studied. Second, our detailed descriptions will help avoid bias in the reporting of the results. We present exactly what researchers have found without filtering the studies or the findings so that they agree with our personal opinions and biases. Other investigators can substantiate our findings and conclusions by simply retrieving the original studies and reviewing them. Finally, these detailed accounts will allow us to comment on each study and point out strengths and weaknesses that could influence the interpretation of the findings.

Some readers, however, may wish to skip the description of individual studies, and go right to the main points. Therefore, we provide a brief summary of the research results at the conclusion of each section, along with tables that summarize the findings that can be quickly scanned. Our objective is to convey a sense of what has been done, where it has been done, and what has been discovered, while using a format that allows readers to examine each study in detail or skim through the research methods and go right to the findings. We hope this review will serve as a stimulus for expanding and improving the research on religion and health in Muslims. As will become evident in the final chapters of this volume, such research is desperately needed to guide healthcare practices and health policy decisions.

We structure our review of this research to parallel that presented among Christians in the last chapter. We first examine research on relationships between

H.G. Koenig and S. Al Shohaib, *Health and Well-Being in Islamic Societies: Background, Research, and Applications*, DOI 10.1007/978-3-319-05873-3_7,

religiosity and mental health (negative emotions and positive emotions), followed by chapters on religiosity and social health, behavioral health, and physical health. We also compare the mental, social, and physical health of Muslims with members of other religious denominations, including Christians (although this is of secondary interest since such comparisons are not particularly useful). We present the studies in chronological order by year of publication to give a sense of how the research has progressed over time. The only exception is when examining the effects of a particular religious activity (e.g., Ramadan fasting) on a health outcome, when grouping the studies together is more logical than discussing them by chronological year. Our goal throughout is to provide an objective picture of the relationship between religiosity and health among Muslims.

Our review of studies is also organized into three groups: (1) studies identified in our 2010 systematic review presented in the two editions of the Handbook of Religion and Health (which provides a benchmark to compare findings in Muslims with those in Christian populations), (2) studies published before 2010 that were missed by our systematic review, and (3) studies conducted since the 2010 systematic review that represent the most recently published research. Studies missed by our 2010 systematic review and those conducted since our 2010 systematic review were identified using Google Scholar (which is probably more comprehensive than either Medline or PsychInfo that were used in compiling the Handbooks, since it picks up studies in smaller non-Western journals). Search terms used were "Muslim," "religion," "religiosity," and the particular health outcome being examined. Typically, the first ten pages (approximately 100 citations) were reviewed to identify eligible quantitative studies relevant to the topic. We stopped searching when no new studies could be located and only those previously identified began to repeat. The reference lists of published reports were also examined for studies missed by the method above. Thus, we feel confident that our review is a comprehensive one that has identified the vast majority of studies published to date on this topic.

Given the important role that Islamic beliefs and practices play in coping with trauma, adaptation to stress, and addressing purpose and meaning in life, the aspect of health most likely to be influenced is mental health. The first area we review is religious coping, followed by research on negative emotions and mental disorders (depression, suicide, anxiety, psychosis, and substance use/abuse).

Religious Coping

Research on religion and coping is key to understanding the mechanism by which religious involvement affects mental health. Because of the importance of this topic, we depart from our usual method of examining only quantitative studies and include here qualitative studies that describe how Muslims view religion as helping them to deal with life stress. Our 2010 systematic review identified 454 studies focused on religious coping and health. Of those, 2.4 % (11) were conducted in Muslim-majority populations, with the first study published in 2002 (Watson et al. 2002). We review seven descriptive (qualitative) reports first and then four quantitative studies.

Descriptive Reports

The first qualitative study of the role that religion plays in coping was conducted in the United Arab Emirates. This study examined how Muslim parents adapt to the stress of having a child with cancer. Eapen and Revesz (2003) surveyed the parents of 38 children (average age 9.6) with acute leukemia, lymphoma, or other serious cancers diagnosed 7–30 months prior to the interview. All parents (100 %) said they relied on their Islamic beliefs to cope.

In a second study, Scholte and colleagues (2004) surveyed a random sample of 1,011 persons aged 15 year or older in the Nangarhar province of eastern Afghanistan (next to western Pakistan) in 2003, asking about sources of emotional support during this war-torn period. Most respondents were of Pashtun ethnicity, over two-thirds had no formal education, and only 41 % had a job. Over half of the sample had directly experienced more than eight traumatic events within the past 10 years, over two-thirds lacked food or water, and nearly three-quarters had no access to medical care. When asked about their main source of support when feeling sad, worried, or tense, 98 % said "Allah." Other sources of support included family (81 %) and in-laws (55 %).

A third study conducted by Hestyanti (2006) interviewed 50 children ages 11–15 who survived the devastating tsunami that hit Indonesia in 2004. These children came from three camps in the Banda Aceh and Great Aceh areas, those most directly affected by the tsunami. The focus of the study was to determine factors associated with emotional resiliency, which was defined as: (1) being involved in at least one community activity, (2) considered by others as good/nice, not a trouble-maker, and (3) having no clinically significant trauma-related symptoms. The results of this study revealed that factors related to resiliency were support from parents, siblings, peers, and social workers, and routine involvement in religious activities. All six children identified as resilient were involved in religious activities such as reading and learning from the Qur'an.

Next, Taleghani and colleagues (2006) interviewed 19 women with newly diagnosed breast cancer in Tehran, Iran, with the goal of identifying themes related to coping with the disease. Results indicated that religious coping behaviors were uniformly used to deal with illness. These included accepting the disease as God's will and considering the disease as a form of test from God that they should "pass with pride." Women noted that God was their only supporter, and that visiting a shrine to worship and saying prayers helped them to relax and stop worrying.

Bataineh and researchers (2006) examined how medical students in Jordan ($n = 145$) coped with the stress of dissecting the human body. Physical and psychological reactions (experienced by nearly one-third) included heart palpitations and recurring visual images of cadavers. Besides using rationalization to deal with the fear (90 %), the most common coping practices were reading religious books (83 %) and praying (79 %). This was especially true for women and those medical students with the most anxiety and fear.

Next, Conrad and colleagues (2007) examined coping behaviors by 24 patients with paranoid schizophrenia in Jordan and 23 patients with the same condition in Germany. Researchers assessed participants at the time of hospital admission and after they had achieved partial remission. All were on antipsychotic medications at the time of evaluation. One aim of the study was to identify factors that patients believed could positively influence their illness. Among patients in Jordan, 29 % spontaneously (without prompting) indicated that religion was such a factor. No other coping factor was more prevalent. Among German patients, none (0 %) mentioned religion.

In the final descriptive study, Errihani and colleagues (2008) surveyed 1,600 Muslim cancer patients in Morocco (mean age 49, 59 % male), assessing religious beliefs and practices and their use in coping with cancer. Participants were divided into two groups based on their religious involvement: 49 % were described as "practicing believers" (active in living out the five pillars of Islam—shahadah, five daily prayers, fasting during Ramadan, zakat, pilgrimage) and 51 % as "non-practicing believers" (did not practice prayers, but did participate in Ramadan fast). Responses to cancer differed in each group. Non-practicing believers reported feeling guilty, believing they were bad Muslims and fearing divine punishment, with some increasing their religious practices but in an extreme way that sometimes conflicted with cancer treatment. Practicing believers reported that cancer was a divine test, resulting in their accepting of the disease, experiencing pride in being selected by God for this test, and continuing to practice their faith. Researchers concluded, "religion plays an important role for Moslem patients, whether practicing or not, in their adjustment to the psychological impact of the disease" (p. 100).

Quantitative

Our 2010 systematic review identified four quantitative studies that examined relationships between religious coping and mental health outcomes in Muslims, three reporting significant positive relationships between religious behaviors and mental health. The first is a study by Watson and colleagues (2002) who examined the relationship between perceived stress and intrinsic religiosity in 231 college students in Tehran, Iran (all Muslim), and 220 college students at the University of Tennessee (Christian). The hypothesis was that intrinsic religiosity would buffer the effects of stressful experiences resulting in lower perceived stress, less depression, less anxiety, and greater self-esteem in those who were more intrinsically religious. In the American sample, intrinsic religiosity was unrelated to anxiety, but inversely related to depression ($r=-0.33$, $p<0.001$), perceived stress ($r=-0.23$, $p<0.01$), and was positively related to self-esteem ($r=+0.34$, $p<0.001$). Similarly, in the Iranian sample, intrinsic religiosity was unrelated to anxiety, but was inversely related to depression (–0.30, $p<0.001$), perceived stress ($r=-0.22$, $p<0.01$), and was positively related to self-esteem ($r=+0.35$, $p<0.001$). Correlations, then, were almost identical in these two religious groups.

Next, Khan and Watson (2006) surveyed 129 college students at the University of Karachi, Pakistan, examining the relationships between religious coping assessed by the Pakistani Coping Practices Scale, intrinsic religiosity, religious interest, and maladjustment (anxiety, depression, and hostility assessed using the Brief Symptom Inventory). No significant correlations were found between religious coping or intrinsic religiosity and anxiety, depression, or hostility. Greater religious interest, however, was related to significantly less depression ($r = -0.21$, $p < 0.05$). Feeling punished or abandoned by God was significantly and positively correlated with depression, anxiety, and hostility (similar to what is usually seen in Christian samples).

The third study, conducted by Aguilar-Vafaie and colleagues (2007) at the University in Tehran, Iran, surveyed 365 college students (56 % women) to determine the psychometric properties of a new 13-item measure of religious coping and to examine relationships with healthy coping behaviors. Religious coping was significantly and positively related to positive reappraisal, seeking guidance and support, problem solving and seeking alternative rewards (all healthy behaviors) in men, with similar though slightly weaker relationships in women. A shortened version (8-item) of the religious coping measure was then administered to a second sample of 176 college students (39 % women). Religious coping was again significantly and positively related to problem solving in men and in women, and to seeking guidance and support, seeking alternative rewards, and acceptance in men (again, all healthy coping behaviors).

Finally, in the only quantitative study to examine adults other than college students, Filazoglu and Griva (2008) surveyed 188 women with breast cancer (90 % Muslim) at three hospitals in Turkey. The purpose was to identify predictors of health-related quality of life (HRQOL), which was assessed using the SF-36. Religious coping was measured using a multi-item subscale of the Ways of Coping Inventory (Lazarus). Regression models examined the relationship between religious coping and physical and mental health components of HRQOL. Religious coping was unrelated to either physical or mental health, although there was a weak trend toward higher religious coping being associated with worse mental health, $B = -0.19$, $p = 0.06$, but only after controlling for healthy coping styles and social support.

Missed Studies. Our 2010 systematic review above did not uncover all studies in Muslims on religious coping, especially descriptive studies. Given the large number of such studies and limited space, however, we will not review missed studies here.

Recent Research. The research on religion and coping among Muslims has increased dramatically since our 2010 review, making it impossible to capture the full richness and diversity of the findings in this area. Two studies, however, illustrate recent findings. First is a study by Nurasikin and colleagues (2013) of 228 outpatients attending a psychiatric clinic at the University of Malaya in Kuala Lumpur. Religious coping was assessed using the 14-item Brief RCOPE, and religiosity was measured using the Duke University Religious Index (DUREL). Also administered was the Depression, Anxiety, and Stress Scale (DASS). Although there was no relationship between positive religious coping and DASS scores, negative religious coping was strongly and positively related to depression, anxiety and stress scores ($r = +0.47$, $p < 0.01$, uncontrolled). In contrast, private religious activities, intrinsic religiosity, and total DUREL scores were related to lower DASS scores (r's $= -0.14$ to -0.19, $p < 0.05$). Regression analyses confirmed these relationships, even after controlling for severity of psychiatric symptoms.

A second study examined the relationships between spiritual coping, religiosity, and quality of life in 362 patients undergoing hemodialysis in Tehran, Iran (Saffari et al. 2013). Spiritual coping was assessed using a 20-item measure adapted for use in Muslims, which was divided into religious and nonreligious coping methods. The DUREL was again used to assess religiosity. Quality of life and overall health status were assessed using a standard measure (EQ-5D-3L). Higher religious coping was related to both greater quality of life ($r = +0.19$, $p < 0.001$) and better health status ($r = +0.12$, $p < 0.05$), as were all three dimensions of religiosity (organized religiosity, private religiosity, and intrinsic religiosity, with correlations ranging from +0.11 to +0.49). All relationships persisted after controlling for other predictors in hierarchical regression models, in particular relationships with religious coping, intrinsic religiosity, and frequency of religious attendance.

Summary. All descriptive studies in Muslims thus far find that religion is consistently and uniformly used to cope with stress and distress, and three-quarters of the few quantitative studies conducted through 2010 report that religious coping and religiosity are related to indicators of successful or healthy coping. Recent studies confirm these findings.

Depression

Depression is the most common mental disorder in the world and the most disabling. Therefore it is appropriate to begin our review of negative emotional states and mental disorders here. In our 2010 systematic review we identified 13 studies, three from Malaysia, four from Iran, and one each from Palestine, Afghanistan, Pakistan, Egypt, Lebanon, and Kuwait, each examining relationships between R/S and depression (or bereavement).

The three studies from the Universiti Sains Malaysia involved randomized clinical trials examining the effects of supplementing standard treatment of depression with Islamic religious psychotherapy, all three showing benefit. In the first study, Azhar and Varma (1995a) randomized 64 Muslims with strong religious beliefs and depression to either (1) standard treatment consisting of weekly psychotherapy and antidepressant medication or (2) standard treatment plus additional Islamic psychotherapy. Subjects were assessed blind to treatment group at 1, 3, and 6 months. Those receiving additional religious psychotherapy improved more quickly than controls at 3 months, but by 6 months there was no difference between treatment groups. A second study by Azhar and Varma (1995b) examined the effects of providing additional Islamic psychotherapy to 30 religious Muslims experiencing bereavement. Subjects were randomized to receive standard treatment (brief psychotherapy plus antidepressant medication) or standard treatment plus additional religious psychotherapy. The additional religious psychotherapy involved "discussions of relevant religious issues." Those receiving the additional religious psychotherapy showed significant improvements over those in the control group at 6 months, based on the Hamilton Depression Scale.

In the third clinical trial, Razali and colleagues (1998) randomized 203 Muslim patients with anxiety/depression to standard care or to standard care plus religious psychotherapy (using cognitive techniques guided by the Qur'an and Hadith). Both groups were followed for 6 months and assessed blind to treatment group using the Hamilton Depression Scale. Patients receiving the additional religious psychotherapy responded significantly faster than those receiving the standard treatment.

The remaining 10 studies are all cross-sectional in design. Ghorbani and colleagues (2000) from the University of Tehran surveyed 178 Muslim university students examining religiosity and depressive symptoms. Religiosity was measured using the Muslim Attitudes Toward Religion Scale (MARS), and depressive symptoms were assessed by the Hopkins Symptom Checklist (Derogatis). Neither the total MARS score nor any of its subscales (personal help, Muslim practices, Muslim worldview) were related to depressive symptoms.

Barber (2001) analyzed data on 6,923 high school students (98 % Muslim) in Palestine, examining the relationship between religiosity and depressive symptoms, among other characteristics. Religiosity was assessed using five items that measured perceived religiosity, religious behavior, and salience of religion. Depressive symptoms were measured using six items from the Child Behavior Checklist-Youth Scale. Controlling for other correlates, religiosity was inversely related to depressive symptoms in both males and females, an association that reached statistical significance in females ($B = -0.12$, $p < 0.001$).

Watson and colleagues (2002), as reviewed above under religious coping, surveyed 227 Muslim university students at the University of Tehran and 220 Christian college students from University of Tennessee, assessing intrinsic religiosity (Allport and Ross) and depressive symptoms. As noted previously, results indicated almost identical inverse correlations between intrinsic religiosity and depressive symptoms in both Muslim ($r = -0.30$, $p < 0.001$) and Christian samples ($r = -0.33$, $p < 0.001$).

Next, Mirzamani and Mohammadi (2003) at Tehran University examined the characteristics of 70 psychiatric outpatients (average age 27), comparing them to a control group of 50 university staff and students (average age 27). Religious values were assessed using a subscale of the Allport, Vernon and Lindzey Study of Values scale, and depression was measured using Derogatis' Symptom Checklist-90 (SCL-90-R). Religious values were lower in psychiatric patients compared to students and university staff, and were inversely related to depressive symptoms in the combined sample ($r = -0.23$, $p = 0.01$, uncontrolled).

In another study described earlier, Cordozo and associates (2004) surveyed a national random sample of 799 adults in postwar Afghanistan, many of whom were very poor and had few resources (100 physically disabled, 699 non-disabled). Religious involvement was assessed using a single item that asked about religious or spiritual practices (reading the Koran, praying, or engaging in traditional religious ceremonies) (yes vs. no). Depressive symptoms were measured using the Hopkins Symptom Checklist-25. Although there was no relationship between religious practices and depressive symptoms in non-disabled subjects, there was a significant inverse relationship between religious activity and depressive symptoms in those who were disabled (65.9 in nonreligious vs. 37.8 in the religiously active, $p=0.01$). Results persisted after adjustment for gender, age, marital status, ethnicity, education, availability of food, and employment.

Also previously described, Khan and Watson (2006) surveyed 129 Pakistani university students, assessing religiosity with the Pakistani Religious Coping Practices Scale, a religious orientation scale (Gorsuch), and the brief RCOPE (Pargament). Depression was measured using the depression subscale from the Brief Symptom Inventory. No relationship was found with any religious measure and depressive symptoms. However, after controlling for negative religious coping, both positive religious coping from the RCOPE ($B=-0.24$, $p<0.01$) and scores on the Pakistani Religious Coping Practices Scale ($B=-0.15$, $p<0.05$) were inversely related to depressive symptoms.

Al-Sabwah and Abdel-Khalek (2006) analyzed data collected on 570 Egyptian women nursing undergraduates (mean age 20, largely Muslim), examining the relationship between religiosity and depressive symptoms. Self-rated religiosity was assessed using a single item with responses ranging from 0 to 10, and "death depression" was measured using a 21-item scale (Templer). Researchers found that religiosity was inversely related to death depression ($r=-0.12$, $p<0.01$, uncontrolled).

Chaaya and colleagues (2007) from the American University of Beirut surveyed a random sample of 750 persons age 60 or over living in three poor urban areas of Lebanon: Burj Barajneh Palestinian camp ($n=246$), Hay El Sellom ($n=118$), and Nabaa ($n=376$). Overall, the sample was 61 % Muslim and 39 % Christian. Three dimensions of religiosity were assessed: organizational (frequency of attendance at mosque), non-organizational (praying and fasting), and subjective religiosity (self-rated religiosity and extent to which religion influences life). Depression was assessed using the 15-item Geriatric Depression Scale. Religious affiliation and religiosity were unrelated to depression after controlling for age, gender, education, marital status, income physical disability, social support, and physical illness. However, in the Burj Barajineh Palestinian Camp (100 % Muslim), those who attended religious services regularly were nearly 60 % less likely to experience depression (OR=0.41, 95 % CI 0.18–0.97, $p<0.05$) compared to less regular attendees.

Vasegh and Mohammadi (2007) from the Tehran University of Medical Sciences surveyed 285 medical students (mean age 24, 97 % Muslim, 53 % male) to examine relationships between religiosity, anxiety, and depression. Religiosity was measured with a new 15-item questionnaire that assessed religious beliefs, religious emotions, and religious behaviors, each measured by 5 questions (total score range 0–71). The Persian version of the 21-item Beck Depression Inventory was used to capture depressive symptoms. Multiple regression determined predictors of depressive symptoms. No significant associations were found between depressive symptoms and either the total religiosity score or subscale scores. However, the religious beliefs subscale was inversely related to depressive symptoms at a trend level ($B=-0.14$, $p=0.06$), which reached statistical significance for anxiety symptoms ($B=-0.16$, $p<0.05$). Individual religious questions significantly and inversely related to depression were "doing five daily prayers" ($B=-0.78$, $p<0.05$) and "doing daily prayers on time" ($B=-0.54$, $p<0.05$).

Finally, Abdel-Khalek (2007) surveyed a random sample of 6,339 Muslim adolescents in Kuwait (mean age 15, 50 % male), examining relationships between religiosity happiness, health, and psychopathology. Self-rated religiosity was measured using a single item with a response range from 0 to 10. The 20-item CES-D was used to assess depressive symptoms. Religiosity was inversely related to depressive symptoms in boys ($r=-0.24$, $p<0.001$) and in girls ($r=-0.26$, $p<0.001$) (uncontrolled). Even after controlling for happiness, mental health, physical health, and anxiety, religiosity remained inversely correlated with depression in girls ($B=-0.11$, $p<0.001$).

Missed Studies. We are sure that our 2010 systematic review did not uncover all studies in Muslims on religiosity and depression published prior to 2010. However, given the space limitations here, we have not identified any further studies.

Recent Research. Since our 2010 review, several studies have examined religiosity and depression in Muslim-majority populations. The following are representative of such studies (again, given the large number, we have not exhaustively reviewed all the studies here, in contrast to other sections below).

Friedman and Saroglou (2010) examined relationships between religiosity, self-esteem, and depressive symptoms among immigrants to Belgium (273 Muslims, 155 mostly Christian non-Muslims, mean age 22). Religiosity was measured with an intrinsic religiosity scale (Gorsuch). Also assessed were acculturation, perceived cultural distance, perceived religious tolerance, feelings of anger, self-esteem (Rosenberg), and depressive symptoms (10-item version of CES-D). Intrinsic religiosity was significantly higher in Muslims compared to non-Muslims ($p<0.001$). In uncontrolled analyses, depression was significantly lower and self-esteem higher in Muslims compared to non-Muslims. While intrinsic religiosity overall was not related to depressive symptoms or self-esteem in either Muslims or non-Muslims, religiosity in Muslims was indirectly related to higher depressive symptoms and lower self-esteem, acting through perceived religious intolerance and anger toward host society.

Abdel-Khalek and Lester (2010) surveyed 192 Muslim college students from Kuwait and 158 largely Christian college students from New Jersey (mean age 21–22), examining relationships between religiosity and mental health (happiness, love of life, anxiety, depression). Religiosity was assessed using two questions (level of religiosity and strength of religious belief) both self-rated on a 0–10 scale. Happiness and love of life were higher, anxiety and depression were lower, and religiosity was lower among American college students compared to Kuwaiti students. Self-rated religiosity and strength of religious belief were significantly and positively related to happiness and love of life in both American and Kuwaiti students. The inverse relationships between religiosity/strength of belief and depression, however, while present in American students ($r=-0.23/-0.19$, both $p<0.01$), did not reach statistical significance in Kuwaiti students ($r=-0.11/-0.10$, both $p=$ns). The findings were the opposite, however for anxiety symptoms, where religiosity was more strongly related to lower anxiety in Kuwaiti students than in American students.

Abdel-Khalek and Eid (2011) analyzed data on 1,937 primary and high school Muslim students in Kuwait and 1,009 students in Palestine (ages 11–17), examining relationships between religiosity, well-being, and depression. Religiosity was assessed with a single-item measure of self-rated religiosity with responses ranging from 0 to 10. Well-being was assessed with two questions assessing happiness and life satisfaction (again, both rated 0–10). Depression was assessed using the 40-item Multidimensional Child and Adolescent Depression Scale (developed by Abdel-Khalek himself). Researchers found that religiosity was positively related to happiness and life satisfaction in both Kuwaiti and Palestinian students, and was also inversely related to depression ($r=-0.23$ in Kuwaiti males, $r=-0.18$ in females, $r=-0.22$ in Palestinian males, $r=-0.20$ in females, all $p<0.01$, uncontrolled).

In the only prospective study (to our knowledge) of religiosity and depression in a Muslim population, Hamdan and Tamim (2011) examined characteristics predicting postpartum depression in 137 pregnant women in Sharjah in the United Arab Emirates (92 % Muslim). Women were followed from their second trimester until 2 months postpartum. Administered at baseline (T1, second trimester) were the Beck Depression Inventory, Beck Anxiety Inventory, Stressful Life Events Inventory, and a measure of religiosity (a 3-item scale assessing self-reported religiosity, observation of the religious commandments, and degree of affiliation with religion). The depression and anxiety inventories were readministered during the third trimester (T2). At 2 months postpartum (T3), the Edinburgh Postnatal Depression Scale (EPDS) was completed and, for those scoring 10 or higher on the EPDS, the MINI neuropsychiatric depression module for major depression was administered. Results indicated that religiosity at T1 was unrelated to depression at T2 or T3. However, 14 of 137 women (10.2 %) experienced postpartum major depression, which was more common in non-Muslims (36.4 %, $n=4$) than in Muslims (7.9 %, $n=10$) ($p=0.015$, uncontrolled).

In the most recent studies, all conducted in students, Kuyel and colleagues (2012) from Istanbul University surveyed 341 Turkish undergraduate college students to determine the association between religiosity (Age Universal Intrinsic-Extrinsic Scale) (Gorsuch) and depression/anxiety (Brief Symptom Inventory) (Derogatis). Intrinsic religiosity was unrelated to either depression or anxiety in this sample, although extrinsic religiosity was related to both greater depression and anxiety ($B=+0.11$, $p<0.05$, uncontrolled). Similarly, Nuraskikin and colleagues (2012) surveyed 173 nursing students at the University Malaysia (95 % Muslim) to determine relationships between religiosity and depressive symptoms. The Malay version of the DUREL assessed religiosity, whereas depressive, anxiety, and stress symptoms were measured using the DASS21. Results indicated an inverse correlation between religiosity and DASS21 scores ($r=-0.16$, $p<0.01$, uncontrolled). Finally, Tavabi and Iran-Pour (2011) examined relationships between religious beliefs and mental health in 200 medical students at the Islamic Azad University in Tehran, Iran. Religious beliefs were assessed using a 26-item measure of religious beliefs, attitudes, behavior, and devotion. Level of depression and anxiety were assessed using the GHQ-28. Strong religious beliefs were associated with significantly lower scores on the GHQ-28 ($p<0.0001$, uncontrolled).

Summary. Based on our 2012 systematic review, we identified three clinical trials from Malaysia and ten cross-sectional studies, most in high school or college students. We also identified seven more recent studies, six of which were cross-sectional and one was prospective. Only one study examined the relationship between religiosity and depressive disorder diagnosed using a standard structured psychiatric interview. Overall, 15 of 20 studies (75 %) found that religious involvement was related to less depression, or that religious interventions (added to standard care) resulted in faster improvement of depression. In one study (5 %) religiosity was found to be related to greater depression, but only indirectly through perceived intolerance and anger toward host society among Muslim immigrants in Belgium (Table 7.1). These negative and positive relationships with depression are similar to those found in Christian populations (61 % and 6 %, respectively). Of three studies that compared Muslims and non-Muslims, two found less depression in Muslims.

Suicide

Suicide is often a consequence of untreated depression. Three studies from Turkey, two from Kuwait, and one study involving 17 Islamic countries have examined relationships between R/S and attitudes toward suicide, suicidal thoughts, suicidal attempts, or completed suicide.

Eskin (2004) surveyed two groups of adolescents in Turkey (99 % Muslim), 206 receiving religious education and 214 receiving secular education in Istanbul (average age 17). Attitudes toward suicide were examined. Participants were asked, "Have you ever thought of killing yourself by committing suicide?" Also administered was a 24-item suicide attitude questionnaire. Finally, adolescents were asked how they would respond to a fictitious close friend who decided to kill himself or herself. Results indicated that adolescents receiving secular education were more likely to have thoughts about killing themselves than those receiving a religious education (41.7 % vs. 24.0 %, $p<0.0005$). The secular education group was also more likely to view suicide as acceptable ($p<0.00001$), view suicide as a mental illness ($p<0.05$), and be open to reporting or discussing suicide factors ($p<0.00001$). The religious group was more likely to say that those who committed suicide would be punished after death ($p<0.00001$), were more likely to communicate suicidal problems ($p<0.00001$), and were more likely to hide suicidal behavior ($p<0.005$). No other variables were controlled in these analyses.

Several years later, Eskin and colleagues (2007) examined the effects of depression, self-esteem, social support, and socioeconomic factors on suicidal behavior in 805 first-year high school students (mean age 15) living in a small town in southwest Turkey. Religiosity was assessed with one question: "What is the depth of your religious faith?" with a response range from 1 to 7. Suicidal ideation, suicidal attempts, and potential for suicide were determined by asking a series of 40 questions. Also assessed were problem-solving abilities, social support, depression, and self-esteem using standard scales. Results indicated that 23 % had thought of killing

Table 7.1 Religiosity, depression, and suicide in Muslims

Authors (year)	Method	Sample size	Participants	Location	Controls	Findings
Depression						
Azhar and Varma (1995a)	RCT	64	Highly religious adults	Malaysia	–	P
Azhar and Varma (1995b)	RCT	30	Highly religious bereaved	Malaysia	–	P
Razali et al. (1998)	RCT	203	Highly religious adults	Malaysia	–	P
Ghorbani et al. (2000)	CS	178	University students	Iran	None	NA
Barber (2001)	CS	6,923	Adolescents	Palestine	MC	P (females)
Watson et al. (2002)	CS	227	University students	Iran	None	P
Mirzamani and Mohammadi (2003)	CS	120	University students, staff	Iran	None	P
Cardozo et al. (2004)	CS	799	Adults in community	Afghanistan	MC	P
Khan and Watson (2006)	CS	129	University students	Pakistan	SC	P
Al-Sabwah and Abdel-Khalek (2006)	CS	570	Nursing students	Egypt	None	P
Chaaya et al. (2007),	CS	750	Older adults	Lebanon	MC	P
Vasegh and Mohammadi (2007)	CS	785	Medical students	Iran	MC	P
Abdel-Khalek (2007)	CS	6,339	Adolescents	Kuwait	MC	P
Friedman and Saroglou (2010)	CS	273	Muslim Immigrants	Belgium	MC	NG
Abdel-Khalek and Lester (2010)	CS	192	University students	Kuwait	None	NA
Abdel-Khalek and Eid (2011)	CS	2,946	Adolescents	Kuwait/Pales	None	P
Hamdan and Tamim (2011)	P	137	Pregnant women	UAE	MC	NA
Kuyel et al. (2012)	CS	341	University students	Turkey	MC	NA
Nuraskikin et al. (2010)	CS	173	Nursing students	Malaysia	None	P
Tavabi and Iran-Pour (2011)	CS	200	Medical students	Iran	None	P

(continued)

Table 7.1 (continued)

Authors (year)	Method	Sample size	Participants	Location	Controls	Findings
Suicide						
Jahangir et al. (1998)	CS	118	Afghan refugees	Pakistan	None	P
Kamal and Loewenthal (2002)	CS	60	Muslim young adults	London, UK	None	NA
Eskin (2004)	CS	420	Adolescents	Turkey	None	P
Eskin et al. (2007)	CS	805	Adolescents	Turkey	None	NA
Gencoz et al. (2007)	CS	330	University students	Turkey	MC	P
Abdel-Khalek and Lester (2007)	CS	460	University students	Kuwait	None	P
Lester and Abdel-Khalek (2007)	CS	460	University students	Kuwait	None	P
Zuraida and Ahmad (2007)	CS	51	Major depression	Malaysia	None	P
Sisask et al. (2010)	CC	502 vs. 632	Suicide attempters vs. controls	Iran	None	P

CS cross-sectional, *P* prospective, *RCT* randomized clinical trial, *NA* no association, *P* significant positive association, *NG* significant negative association, *MC* multiple controls, *SC* some controls, *UAE* United Arab Emirates

themselves at some time in their lives (29 % of girls, 15 % of boys) and 11 % within the past 12 months (14 % girls, 6 % boys). With regard to suicide attempts, 2.4 % had done so at some time during their lives (3.0 % girls, 1.7 % boys) and 1.3 % had attempted within the past 12 months (1.8 % girls, 0.5 % boys). Depressive symptoms and low self-esteem were strongly related to suicidal ideation and suicide attempts. Religious belief (surprisingly) was not related to suicidal ideation or suicide attempts in either girls or boys.

Gencoz and colleagues (2007) administered a questionnaire examining religion and suicide attitudes to 330 undergraduate students at five universities in Turkey and 419 undergraduate students from two universities on the East Coast of the USA. The mean age of both samples was 21 years, although 51 % of participants were male in the Turkish sample and 25 % were male in the American sample. A standard 30-item suicide ideation scale was administered, along with a 14-item intrinsic–extrinsic religiosity scale (Gorsuch and McPherson) and a measure asking whether the respondent believed that life belongs to the individual, to the state, or to God (Ross and Kaplan). Also assessed were hopelessness, manic-depressive symptoms, perceptions of the causes of suicide, and social distance, all using standard scales. Results indicated that compared to American students, Turkish students experienced significantly higher hopelessness, suicidal ideation, and depression, lower intrinsic religiosity, greater stigma against those who attempted suicide, were less likely to attribute suicide to interpersonal causes and more likely to attribute it to societal causes. Controlling for other predictors, correlates of suicidality in Turkish students were younger age, greater hopelessness and depression, greater state or self-ownership of life, and lower intrinsic religiosity. Correlates in American students were similar (younger age, greater hopelessness and depression, lower intrinsic religiosity).

Abdel-Khalek and Lester (2007) examined religiosity and psychopathology (including suicidal ideation) in 460 Kuwaiti (all Muslim) and 274 American college students (primarily Catholic). Mean age (23) and gender (78 % female) were similar in the two groups. Single items were used to assess overall level of religiosity, estimation of mental health, and estimation of physical health, each on a 0–10 scale. Also administered were standard scales assessing optimism and pessimism, anxiety, obsessive-compulsive symptoms, ego grasping, death obsession, and suicidal ideation (30-item scale). Compared to American students, Kuwaiti students scored significantly higher on overall religiosity, pessimism, anxiety, obsessive-compulsive symptoms, death obsession, and ego grasping, but significantly lower on ratings of mental health and optimism, although there was no difference on suicidal ideation. In uncontrolled analyses, religiosity was inversely related to suicidal ideation in both Kuwaiti ($r = -0.15$, $p < 0.01$) and American students ($r = -0.23$, $p < 0.001$). In analyses that controlled for symptoms of psychopathology, a significant inverse relationship between religiosity and suicidal ideation was present only in American students.

Lester and Abdel-Khalek (2007) also published a separate paper on the correlation between a Taoist orientation (measured by the Ego Grasping Scale) and mental health in the same sample. Having a Taoist orientation to life (rather than an Ego Grasping) involves seeing the interrelated oneness of life and going beyond rational, self-centered thinking to a more intuitive view. In both Kuwaiti and American students, having a Taoist orientation was associated with less suicidal ideation (uncontrolled correlations).

Finally, Pritchard and Amanullah (2007) analyzed mortality data from the World Health Organization (based on death certificates) to compare suicide rates and other violent deaths (OVD) in the UK with those in 17 Islamic countries. They noted that "hidden" suicides often get placed in the OVD category to spare family undue distress, and hypothesized that this might be particularly true in Islamic countries where there is strong stigma against committing suicide. Mortality data were analyzed stratified by age and gender. Islamic countries were grouped by degree of religious practice, from least (former USSR republics of Azerbaijan, Kazakhstan, Kyrgyzstan, Tajikistan, Turkmenistan, Uzbekistan) to moderate (Eastern European countries of Albania, Bosnia, Turkey) to more religious (South Asian countries of Malaysia and Pakistan) to most religious (Middle Eastern countries of Bahrain, Egypt, Kuwait, Iran, Qatar, Syria). Researchers found that the highest suicide rates were in the least religious Islamic countries [e.g., Kazakhstan with 506 per million (pm) for men and 89 pm for women], and the lowest suicide rates were in the most religious countries (Qatar, Egypt, Iran, Pakistan, Syria, and Turkey, where the rate was less than 5 pm for men and women). For example, the suicide rate in Egypt was reported as 1 pm in men (36 suicides in men in a population of 33.8 million) and 0 pm in women, and the rate in Qatar was 0 pm for both men and women. In comparison, the UK suicide rate was 116 pm in men and 31 pm in women.

When examining OVD rates, the lowest rate for men was reported in Pakistan (0 pm) and the highest rate in Qatar (420 pm), whereas rates were intermediate in other Middle Eastern countries (132 pm) and Malaysia (166 pm). For comparison, the OVD rate in the UK was 50 pm for men and 21 pm for women. When comparing ratios of OVD rates to suicide rates (where high OVD/suicide ratios suggests under-reporting of suicide), ratios were highest in Middle Eastern countries (average 13.2) and in Malaysia (13.8), and were lowest in European (0.7) and former USSR Islamic countries (0.9). In comparison, the OVD/suicide ratio in the UK was 2.3 for men and 1.5 for women. Researchers concluded that in more religious Islamic countries, suicide rates may go under-reported and instead categorized as OVD, which has less stigma for the deceased person and family.

Missed Studies. We also identified several studies published prior to 2010 but missed by our systematic review. Levav and Aiesenberg (1989) examined completed suicides in Israel by Jews, Muslims Arabs, Christians, and Druze over a 10-year period from 1976 to 1985. Suicide rates per 100,000 among men were lowest in Muslim Arabs (3.6) compared to Christians (4.2), Jews (12.3) and Druze (12.5) ($p<0.001$). Similar results were reported for women, with Muslims and Druze having the lowest rates (2.8 and 1.9, respectively) compared to Christians (5.7) and Jews (6.4), although differences were not statistically significant. Religiosity was not examined.

In a study of 118 depressed Afghan refugees being seen at a psychiatric facility in Peshawar, Pakistan, Jahangir and colleagues (1998) had two clinical psychiatrists rate patients on a 4-point scale (absent to severe) regarding suicidal attempts, suicidal plans, and wishes for death. The same psychiatrists also rated patients for degree of religiosity on a similar 4-point scale. Results indicated that degree of religiosity was inversely related to all three indicators of suicide tendency with p values ranging from 0.005 to 0.0001 (uncontrolled). Although this study suffers from potentially serious bias, since both suicide and religiosity were rated by the same interviewers, the findings are still noteworthy.

Kamal and Loewenthal (2002) surveyed 40 Hindu and 60 Muslim young adults (mean age 23) in London, UK, examining relationships between religion, gender, reasons for living, and suicidal thoughts, plans, and attempts. Religiosity was measured using a 3-item measure that assessed frequency of prayer, religious study, and religious attendance. Religiosity was not related to any measure of suicide or reason for living, except moral (religious) reasons for living. Furthermore, there was no difference between Hindus and Muslims on suicidal thoughts, plans, or attempts.

Finally, Zuraida and Ahmad (2007) examined correlates of suicidal ideation in 51 patients with major depression or in the depressed phase of bipolar disorder. All participants were hospitalized in Kuala Lumpur, Malaysia. Suicidal ideation was measured using a standard scale. Religious salience was measured by asking patients to choose the three domains of life they considered most important: good income, harmonious family life, good health, meaningful pastimes, good marital life, a strong faith, or many friends. Religion was considered salient for those who selected "a strong faith" (19 patients). Suicidal ideation was significantly lower among those for whom religion was salient (4.4 vs. 9.9, $p<0.05$, uncontrolled).

Recent Research. After reviewing the literature on suicide rates in Middle Eastern countries, Rezaeian (2010) concluded that there was an increasing rate of suicide or attempted suicide among young women in this region of the world. Reasons given for this were greater availability of methods to commit suicide, increasing mental disorder with limited access to mental healthcare, marriage (a risk factor for committing suicide), and masculine role (young women forced into marriage). Exposure to Western culture through TV and the Internet might also cause younger women to feel that they are missing something due to cultural restrictions.

Since our review in 2010, one study has examined religiosity and suicide in Muslims, and several studies have compared suicide rates in Muslims and other religious denominations. Sisask and colleagues (2010) compared 2,819 suicide attempters with 5,484 community controls by religious denomination, self-rated religiosity, and frequency of religious attendance in seven countries (Brazil, Estonia, Iran, Sri Lanka, India, South Africa, Vietnam). Controlled for were age, gender, marital status, employment status, and education. In Iran (the only Muslim-majority country), those who attempted suicide were significantly less likely to attend religious services regularly or consider themselves religious (differences were significant at $p<0.005$). Only in Brazil (a highly religious Catholic country) were relationships between religiosity and suicide attempts as strong as in Iran.

Shah and Chandia (2010) analyzed data on general population suicide rates available from the World Health Organization from 1991 to 2002 for 27 countries, examining the relationship between suicide rate and percentage of adherents to Islam. The median rates of suicide for men and women across all countries was 19.8 (range 0–47.7) for men and 4.7 (0–17.9) for women per 100,000. When suicide rate was correlated with percentage of the population adherent to Islam, a significant inverse relationship emerged in both men ($r=-0.53$) and women ($r=-0.46$) ($p<0.05$ for both). Suicide rates per 100,000 in Bahrain (7.2 for male, 0.3 for women), Egypt (0.1 and 0.0), and Qatar (7.5 and 0.0) were far below the 19.8 in men and 4.7 in women across all countries examined.

Gal and colleagues (2012) compared suicide rates among Muslims and Jews in Israel based on national records from 2003 to 2007. Rate of completed suicide was lower in Muslims (3.0 per 100,000) compared to Jews (8.2 per 100,000). However, self-reported lifetime suicide attempts in Muslims were higher than in Jews (2.8 % vs. 1.2 %, respectively). Researchers concluded that Muslims in Israel have relatively low suicide rates, but not as low as reported by those living in Arab countries.

Summary. The majority of studies (7 of 9) find that religiosity in Muslims is related to negative attitudes toward suicide, fewer suicide attempts, and less completed suicide (Table 7.1). As with depression, these findings are similar to those in Christians (where 79 % of studies report inverse relationship between suicide and religiosity). Muslim-majority countries have some of the lowest suicide rates in the world, although there is some question of under-reporting given the strong religious and culture prohibitions against suicide. In seven studies that compared Muslims and non-Muslims, three found more negative attitudes, fewer attempts or lower suicide rates in Muslims and one found the opposite. There is concern about increasing rates of suicide in young female Muslims, and if that is confirmed, then more research is needed to better understand why this is occurring and how to prevent it.

Physician-Assisted Suicide. Although our 2010 systematic review failed to locate any studies on relationships between religiosity and physician-assisted suicide (PAS) or euthanasia in Muslim-majority countries, we have now identified several studies that examined attitudes of Muslim physicians and medical students in this regard. Curlin and colleagues (2009) assessed attitudes in 33 Muslim physicians in the USA, finding that 79 % objected to PAS, which was similar to Catholic (79 %), Protestant (75 %), and Hindu (74 %) physicians, but more than in Jewish physicians (50 %) or those with no affiliation (39 %). Ahmed and Kheir (2006) examined attitudes of 141 Muslim medical students in their final year at the University of Khartoum (Sudan), finding that 77 % objected to euthanasia and believed it should not be legalized. These findings are not surprising given a recent review by Van den Branden and Broeckaert (2011) of 32 English Sunni e-fatwas on active termination of life by physicians, all of which firmly oppose it. Attitudes, however, may be changing among younger physicians. For example, a 2010 study of 321 medical interns and residents in Tehran, Iran, found that only 18 % completely opposed euthanasia, whereas 33 % opposed it but not strongly and 49 % supported it (Zarghami et al. 2010).

Anxiety

Given the emphasis placed in Islam on the weighing of good and bad deeds as an important determinant of whether a Muslim goes to heaven or hell, one might expect that increasing religiosity would increase anxiety, especially anxiety related to death. In contrast, the opposite finding might be anticipated in Christians because of the belief that Jesus died for their sins and that faith in the death and resurrection of Jesus assures them of eternal salvation, regardless of what they have done—even if that includes some very bad deeds. Theoretical expectations, however, are not always confirmed in the real world.

Our 2010 systematic review uncovered 23 studies published up through 2010 that examined relationships between R/S and anxiety in Muslim-majority countries. These studies were conducted in Kuwait ($n=6$), Iran ($n=4$), Turkey ($n=3$), Malaysia ($n=3$), Pakistan ($n=3$), and India, Afghanistan, Egypt, and Algeria (one each).

The first such study was conducted in Muslims living in India in 1982. Beg and Zilli (1982) surveyed 100 English-speaking Muslim university students ages 20–30 and 100 older adults ages 40–60 from the Muslim university staff. Religiosity was assessed using the Religious Ideology Scale (Putney and Middleton), whereas anxiety was measured using the Death Anxiety Scale (Templer). Low and high religiosity groups based on religiosity score (below 22nd percentile and above 66th percentile) were created in the younger and the older samples, resulting in four groups with 20 persons each: high religious young, low religious young, high religious old, and low religious old. Results indicated that only age (not religiosity) was related to death anxiety, being higher in the younger group and lower among older participants. Although researchers indicated that death anxiety was higher in younger persons who were more religious, no statistic of association or significance level was provided. They concluded, "These results tend to set aside the view of Templer (1972) that death anxiety is considerably alleviated through deep involvement in religious" (p. 123).

Next, three clinical trials from researchers at the Universiti Sains Malaysia examined the effects of adding Islamic psychotherapy to standard treatment for anxiety disorder. In the first study, Azhar and colleagues (1994) randomly assigned 62 highly religious Muslims with DSM-III-R generalized anxiety disorder (GAD) to standard care (medication and weekly supportive psychotherapy for anxiety) ($n=31$) or standard care plus religious psychotherapy ($n=31$). Religious therapy involved "additional psychotherapy in the form of discussion of religious issues specific to the patients (such as the reading of verses of the Holy Koran and the encouragement of prayers)." Patients were rated by a psychiatrist blind to treatment group using the Hamilton Anxiety Rating Scale at the start of treatment and again at the end of the third and sixth month. Results indicated that there was no difference between groups at baseline, although by 3 months the religious intervention group did significantly better than the standard treatment group ($p<0.001$). This difference, however, disappeared by the sixth month when both groups had minimal anxiety symptoms. Researchers concluded that adding religious psychotherapy to the treatment regimen increased the speed of remission for GAD.

In the second study, reviewed previously under depression, Razali and colleagues (1998) randomly assigned 103 religious Muslim patients with generalized anxiety and 100 religious Muslims with depression to either a religious intervention group or a control group. Both groups received standard treatment (medications and psychotherapy), although the religious intervention group received additional religious–sociocultural psychotherapy. This religious psychotherapy included encouraging patients to be close to God, pray regularly, read the Qur'an, and change their lifestyle to conform to the life of the Prophet Muhammad. Subjects were followed for 6 months and patients with GAD were assessed blind to treatment group using the Hamilton Anxiety Rating Scale. Results indicated that patients receiving the additional religious psychotherapy improved significantly faster, although by 6 months there were again no differences between treatment groups.

In the third Malaysian study, Razali and colleagues (2002) randomized 85 religious and 80 nonreligious Muslims with GAD to either standard treatment or standard treatment plus additional religious–cultural psychotherapy (RCP). As in the 1998 study, the additional RCP involved encouraging closeness to God, prayer, reading the Qu'ran, and following the Prophet's lifestyle. Patients were assessed weekly for the first four weeks, every other week for the next 8 weeks, and then monthly using the Hamilton Anxiety Rating Scale by a psychiatrist blind to treatment group. Compared to religious patients assigned to standard treatment alone ($n=40$), religious patients assigned to the additional RCP group ($n=45$)

experienced a more rapid decrease in anxiety symptoms at 4 and 12 weeks (both $p<0.01$). By 26 weeks, however, symptoms were minimal in both groups and the difference between groups disappeared. In nonreligious Muslims (42 in the additional RCP group and 38 in the standard treatment group), there was no difference between groups at any point in time during the 6-month follow-up. This was an important study, since it showed no benefit for additional religious psychotherapy in nonreligious Muslims.

The remaining 19 studies were all cross-sectional. As described earlier, Ghorbani and colleagues (2000) surveyed 178 Iranian college students examining the relationship between religiosity and emotional symptoms, including anxiety. Religiosity was measured using the MARS, and anxiety symptoms by the Hopkins Symptom Checklist. Neither the total MARS score nor any of its subscales were related to anxiety symptoms.

Next, Suhail (2001) reported no relationship between religiosity and death anxiety in 132 adults in Lahore, Pakistan. Higher death anxiety was reported in this sample compared to other population groups, causing the researcher to conclude that among Muslims without strong religious beliefs, religion may induce greater death anxiety through the concept of punishment in the afterlife (few details are available on this report). In the second report on this sample published 1 year later (with more details), Suhail and Akram (2002) surveyed 132 adults in Lahore, equally divided between men and women, young (ages 16–30) and older people (age 55 or over). Religiosity was measured using the 18-item Scale of Religious Index (SRI) that assessed Islamic beliefs and practices. Participants were divided into high and low religious groups at the median score on the SRI. Anxiety was assessed using the 15-item Death Anxiety Scale (Templer) and the Fear of Death Scale (Lester). Results indicated that those in the high religious group experienced lower levels of anxiety on both anxiety scales, but this reached statistical significance only on the Fear of Death Scale (20.2 vs. 24.4, $p<0.05$, no controls).

Tek and Ulug (2001) surveyed 45 psychiatric outpatients with obsessive-compulsive disorder (OCD) from Ankara, Turkey, examining the relationship with religiosity. OCD symptoms were assessed using several standard measures, and religiosity was measured using the Muslim Religious Practices Index, a scale developed specifically for this study. Over one-third of patients (42 %) had religious obsessions as part of their psychopathology. These patients were compared to patients without religious obsessions on level of religiosity. Results indicated that there was no difference on religiosity between patients with and without religious obsessions (uncontrolled). Thus, Muslims with OCD and religious obsessions appeared to be no more religious than Muslims with OCD but no religious obsessions.

Several studies described earlier also explored religiosity and anxiety in Muslims. Watson and colleagues (2002) examined the correlation between anxiety and intrinsic religiosity in 231 Iranian college students and 220 American college students. Intrinsic religiosity was not related to anxiety in either group. However, higher scores on scales measuring extrinsic religiosity (use of religion to achieve goals more important than religion) were related to significantly higher anxiety in both groups. In another study described earlier, Mirzamani and Mohammadi (2003) surveyed 70 psychiatric outpatients in Tehran, comparing them to a control group of 50 university staff and students of similar age. Religious values (Allport Values Scale) were inversely correlated with anxiety symptoms (SCL-90-R) in the combined sample ($r = -0.26$, $p < 0.01$, uncontrolled). Cardoza and colleagues (2004) also found that anxiety symptoms were significantly lower in non-disabled community-dwelling Afghan Muslims who were more religious compared to others (58.5 vs. 80.0, $p = 0.01$, controlled for sex, age, marital status, ethnicity, education, availability of food, and employment).

In the year 2006, several studies examining religiosity and anxiety were conducted in college or high school students. As reviewed earlier, Khan and Watson (2006) found that religious interest (measured using a single item with responses ranging from 0 to 9) was inversely correlated with anxiety symptoms (assessed by Brief Symptom Inventory) in 129 Pakistani university students ($r = -0.21$, $p < 0.05$, uncontrolled). Negative religious coping, in contrast, was positively related to anxiety ($r = +0.32$, $p < 0.01$) in that study. Likewise, Al-Sabwah and Abdel-Khalek (2006) found an inverse correlation between religiosity (single item) and death anxiety (Templer) in 570 Egyptian female nursing undergraduates ($r = -0.14$, $p < 0.01$). Similarly, in a survey of 941 Kuwaiti high school students, Baroun (2006) found that all three measures of religiosity (10-item Hoge Intrinsic Religiosity Scale, and two items assessing strength of religious belief and self-rated level of religiosity on a 0–10 scale) were inversely related to anxiety (20-item Kuwait University Anxiety Scale) ($r = -0.24$, $r = -0.24$, and $r = -0.21$, respectively, all $p < 0.001$, uncontrolled).

A number of additional studies led by Abdel-Khalek from Kuwait University have examined relationships between religion and anxiety, again primarily among high school or college students. First, Abdel-Khalek (2002) analyzed data on 2,453 adolescents attending high schools in Kuwait (mean age 16; half female). Religiosity was assessed with a single item (0–10 scale), and anxiety was measured using the Kuwait University Anxiety Scale. Uncontrolled correlations between religiosity and anxiety were $r = -0.22$ ($p < 0.01$) in both boys and girls analyzed separately. In a second study, Abdel-Khalek (2007) surveyed a random sample of 6,339 high school students from Kuwait, examining the relationship between religiosity (single item, 0–10) and anxiety (Kuwait Scale). Religiosity was again associated with lower anxiety in both boys ($r = -0.22$, $p < 0.001$) and girls ($r = -0.25$, $p < 0.001$). After controlling for happiness, mental health, physical health, and depression in a regression model, the inverse relationship between religiosity and anxiety persisted only in boys ($B = -0.10$, $p < 0.001$). In a third study, Lester and Abdel-Khalek (2007) found that a "Taoist orientation" was related to lower death anxiety in 460 Kuwaiti college students (uncontrolled correlations ranging from −0.19 to −0.32, $p < 0.01$) and in 274 American college students (correlations ranging from −0.13 to −0.25, $p < 0.05$). In a fourth study, Abdel-Khalek and Naceur (2007) surveyed 244 Muslim college students in Algeria (55 % female) using a similar methodology as in previous studies. They found that religiosity (single item, 0–10 scale) was inversely related to anxiety (Kuwait Scale) in men ($r = -0.43$, $p < 0.001$, uncontrolled), but not in women ($r = -0.17$, $p = \text{ns}$).

At least two studies by Abdel-Khalek's research group, however, have not found a relationship between religiosity and anxiety. Abdel-Khalek and Maltby (2008) analyzed data from 271 college students in Kuwait and 205 students in the UK that included measures of religiosity (single item, 0–10 scale) and anxiety (Kuwait Scale). Religiosity was not related to anxiety in either group, although anxiety was higher in Kuwaiti than in the UK students. Similarly, Abdel-Khalek (2009) surveyed 152 Kuwaiti Muslim college students (80 % women), administering two death anxiety scales (Templer, Lester) and three religiosity scales (Hoge Intrinsic Religiosity Scale, and two single items assessing self-rated religiosity and strength of religious belief). No significant correlations between religiosity scales and death anxiety scales were found.

In a previously described study, Vasegh and Mohammadi (2007) examined relationships between religiosity (15-item Religious Questionnaire) and anxiety (Beck Anxiety Inventory) in 285 Iranian medical students. In uncontrolled analyses, significant inverse associations were found between anxiety symptoms and both a religious beliefs subscale ($r = -0.17$, $p < 0.01$) and the total Religious Questionnaire score ($r = -0.15$, $p < 0.05$). When multiple regression was used to examine religious predictors of anxiety symptoms, higher scores on the religious beliefs subscale continued to predict lower anxiety symptoms ($B = -0.16$, $p < 0.05$). Individual items on the Religious Questionnaire related to lower anxiety were religious commitment (extent to which individual believed that religious commands should be completely or absolutely obeyed) ($B = -0.63$, $p < 0.01$), frequency of "daily asking" from God ($B = -0.60$, $p < 0.05$), and frequency of saying monthly special prayers ($B = -0.37$, $p < 0.05$). Analyses were controlled for family disease, history of family depression, and substance use.

Two studies have focused on religiosity and anxiety in Muslims from Turkey. Tuncay and colleagues (2008) surveyed 151 adults with diabetes (mean age 49), examining relationships between coping behaviors and anxiety. Among coping behaviors assessed was religious coping based on a 2-item scale derived from the Brief COPE (Carver). "Acceptance" and religion were the two most common coping behaviors used by participants in this sample. Anxiety was measured using the State-Trait Anxiety Scale (Spielberger). Religious coping was inversely related to trait anxiety ($r = -0.39$, $p < 0.01$, uncontrolled). Among coping behaviors, psychological, medical, and sociodemographic characteristics, no other factor (except overall emotional status) was as strongly and inversely correlated with anxiety as religious coping.

The second study from Turkey, by Yorulmaz and colleagues (2009), examined religiosity and OCD symptoms in 115 Muslim college students from the Middle East Technical University in Ankara and in 104 Christian college students from the University of British Columbia. OCD symptoms were assessed using the 44-item Obsessive-Compulsive Beliefs Questionnaire and four other OCD symptom scales (all of these OCD scales are likely contaminated by items assessing conservative religious values). Religiousness was assessed using a 7-item scale that measured religious involvement, impact of religious principles, and religious activities. Religiosity was similar in Muslims and Christians, although OCD symptoms were higher in Muslims (42.5 vs. 24.3, $p < 0.001$). Students were then dichotomized into high and low religiosity groups. Although total OCD symptom score was the same in high vs. low religious groups (Muslims and Christians combined, $F=1.86, p=\text{ns}$), individual symptoms did vary. Highly religious participants were more likely to emphasize the importance of controlling thoughts, endorse thought-action fusion items in the mortality dimension (TAF-mortality), and endorse obsessional thoughts of harm and checking. When examined by religious denomination, religiosity in Christians was correlated with TAF-mortality and belief in controlling thoughts. In Muslims, religiosity was correlated only with TAF-mortality. Researchers concluded that these results supported the association between religiosity and OCD in Christians and Muslims. Given the likely contamination of OCD measures with conservative religious beliefs and values, we would disagree with them.

Finally, one additional report discusssed differences in anxiety in Spain (a Christian country) compared to anxiety in Muslim Arab countries. We did not include this in our systematic review because the study did not directly compare Muslims and Christians. Tomas-Sabado and Gomez-Benito (2004) summarized the results from several studies showing higher death anxiety among college students in Arab countries compared to death anxiety among students in Spain. The first report by Abdel-Khalek (2003) compared scores on the Templer Death Anxiety Scale among 187 college students (79 % female) in Spain with those obtained from 270 students in Egypt (50 % female), 270 students in Kuwait (54 % female), 220 students in Qatar (50 % female), 344 students in Lebanon (51 % female), and 709 students in Syria (50 % female). Death anxiety scores were lowest among students in Spain. Similar findings were reported by these researchers when comparing nursing undergraduates in Egypt and Spain across five different anxiety scale, both Arabic and English versions (Abdel-Khalek and Tomas-Sabado 2005). Tomas-Sabado and Gomez-Benito concluded that lower anxiety in Spanish samples was due to the secularization of the country and adoption of Western values that attempt to hide and ignore death.

Missed Studies. We are sure that our 2010 systematic review did not uncover all studies in Muslims on religiosity and anxiety published prior to 2010. However, given the space limitations here, we did not identify any further studies.

Recent Research. Since our 2010 review, several studies have examined religiosity and anxiety in Islamic countries.

Azaiza and colleagues (2010) studied risk factors for increased death anxiety among 145 Muslim Arabs age 60 or older (average age 74) living in northern Israel. This is one of the few studies in mature adults that has examined the religion–anxiety relationship in Muslims. Religiosity was assessed by a single item with responses ranging from 1 (secular) to 4 (very religious). Self-esteem (Rosenberg), social support (Carmel), and anxiety (12-item Death and Dying Anxiety scale) were also assessed. Religiosity was unrelated to anxiety among elders living in nursing homes ($n=65$), those living the community ($n=80$), or in the combined sample. However, among community-dwelling older Muslims, greater religiosity was related to lower self-esteem ($r=-0.22, p<0.05$).

Abdel-Khalek (2011) surveyed 499 Muslim Kuwaiti adolescents (mean age 17) examining relationships between religiosity, well-being, self-esteem, and anxiety. Methods were similar to those used in earlier studies (self-rated religiosity and strength of religious belief were assessed on a 0–10 scale, and anxiety measured using the Kuwait Scale). Religiosity and strength of religious belief were inversely related to anxiety ($r=-0.22$ and $r=-0.20$, both $p<0.01$, uncontrolled). Similar relationships, although stronger and positive in direction, were found with self-esteem, life satisfaction, and happiness (with r's ranging from +0.41 to +0.50).

Khamis (2012) examined relationships between religiosity, anxiety, and war trauma in 600 Muslim adolescents ages 12–16 living in the Gaza Strip (Palestine) and southern Lebanon (300 adolescents from each region). Religiosity was assessed using at 17-item Muslim religious beliefs and practices scale. Post-traumatic stress disorder (PTSD) was diagnosed using a structured psychiatric interview based on DSM-IV criteria. Anxiety symptoms were measured using the Revised Children's Manifest Anxiety Scale. Analyses were controlled for type of trauma, family member killed/injured, house demolished, economic pressure, and *ideological commitment* (including commitment to religion as faith and practice). In the combined sample, religiosity was inversely related to anxiety ($r=-0.24$, $p<0.001$, uncontrolled), but was unrelated to PTSD diagnosis. In separate regression models developed in Palestinians and Lebanese adolescents, religiosity was negatively related to anxiety in Lebanese ($B=-0.19$, $p<0.01$), but positively related to anxiety in Palestinians ($B=+0.20$, $p<0.0001$). Note, however, that ideology was strongly and inversely related to anxiety ($B=-0.47$, $p<0.0001$) in Palestinians, and only when ideological commitment was controlled for did the positive relationship with anxiety emerge.

In more recent research, Yuniarti and colleagues (2013) examined religiosity and psychosocial factors in 78 type II diabetics ages 40–70 in Indonesia (94 % Muslim). Religiosity was measured using a multidimensional scale that assessed faith, worship, charity, deeds, and "science." Anxiety was assessed by a scale that was not described, except that scores were based on anxiety manifested in both the physical and psychological realm. Religiosity was inversely related to anxiety ($r=-0.59$, $p<0.05$) and positively associated with self-acceptance ($r=+0.51$, $p<0.01$) (no controls).

In the latest randomized clinical trial testing the effects of a religious intervention on anxiety, Hosseini and colleagues (2013) randomized 66 patients undergoing coronary artery bypass grafting in Iran to receive either a preoperative Shia Muslim spiritual/religious (S/R) training intervention or to standard preoperative care. The S/R intervention was administered in a group format (5–7 participants) for 45–60 min on each of five consecutive days before surgery. The S/R intervention focused on the Qur'an and Hadith, and on trusting and relying on Allah. Anxiety was assessed at baseline (1 week prior to surgery) and 2 h prior to surgery using the 14-item Hamilton Anxiety Scale (HAS). [Although the HAS is a clinician-rated scale, researchers did not specify whether it was clinician-rated or self-rated in this study, and if clinician-rated, whether the clinician was blind to treatment group.] Standard care in the control group involved routine preoperative nursing care (but, some control patients received spiritual care prior to surgery, as required by the ethics committee). There were no differences in anxiety between groups at baseline. However, anxiety levels dropped in patients receiving the S/R intervention (from 31.9 to 19.5, $p < 0.001$) and increased in the control group (from 31.0 to 43.3, $p < 0.001$). Only pre-post comparisons were done, rather than a more standard group by time analysis.

Ellis and colleagues (2013) examined fear of death among 2,125 college students in Malaysia (62 % Muslim), 265 in Turkey (100 % Muslim), and 1,291 in the USA (2 % Muslim). Seven items were used to measure religiosity, each on a 0–10 scale of agreement (belief in God, belief in immortality, importance of religion, religious fundamentalism, obey religious teachings, active in religious observances, parental religious strictness). Fear of death was measured using a single item rated from 0 (none at all) to 10 (extreme degree). Results (uncontrolled) indicated that fear of death was positively related to all seven religious items in Malaysia (r's ranging from 0.22 to 0.25, $p < 0.001$), in five of the seven religious items in Turkey (r's ranging from 0.01 to 0.31), and all seven religiosity items in the USA (r's ranging from 0.08 to 0.14, most $p < 0.001$). Furthermore, Muslim students experienced significantly greater fear than students from other religious groups. Researchers concluded that these results were consistent with a new "death apprehension theory," which predicted that religiosity would be positively correlated with fear of death.

Finally, we describe here a single case report that illustrates the interaction between religion and anxiety. Bragazzi and Del Puente (2012) presented the case of a 19-year-old Muslim girl from Tunisia who was seen by a psychiatrist for anxiety and panic attacks because she believed that she was possessed by jinn. She reported seeing jinn on several occasions, when she would immediately begin reading the Qur'an and praying to keep the jinn from entering her brain. In explaining her condition, she said "Maybe all this happens because Allah is punishing me for not being a real Muslimah." The psychiatrist treated her with fluoxetine (Prozac) and the assistance of an ulama (a Muslim scholar well informed on Islam), who helped with religious restructuring and reframing of her beliefs. After 4 weeks of treatment her anxiety symptoms and panic attacks decreased, and after 1 year of follow-up, her panic attacks had not returned. Note, however, that belief in jinn, black magic, and the evil eye are widespread among Muslims without psychiatric disorder, especially among women and those with less education.

Summary. In conclusion, a clear majority (68 %) of the research (19 out of 28 studies) finds lower anxiety among Muslims who are more religious and significant benefits from religious interventions (Table 7.2). Many of these studies (57 %) were in grade school, high school, or college students, although a significant proportion have been in adults, especially more recent studies. Most of these reports (71 %) presented uncontrolled correlations that did not take into account other factors that could confound the relationship between religiosity and anxiety. However, all randomized clinical trials to date that have tested R/S interventions in Muslim patients (four, including the latest study in cardiac surgery patients) reported a decrease in anxiety among those receiving the Islamic intervention.

Table 7.2 Religiosity and anxiety in Muslims

Authors (year)	Method	Sample size	Participants	Location	Controls	Findings
Beg and Zilli (1982)	CS	200	50% adults ages 40–60	India	None	NA
Azhar et al. (1994)	RCT	62	Highly religious adults	Malaysia	–	P
Razali et al. (1998)	RCT	103	Religious adults	Malaysia	–	P
Razali et al. (2002)	RCT	165	52% religious adults (RA)	Malaysia	–	P (RA only)
Ghorbani et al. (2000)	CS	178	University students	Iran	None	NA
Suhail (2001)	CS	132	Adults in community	Pakistan	None (?)	NA
Suhail and Akram (2002)	CS	132	50% older adults	Pakistan	None	P
Watson et al. (2002)	CS	221	University students	Iran	None	NA
Mirzamani et al. (2003)	CS	120	Psychiatric patients, staff	Iran	None	P
Cardozo et al. (2004)	CS	799	Adults in community	Afghanistan	MC	P (ND)
Khan and Watson (2006)	CS	129	University students	Pakistan	None	P
Al-Sabwah and Abdel-Khalek (2006)	CS	570	University students	Egypt	None	P
Baroun (2006)	CS	941	Adolescents	Kuwait	None	P
Abdel-Khalek (2002)	CS	2,453	Adolescents	Kuwait	None	P
Abdel-Khalek (2007)	CS	6,339	Adolescents	Kuwait	MC	P (M only)
Lester and Abdel-Khalek (2007)	CS	460	University students	Kuwait	None	P
Abdel-Khalek and Maltby (2008)	CS	244	University students	Algeria	None	P (M only)
Abdel-Khalek and Maltby (2008)	CS	271	University students	Kuwait	None	NA
Abdel-Khalek (2009)	CS	152	University students	Kuwait	None	NA
Vasegh et al. (2007)	CS	285	Medical students	Iran	MC	P
Tuncay et al. (2008)	CS	151	Diabetics	Turkey	None	P
Yorulmaz et al. (2009)	CS	115	University students	Turkey	None	NG
Azaiza et al. (2010)	CS	145	Older adults	N. Israel	None	NA

(continued)

Table 7.2 (continued)

Authors (year)	Method	Sample size	Participants	Location	Controls	Findings
Abdel-Khalek (2011)	CS	499	Adolescents	Kuwait	None	P
Khamis (2012)	CS	600	Adolescents	Palest/Leban	MC	P (Lebanon)
Yuniarti et al. (2013)	CS	78	Diabetics	Indonesia	None	P
Hosseini et al. (2013)	RCT	66	Cardiac surgery patients	Iran	–	P
Ellis et al. (2013)	CS	1,762	University students	Malay, Turk	None	NG

CS cross-sectional, *RCT* randomized clinical trial, *F* female, *M* male, *NA* no association, *P* significant inverse or negative association, *NG* significant positive association, *MC* multiple controls, *SC* some controls, *ND* non-disabled

Five studies, however, suggested that anxiety levels are higher in Muslim compared to Christian populations. To confirm this, we decided to review this area again, specifically focused on identifying Muslim–Christian differences in anxiety. Two additional studies were uncovered. One found no difference in anxiety between community-dwelling adult Christians and Muslims in Ethiopia (Awas et al. 1999), and the other study (one that compared Muslim college students in Turkey and Christian college students in Canada) found higher anxiety in Turkish students (Inozu et al. 2012).

Six out of seven studies, then, have found higher anxiety in Muslims. Muslims, however, tend to be more religious than Christians, and greater religiosity is consistently related to less anxiety in Muslims (68 % of studies), even more so than in Christians (49 % of studies). Thus, Muslims who are not very religious may be at particular high risk for anxiety (given the importance placed on strong faith and good deeds in Islam). Risk of anxiety may be lower in less religious Christians, who take their religion less seriously due to Western secularization, or in highly religious Christians due to beliefs that salvation is guaranteed regardless of works.

Psychosis

Our systematic review uncovered only two published reports in Muslim populations on R/S and psychotic symptoms. One study examined the role of religion in coping with psychotic symptoms (Wahass and Kent 1997) and the other assessed the effect of spiritual healing on relapses in patients with schizophrenia (Salib and Youakim 2001).

Wahass and Kent (1997) were the first to examine how Muslim patients cope with psychotic symptoms. They recruited male and female outpatients and inpatients with schizophrenia from the UK ($n=33$) and Saudi Arabia ($n=37$), examining factors that enabled patients to deal with hallucinations (especially hearing voices).

All participants were prescribed antipsychotic medication, were between the ages 20 and 65, and were diagnosed with schizophrenia (ICD-10) for at least 4 years. There was no significant difference between the UK and Saudi patients in terms of age, gender, age at onset, marital status, or whether they were inpatients or outpatients. Qualitative analyses demonstrated that coping methods could be categorized into six types. Coping types were (1) religious activities (behavior related to relationship with God, prayer, reading Bible or Koran, listening to religious cassettes, etc.), (2) distraction (watching TV or listening to music on radio), (3) individualistic (sleeping, reading, working), (4) cessation techniques (thought stopping, crying, screaming), (5) social changes (talking to others or social withdrawal), and (6) physiological methods (engaging in sports, taking medication, using alcohol). Nearly one-half (43 %) of Saudi patients coped using religious activities, compared to only 3 % of the UK patients ($p < 0.01$). With regard to how they coped with specific symptoms, Saudis were more likely than the UK patients to use religion to stop voices (57 % vs. 3 %, respectively), lessen distress (51 % vs. 0 %), ignore voices (43 % vs. 0 %), reduce the loudness of voices (35 % vs. 0 %), and disbelieve in the voices (41 % vs. 0 %).

Salib and Youakim (2001) from Hollins Park Hospital (UK) examined spiritual healing practices and occurrence of psychotic relapse in 40 elderly patients with schizophrenia hospitalized in Cairo, Egypt. This case–control study compared 20 schizophrenic patients over age 60 who had received spiritual healing prior to the study and planned to receive it afterwards (cases) with 20 schizophrenic patients who had not received nor planned to receive spiritual healing (controls), matching them by age, sex, and duration of illness. Relapses (readmission to hospital) were determined over the next 18 months and compared in cases and controls. "Spiritual healing" was defined as "excessive use of prayers; reading verses of the Koran or the Bible as a form of counseling based on religious relevance (at least an hour a day); excessive attendance at Mosques or Churches for solitary or group meditation (more than five times a week); attending sessions that included the use of witchcraft or related methods (ever) and attending rituals including exorcism and Zar processions (ever)" (p. 367). After controlling for other predictors of relapse, cases were three and one-half times more likely to relapse compared to controls (adjusted $OR = 3.5$, $p < 0.05$). Those most likely to relapse used Zar or exorcism (five cases), and these individuals were four times more likely to relapse compared to those who relied on excessive prayers.

Missed Studies. We also identified several additional studies not included in our 2010 systematic review. The first study ever to examine the nature of psychotic symptoms in a Muslim country was conducted by Ahmad and Naeen (1984), who compared first rank symptoms (FRS) of schizophrenia among Muslim psychiatric patients in Pakistan with those of Muslim patients in Saudi Arabia and non-Muslim patients in the UK. Although the incidence of FRS in Pakistani and Saudi patients were similar (and different in religious content from those in the UK), individual symptoms varied, making researchers conclude that cultural factors were more important than religion in determining the type of psychotic symptoms patients experienced. Azhar and colleagues (1995) surveyed 270 patients with schizophrenia in Malaysia, finding a high prevalence of religious and culture-related delusions in these patients, concluding that both religious and cultural factors influenced the presentation of psychotic symptoms.

Atallah and colleagues (2001) conducted a 22-year retrospective analysis of the medical records of 5,275 psychotic inpatients seen at Behman psychiatric hospital in Cairo, Egypt, from 1975 to 1996. Among those patients, 632 (12 %) had "religious symptoms" (delusions, hallucinations, preoccupations) documented in their medical records (70 % Muslim, 30 % Christian). The most common religious symptoms involved God (36 %) followed by those related to the devil (14 %), sheikhs or priests (12 %), Jesus (11 %), the Prophet Muhammad (9 %), and "ghosts or afreet" (9 %). The most frequent religious behaviors were talking/preaching (21 %), praying (20 %), and increased religiosity in general (19 %). Delusional themes most commonly documented were having special knowledge or power from God (19 %), being cursed by black magic (15 %), and being controlled by an evil spirit (13 %). Religious hallucinations were auditory in 21 % of those with religious symptoms and visual in 17 %. Patients with religious psychotic symptoms were compared to 281 psychiatric inpatients without them. Average age of those with religious symptoms was slightly younger (32.5 vs. 34.3, $p<0.05$), affiliation was more likely Christian than Muslim (30.1 % vs. 23.8 %, respectively, $p<0.05$), and nationality was more likely to be Egyptian (86.1 % vs. 79.4 %, $p<0.05$), although differences between groups were small.

Farooqi (2006) interviewed 87 Muslim psychiatric patients treated at public hospitals in Lahore, Pakistan, examining traditional healing practices that patients sought for psychiatric illness and discussing the role that Islam played in Pakistani patients' perceptions of health and healing. The typical practice of faith healers in Pakistan is to recite verses from the Qur'an that are related to the patient's symptoms and then breathe into a piece of cloth or paper or container of water or onto a piece of food or amulet that is then considered blessed. The patient keeps this blessed article, is promised healing, is given a schedule of daily chores and prayers, and is advised to never give up hope in Allah. This process may be repeated more than once for those with severe illness. The majority of patients in this study had diagnoses of affective disorders or schizophrenia. Islamic faith healing practices were most commonly sought by those with schizophrenia (18 %), somatoform disorders (18 %), and affective disorders (9 %). The effect of Islamic faith healing practices on severity of psychotic symptoms or frequency of relapse, however, was not examined. There is some evidence that Muslim psychiatric patients are more likely to see a religious healer than either Christians or Hindus in South Asia.

Finally, Johnstone and Tiliopoulos (2008) examined 114 adult Muslims from 18 countries to determine the relationship between schizotypal personality traits and religious attitudes. Participants were administered the Brief Schizotypal Personality Questionnaire. Religiosity was assessed with by the Sahin-Francis Scale of Attitude Toward Islam, frequency of prayer, and mosque attendance. All three measures of religiosity were weakly but negatively related to schizotypal traits (details are limited since only abstract of study was available).

Recent Research. Several relevant studies on this topic have been published since our 2010 review. Suhail and Ghauri (2010) surveyed 53 Muslim patients with schizophrenia from three psychiatric units in Lahore, Pakistan. A standard psychiatric interview (Present State Examination) and a 27-item religiosity scale (15 items that assessed belief and 12 items that assessed practices) were administered. Among patients with delusions, grandiose (76 %) and religious (62 %) delusions were the most common types. Participants were dichotomized into less religious and more religious groups based on their median score on the religiosity scale. Religious patients were more likely than less religious patients to have delusions of grandiose ability (89 % vs. 60 %), grandiose identity (64 % vs. 36 %), and of a religious nature (75 % vs. 48 %), but were less likely to have delusions of reference or delusion of alien forces penetrating or controlling mind/body. With regard to delusion interpretations, religious patients were more likely than the less religious to have explanations that involved spirits, jinn, or ghosts (78.6 % vs. 48 %). Types of hallucination also varied by degree of religiosity, with verbal hallucinations (voices from supernatural agents), dissociative hallucinations, and visual hallucinations (of paranormal agents) more common in those who were more religious. Authors concluded that patients who were more religious had significantly greater number of delusions and hallucinations, but that religion was also often used to cope with psychotic symptoms.

Ndetei and researchers (2012) from University of Nairobi administered the WHO Composite International Diagnostic Interview to 2,963 college students (mean age 21) attending seven institutions across Kenya. Religious affiliation of respondents was Protestant ($n=1{,}779$), Catholic ($n=851$), Muslim ($n=131$), or other ($n=202$). Muslims were 38 % less likely than Protestants to have psychotic experiences and 22 % less likely to have visual hallucinations, although these differences did not reach statistical significance.

Amr and associates (2013) from Mansoura University examined spirituality and medication adherence in 92 psychiatric outpatients with schizophrenia at the Mansoura University Hospital in Egypt. R/S was assessed using the 16-item Daily Spiritual Experiences Scale (DSES). Medication adherence was measured using the Morisky Medication Adherence Scale, and based on that score, participants were categorized into adherent ($n=24$) and non-adherent ($n=68$) groups. Adherent patients scored significantly higher than non-adherent patients on the DSES (40.8 vs. 37.3, $p<0.05$). Thus, no evidence was found that R/S interfered with psychiatric treatment, and in fact, may have actually improved compliance with psychiatric medication.

Summary. Only four studies have examined the relationship between religiosity and psychotic symptoms in Muslims, two reporting positive and two reporting negative associations (Table 7.3). There is a relatively high prevalence of religious delusions among Muslim patients with schizophrenia. Although religious delusions appear to be more frequent among Muslim patients who are more religious, these patients report that religious beliefs and practices are used to cope with distressing psychotic symptoms (thus, the claim that religiosity worsens delusions cannot be made).

Table 7.3 Religiosity and psychosis, alcohol and drug use in Muslims

Authors (year)	Method	Sample size	Participants	Location	Controls	Findings
Psychosis						
Salib and Youakim (2001)	CC	20 vs. 20	Psychiatric patients>60	Egypt	–	NG
Johnstone and Tiliopoulos (2008)	CS	114	Adults	18 countries	(?)	P
Suhail and Ghauri (2010)	CS	53	Psychiatric inpatients	Pakistan	None	NG
Amr et al. (2013)	CS	92	Psychiatric patients	Egypt	None	P
Alcohol use/abuse						
Uddin (2007–2008)	CS	391	Adults	Bangladesh	(?)	P
Diamond et al. (2008)	CS	1,261	Bedouin adults	Israel	None	P
Ozbay (2008)	CS	974	University students	Turkey	MC	P
Ghandour et al. (2009)	CS	689	University students	Lebanon	SC	P
Burazeri and Kark (2010)	CS	473	Adults	Albania	SC	P
Badr et al. (2013)	CS	52	Adolescents	Lebanon	None	P
Drug use/abuse						
Uddin (2007–2008)	CS	391	Adults	Bangladesh	(?)	P
Diamond et al. (2008)	CS	1,261	Bedouin adults	Israel	None	P
Ozbay (2008)	CS	974	University students	Turkey	MC	P
Ghandour et al. (2009)	CS	689	University students	Lebanon	SC	P
Burazeri and Kark (2010)	CS	473	Adults	Albania	SC	P
Badr et al. (2013)	CS	52	Adolescents	Lebanon	None	P

CC case control, *CS* cross-sectional, *NA* no association, *P* significant positive association, *NG* significant negative association, *MC* multiple controls, *SC* some controls

Although spiritual healing or excessive religious practices appear to be associated with a greater relapse in older patients with schizophrenia, what this means is not clear. Rather than religious practices causing a worsening of psychosis or an increase in the risk of relapse, it could be that excessive religious practices simply represent an indicator of illness severity and of desperate attempts by religious individuals to cope with disturbing symptoms using their religion. There is no evidence that psychotic symptoms are any more frequent among Muslims than in members of other major religious traditions, although there is some evidence that Muslims are more likely than Christians or Hindus to seek help from a traditional religious healer.

Alcohol Use/Abuse

We found only two studies in our 2010 systematic review that examined the relationship between religiosity and alcohol use or abuse in Muslim-majority countries (Turkey, Lebanon). These studies represent less than 1 % of the 278 studies on R/S and alcohol use/abuse published worldwide. In fact, no studies on this topic were conducted in Muslim countries prior to 5 years ago. In contrast, a number of studies have compared alcohol use in Muslims and non-Muslims.

Religiosity. Ozbay (2008) analyzed data from a 2004 survey of 974 students at Nigde University, Turkey, to identify factors related to social capital including religion and alcohol use. Religion was assessed by two questions that asked whether (a) students talked with friends on the topic of religion in the past year or (b) student's family talked with friends/neighbors about religion (admittedly, not very strong measures of religiosity). Alcohol use was measured by a single question (yes or no). In this overwhelmingly Muslim population, one-third (34 %) of students answered yes to the alcohol question on use. If family talked with friends/neighbors about religion, however, the likelihood that students used alcohol was significantly lower (after controlling for multiple other predictors).

Ghandour and colleagues (2009) surveyed 1,837 students at two major private universities in Beirut, Lebanon. One university followed the American system (University A), where close to 60 % of students were Muslim, and the other followed the French system (University F), where the majority were Christian. A total of 689 Muslim students participated. This is the first study explicitly intending to examine the relationship between religiosity and alcohol use/abuse in a Muslim-majority population (University A). Religiosity was assessed by two questions: belief in God and practice of faith by participating in religious activities such as praying, going to church or mosque. Alcohol use was assessed by several questions asking about lifetime alcohol use, abuse, and dependence based on DSM-IV criteria. Results indicated that fewer Muslim students had a lifetime history of alcohol use than either Druze or Christian students (43.8 % vs. 67.4 % or 87.5 %, respectively); the same relationships were found for lifetime alcohol abuse and dependence, both statistically significant. Religiosity, especially engagement in religious practices, was also inversely related to alcohol use, abuse, and dependence in both Muslim and Christian students, but especially in Muslim students (adjusted for age, gender, university, and major of study).

Muslims vs. Non-Muslims. Several studies have compared alcohol use in Muslims and non-Muslims, especially in Nigeria. Adelekan and colleagues (1993) compared current and lifetime use of alcohol between 483 Christian and 137 Muslim students at a Nigerian university in 1988. Christians had higher current alcohol use than Muslims (45 % vs. 25 %, respectively) and lifetime use (82 % vs. 62 %). Comparing Christian and Muslim students again in 1993 (another cross-sectional survey), Ndom and Adelekan (1996) found that Christian students at the Nigerian university continued to be more likely than Muslim students to use alcohol, although the difference had narrowed (30 % vs. 20 % current use, respectively). Finally, Fatoye (2003) examined substance use by 557 high school seniors in southwestern Nigeria, comparing current and lifetime use between Muslims ($n=46$) and Christians ($n=511$). Current and lifetime use of alcohol were acknowledged by 13 % and 24 % of Muslim students, respectively, and 14 % and 27 % of Christian students. These differences were not statistically significant, although number of Muslims in this sample was small. Religiosity (self-rated) was significantly and inversely related to both current and lifetime alcohol use in the combined sample.

Two studies compared alcohol use in Muslims and non-Muslims in other non-Muslim-majority populations. Chaturvedi and colleagues (2003) compared alcohol use in Muslims, Hindus, and Christians in northeastern India ($n=1,831$, mean age 30 years). Muslim, Hindu, and Christian adults were equally likely to use alcohol (ranging from 7 to 13 %). In a prospective study, Bradby and Williams (2006) compared Christian, Muslims, and Hindu/Sikh high school students in Scotland on lifetime alcohol use at ages 14–15 ($n=620$) and at 18–20 years old ($n=375$). At age 14–15, Christian boys were more likely (71 %) than Muslims (12 %) or Sikh/Hindu (41 %) to have ever used alcohol. Four years later, Christians at age 18–20 were again more likely (98 %) than Muslims (18 %) or Sikh/Hindu (82 %) to have ever used alcohol. Among women, Christian girls at age 14–15 were also more likely (85 %) than Muslims (13 %) and Sikh/Hindu (27 %) to have used alcohol, a pattern that continued when they were 18–20 years old (99 % Christian, 14 % Muslim, 64 % Sikh/Hindu).

Studies Missed. Several studies were missed in our 2010 systematic review. The following are examples of such studies (but again these do not represent an exhaustive review of the published research as we have done in other sections). Pedersen and Kolstad (2000) surveyed 3,424 10th grade students (10 % Muslim) in Oslo, Norway, examining relationships between religious affiliation, religiosity, and alcohol use. Muslim students were significantly more likely to abstain from alcohol than Christian, other religious groups, or those with no religious affiliation (57.5 % vs. 11.8 %, 23.8 %, and 11.2 %, respectively, $p<0.0001$). Religiosity in the overall sample was positively related to abstaining from alcohol ($p<0.0001$) (relationships were confirmed in multivariate analyses).

Uddin (2007–2008) examined moderate and chronic "arrack" drinking (alcohol) in a random sample of 391 Muslims, Hindus, Santal, and Oraon adults in Bangladesh, finding that Muslims were less likely than other groups to drink arrack, and if they did, these individuals were less involved in Islamic religious activities. Similar findings were reported by Diamond and colleagues (2008), who surveyed a representative sample of 821 adult and 440 adolescent Bedouins (mostly Muslim) in the Negev (Israel). Religiosity was strongly and inversely related to alcohol use in both adults (57.2 % of secular used alcohol vs. 4.4 % of devout, $p<0.001$) and adolescents (39.4 % of secular vs. 16.8 % of devout, $p<0.01$).

Recent Research. In a study of alcohol consumption at the country level, Inelmen and colleagues (2010) analyzed data from a WHO 2004 and 2008 database. They found that the five top countries with the highest alcohol consumption were all Christian-majority European nations (Luxembourg, Czech Republic, Ireland, Modova, France), whereas four of the five countries with the lowest alcohol consumption were Muslim-majority countries (Kuwait, Iran, Egypt, Jordan).

Kabiru and associates (2010) examined alcohol use and drunkenness in a random sample of 9,819 adolescents ages 12–19 living in four sub-Saharan African countries (Burkina Faso, Ghana, Malawi, Uganda), one of which is a Muslim-majority country (Burkina Faso, which comprised 28.7 % of the overall sample). The country with the lowest rate of drunkenness within the past 12 months was Burkina Faso (4.3 % vs. 8.9 % in Ghana, 4.9 % in Malawi, and 11.4 % in Uganda). Controlling for other variables in a regression model, the odds of drunkenness in the past 12 months were from 2.0 to 3.7 times greater in the other three countries compared to Burkina Faso (all statistically significant, except for the comparison with women in Malawi). Importance of religion was inversely related to drunkenness among males in the overall sample.

Burazeri and Kark (2010) examined determinants of binge drinking in a middle-aged population (age 35–70) of 450 men and 235 women in post-communist Albania (69 % Muslim, 30 % Christian). Binge drinking was defined as "ever got drunk or had hangovers, or had short drinking session with more than two drinks." Besides religious affiliation, religiosity was also assessed with a single question asking if respondents were totally secular, mild/moderately religiously observant, or observant. Age-adjusted results indicated no difference in binge drinking between Christians and Muslims. However, religiously observant Christians and Muslims were both much less likely to binge drink than those who were secular (Christians 84 % less likely and Muslims 80 % less likely, adjusting for age).

Finally, Badr and colleagues (2013) analyzed data on 103 Lebanese adolescents ages 13–18 (51 Christians and 52 Muslims), half of whom were from Beirut, Lebanon, and half from Los Angeles. The goal was to determine the role of spirituality, religion, and culture on rates of substance use (alcohol and illegal drugs). Besides religious affiliation, a single question asked about degree of attachment to God. In the Los Angeles sample, attachment to God was significantly higher in Muslims compared to Christians, although there was no difference in the Beirut sample. Use of alcohol and drugs was assessed using a standard scale. Results indicated that both alcohol and drug use were significantly higher among Christians than in Muslims in both Los Angeles and Beirut. Attachment to God predicted lower alcohol and drug use in both Christians and Muslims at both locations with similar strength.

Summary: Active religious involvement is related to less alcohol use and abuse (6 of 6 studies) among Muslims (Table 7.3), and the strength of this relationship appears to be similar in Muslims and Christians. In general, alcohol use and abuse is lower in Muslims than in Christians or other religious groups (9 of 12 studies).

Drug Use/Abuse

Our 2010 systematic review identified only one study that examined the relationship between religiosity and illicit drug use/abuse in a Muslim-majority population.

Rodek and colleagues (2009) surveyed 27 weightlifting/powerlifting Muslim athletes from Bosnia and Herzegovina to determine factors related to doping behavior, including religious involvement. Participants ranged in age from 20 to 37, were regularly engaged in training and competition, typically had only a high school education, or were currently in school (81 %). Over 70 % used alcohol, over 40 % smoked, 18 % used pain killers often or regularly, 22 % used cannabis or hashish, and 68 % used doping (performance enhancing drugs) from time to time or regularly. With regard to religiousness, 30 % were Muslim and regularly attended mosque; 33 % were Muslim but rarely or never attended mosque; and 37 % were not religious. Religiousness was inversely related to attitudes toward the prevalence of doping in the sport of weightlifting (–0.62, $p<0.05$, uncontrolled) and personal doping behavior (–0.58, $p<0.05$).

Muslims vs. Non-Muslims. Several studies have compared Muslims with members of other religious denominations in non-majority Muslim countries. Dube et al. (1975) examined the patterns of drug use in hospitalized psychiatric patients in northern India, comparing marijuana use between 512 Hindu and 53 Muslim male patients. Hindus were more likely to use (25.8 %) than Muslims (3.8 %). Adelekan et al. (1993) compared lifetime use of marijuana between 483 Christian and 137 Muslim students at a Nigerian university in 1988. Christians were no more likely than Muslims to have used marijuana (7 % vs. 10 %, respectively). Comparing marijuana use again between Christians and Muslims students at the same Nigerian university in 1993, Ndom and Adelekan (1996) found that Christian students were again no more likely than Muslim students to have used marijuana (4 % vs. 2 %). Fatoye (2003) examined drug use by 557 high school seniors in southwestern Nigeria, comparing use between Muslims ($n=46$) and Christians ($n=511$). Current and lifetime use of stimulants were acknowledged by 24 % and 46 % of Muslim students, respectively, and 21 % and 37 % of Christian students. Similarly, current and lifetime use of sedatives were 11 and 20 % of Muslims students and 9 and 14 % of Christian students. These differences were not statistically significant.

Finally, Bradby and Williams (2006) compared Christian, Muslims, and Hindu/Sikh high school students in Scotland on whether they had ever tried drugs at ages 14–15 ($n=620$) and then again at 18–20 years old ($n=375$). Among males, Christian boys were more likely (35 %) than Sikh/Hindu (24 %) or Muslims (16 %) to have tried drugs by age 14–15; likewise, Christian boys at age 18–20 were more likely (60 %) than Sikh/Hindu (47 %) or Muslims (29 %) to have tried drugs. Among females, Christian girls at age 14–15 were also more likely (49 %) than Sikh/Hindu (18 %) or Muslims (12 %) to have tried drugs, a pattern that continued when they were 18–20 years old (69 % for Christian, 9 % for Sikh/Hindu, and 18 % for Muslim).

In a study we missed in our 2010 review, Khan and colleagues (2006) analyzed data from a random sample of 4,297 men ages 15–54 living in Bangladesh, examining rates of cigarette smoking and illicit drug use by religious denomination and other factors (we include this study here rather than below because it compares Muslims and non-Muslims). Muslim men were less likely than non-Muslims to chew tobacco leaves or shada pata or gul (5.0 % vs. 12.5 %, $p < 0.001$, uncontrolled), and were less likely to be taking any illicit drug (3.8 % vs. 5.8 %, $p < 0.05$).

Studies Missed. Several additional studies were found that we originally missed in our 2010 systematic review, all examining religiosity and drug use. Noon and colleagues (2003) surveyed 2,869 Malaysian teenagers (69 % Muslim) on religiosity and its relationship to drug use and other social problems. Religiosity was assessed using a questionnaire that measured five aspects of religious involvement: ritualistic, experiential, ideological, consequential, and intellectual. Although unrelated to drug use in non-Muslims, religiosity was inversely related to drug use in Muslim teenagers ($r = -0.06$, $p < 0.05$, uncontrolled).

Aliverdinia and Pridemore (2007) examined factors related to drug involvement in 342 drug offenders in an Iranian prison. Family attachment was assessed using a 10-item scale and religious attachment by a 12-item scale, both developed specifically for this study. Drug involvement was measured using a 9-item scale that assessed drug use before being arrested. Scores on the combined measure of family and religious attachment were significantly and inversely related to drug involvement, acting indirectly through less peer drug involvement and higher self-esteem as mediators.

Finally, in a study cited earlier, Diamond and colleagues (2008) examined correlates of drug use among a random sample of 821 adult and 440 adolescent Arabic Bedouins living in the Negev, Israel. Religiosity was assessed using a single question that identified participants as devout, practicing, or secular. Drug use was assessed as any drug use, cannabis, prescription drugs, and other drugs. Religiosity was strongly and inversely related to all forms of drug use in both adults and adolescents. For adults, 30.4 % of those who were secular used any drugs, compared to 5.6 % of those who were devout ($p < 0.001$, uncontrolled). For adolescents 47.7 % of secular and 19.0 % of the devout used any drugs ($p < 0.001$).

Recent Research. We've identified two additional studies published since our 2010 review, both examining religiosity and drug use. The first study by Khoshtinat (2012) examined the impact of Islamic belief on drug use in 400 students at Payame Noor University in Iran. Religiosity was assessed using a 45-item measure of Islamic belief and practice that was developed for this study. Religiosity was significantly and inversely related to drug use ($r = -0.34$, uncontrolled). A second study (Kagimu et al. 2012) examined HIV-status, drug use and the "sujda," a hyperpigmented spot on the forehead due to repeated prostration during prayers and worship (an objective indicator of religious practice) among 1,145 Muslims ages 15–24 seen at an HIV clinic in Uganda. Among 481 patients with a Sujda, 13 (3 %) had ever used narcotic drugs compared to 37 (6 %) among 664 patients without a Sujda ($p = 0.02$, uncontrolled).

Summary: Thus, combining studies from our systematic review with those from studies missed by that review and recent studies since 2010, we found six studies that examined religiosity and drug use in Muslim-majority populations. All six (100 %) found significant inverse relationships (Table 7.3). Six studies also compared drug use in Muslims and Christians or other non-Muslims. Three of those studies found significantly less drug use in Muslims (from Scotland, India, and Bangladesh), whereas the other three studies of Christians and Muslims in Nigeria found no difference in drug use.

Summary and Conclusions

When Muslims experience stress or loss or must confront physical illness, most turn to their religious beliefs to cope. Religious coping, in turn, and religious involvement in general, is related to fewer negative emotions in the vast majority of studies that have examined this relationship in Muslim populations. Fewer negative emotions mean fewer depressive symptoms, less suicide and more negative attitudes toward suicide, lower anxiety, and less alcohol and drug use and abuse.

In almost every one of these areas, however, more research and better-designed studies are needed. Compared to Christian populations, only a tiny fraction of the research overall has been conducted in samples where the majority of participants are Muslim. Of particular concern is that most of the research in Muslim populations has been done in college students, not in the general community population, and has seldom controlled for other relevant factors that might influence relationships with mental health. So far, though, relationships between religiosity and mental health states appear quite similar (if not more favorable) in Muslims compared to Christians. There also appear to be few differences in mental health when Muslims and Christians are directly compared with each other. Given similarities in belief, practices, and moral values between the two traditions, these findings are not surprising.

References

Abdel-Khalek, A. M. (2002). Age and sex differences for anxiety in relation to family size, birth order, and religiosity among Kuwaiti adolescents. *Psychological Reports, 90*(3, Pt. 1), 1031–1036.

Abdel-Khalek, A. M. (2003). Death anxiety in Spain and five Arab countries. *Psychological Reports, 93*, 527–528.

Abdel-Khalek, A. M., & Tomas-Sabado, J. (2005). Anxiety and death anxiety in Egyptian and Spanish nursing students. *Death Studies, 29*, 157–169.

Abdel-Khalek, A. M. (2007). Religiosity, happiness, health, and psychopathology in a probability sample of Muslim adolescents. *Mental Health, Religion and Culture, 10*(6), 571–583.

Abdel-Khalek, A. M., & Lester, D. (2007). Religiosity, health, and psychopathology in two cultures: Kuwait and USA. *Mental Health, Religion and Culture, 10*(5), 537–550.
Abdel-Khalek, A. M., & Naceur, F. (2007). Religiosity and its association with positive and negative emotions among college students from Algeria. *Mental Health, Religion and Culture, 10*(2), 159–170.
Abdel-Khalek, A. M., & Maltby, J. (2008). The comparison of predictors of death obsession within two cultures. *Death Studies, 32*(4), 366–377.
Abdel-Khalek, A. M. (2009). Religiosity and death anxiety: no association in Kuwait. *Psychological Reports, 104*, 770–772.
Abdel-Khalek, A. M., & Lester, D. (2010). Constructions of religiosity, subjective well-being, anxiety, and depression in two cultures: Kuwait and USA. *International Journal of Social Psychiatry, 58*(2), 138–145.
Abdel-Khalek, A. M. (2011). Religiosity, subjective well-being, self-esteem, and anxiety among Kuwaiti Muslim adolescents. *Mental Health, Religion and Culture, 14*(2), 129–140.
Abdel-Khalek, A. M., & Eid, G. K. (2011). Religiosity and its association with subjective well-being and depression among Kuwaiti and Palestinian Muslim children and adolescents. *Mental Health, Religion and Culture, 14*(2), 117–127.
Adelekan, M. L., Abiodun, O. A., Imouoklhome-Obayan, A. O., Oni, G. A., & Ogunremi, O. O. (1993). Psychosocial correlates of alcohol, tobacco and cannabis use: Findings from a Nigerian university. *Drug and Alcohol Dependence, 33*, 247–256.
Aguilar-Vafaie, M. E., & Abiari, M. (2007). Coping Response Inventory: Assessing coping among Iranian college students and introductory development of an adapted Iranian Coping Response Inventory (CRI). *Mental Health, Religion and Culture, 10*(5), 489–513.
Ahmed, A. M., & Kheir, M. M. (2006). Attitudes towards euthanasia among final-year Khartoum University medical students. *Eastern Mediterranean Health Journal, 12*(3/4), 391–397.
Ahmed, H., & Naeen, S. (1984). First rank symptoms and diagnosis of schizophrenia in developing countries. *Psychopathology, 17*, 275–279.
Aliverdinia, A., & Pridemore, W. A. (2007). A first glimpse at narcotics offenders in an Islamic republic: A test of an integrated model of drug involvement among a sample of men incarcerated for drug offenses in Iran. *International Criminal Justice Review, 17*, 27–44.
Al-Sabwah, M. N., & Abdel-Khalek, A. M. (2006). Religiosity and death distress in Arabic college students. *Death Studies, 30*(4), 365–375.
Amr, M., El-Mogy, A., & El-Masry, R. (2013). Adherence in Egyptian patients with schizophrenia: The role of insight, medication beliefs and spirituality. *Arab Journal of Psychiatry, 24*(1), 60–68.
Atallah, S. F., Ar, E.-D., Coker, E. M., Nabil, K. M., & El-Islam, M. F. (2001). A 22-year retrospective analysis of the changing frequency and patterns of religious symptoms among inpatients with psychotic illness in Egypt. *Social Psychiatry and Psychiatric Epidemiology, 36*, 407–415.
Awas, M., Kebede, D., & Alem, A. (1999). Major mental disorders in Butajira, southern Ethiopia. *Acta Psychiatrica Scandinavica, 100*, 56–64.
Azaiza, F., Ron, P., Shoham, M., & Gigini, I. (2010). Death and dying anxiety among elderly Arab Muslims in Israel. *Death Studies, 34*, 351–364.
Azhar, M. Z., Varma, S. L., & Dharap, A. S. (1994). Religious psychotherapy in anxiety disorder patients. *Acta Psychiatrica Scandinavica, 90*, 1–3.
Azhar, M. Z., & Varma, S. L. (1995a). Religious psychotherapy in depressive patients. *Psychotherapy and Psychosomatics, 63*, 165–173.
Azhar, M. Z., & Varma, S. L. (1995b). Religious psychotherapy as management of bereavement. *Acta Psychiatrica Scandinavica, 91*, 233–235.
Azhar, M. Z., Varma, S. L., & Hakim, H. R. (1995). Phenomenological differences of delusions between schizophrenic patients of two cultures of Malaysia. *Singapore Medical Journal, 36*, 273–275.
Badr, L. K., Taha, A., Dee, V. (2013). Substance abuse in middle eastern adolescents living in two different countries: Spiritual, cultural, family and personal factors. *Journal of Religion and Health* [Epub ahead of print]. http://link.springer.com/article/10.1007%2Fs10943-013-9694-1.

Barber, B. K. (2001). Political violence, social integration, and youth functioning: Palestinian youth from the Intifada. *Journal of Community Psychology, 29*(3), 259–280.
Baroun, K. A. (2006). Relations among religiosity, health, happiness, and anxiety for Kuwaiti adolescents. *Psychological Reports, 99*(3), 717–722.
Bataineh, Z. M., Hijazi, T. A., & Hijleh, M. F. (2006). Attitudes and reactions of Jordanian medical students to the dissecting room. *Surgical and Radiologic Anatomy, 28*(4), 416–421.
Beg, M. A., & Zilli, A. S. (1982). A study of the relationship of death anxiety and religious faith to age differentials. *Psychologia, 25*, 121–125.
Bradby, H., & Williams, R. (2006). Is religion or culture the key feature in changes in substance use after leaving school? Young Punjabis and a comparison group in Glasgow. *Ethnicity & Health, 11*(3), 307–324.
Bragazzi, N. L., & Del Puente, G. (2012). Panic attacks and possession by djinns: lessons from ethnopsychiatry. *Psychology Research and Behavior Management, 5*, 185–190.
Burazeri, G., & Kark, J. D. (2010). Prevalence and determinants of binge drinking in middle age in transitional post-communist country: A population-based study in Tirana, Albania. *Alcohol and Alcoholism, 45*, 180–187.
Cardozo, L. B., Bilukha, O. O., Gotway Crawford, C. A., Shaikh, I., Wolfe, M. I., Gerber, M. L., et al. (2004). Mental health, social functioning, and disability in postwar Afghanistan. *Journal of the American Medical Association, 292*(5), 575–584.
Chaaya, M., Sibai, A., Fayad, R., & El-Roueiheb, Z. (2007). Religiosity and depression in older people: Evidence from underprivileged refugee and non-refugee communities in Lebanon. *Aging & Mental Health, 11*(1), 37–44.
Chaturvedi, H., Phukan, R., & Mahanta, J. (2003). The association of selected sociodemographic factors and differences in patterns of substance use: A pilot study in selected areas of Northeast India. *Substance Use & Misuse, 38*(9), 1305–1322.
Conrad, R., Schilling, G., Najjar, D., Geiser, F., Sharif, M., Liedtke, R., et al. (2007). Cross-cultural comparison of explanatory models of illness in schizophrenic patients in Jordan and Germany. *Psychological Reports, 101*(2), 531–546.
Curlin, F. A., Nwodim, C., Vance, J. L., Chin, M. H., & Lantos, J. D. (2009). To die, to sleep: US physicians' religious and other objections to physician-assisted suicide, terminal sedation, and withdrawal of life support. *American Journal of Hospice and Palliative Medicine, 25*, 112–120.
Diamond, G. M., Farhat, A., Al-Amor, M., Elbedour, S., Shelef, K., & Bar-Hamburger, R. (2008). Drug and alcohol use among the Bedouin of the Negev: Prevalence and psychosocial correlates. *Addictive Behaviors, 33*, 143–151.
Dube, K. C., Jain, S. C., Basu, A. K., & Kumar, N. (1975). Patterns of the drug habit (cannabis) in hospitalized psychiatric patients. *Bulletin on Narcotics, 27*(2), 1–10.
Eapen, V., & Revesz, T. (2003). Psychosocial correlates of paediatric cancer in the United Arab Emirates. *Supportive Care in Cancer, 11*(3), 185–189.
Ellis, L., Wahab, E. A., & Ratnasingan, M. (2013). Religiosity and fear of death: A three-nation comparison. *Mental Health, Religion and Culture, 16*(2), 179–199.
Errihani, H., Mrabti, H., Boutayeb, S., El Ghissassi, I., El Mesbahi, O., Hammoudi, M., Chergui, H., & Riadi, A. (2008). Impact of cancer on Moslem patients in Morocco. *Psychooncology, 17*(1), 98–100.
Eskin, M. (2004). The effects of religious versus secular education on suicide ideation and suicidal attitudes in adolescents in Turkey. *Social Psychiatry and Psychiatric Epidemiology, 39*(7), 536–542.
Eskin, M., Ertekin, K., Dereboy, C., & Demirkiran, F. (2007). Risk factors for and protective factors against adolescent suicidal behavior in Turkey. *Crisis, 28*(3), 131–139.
Farooqi, Y. N. (2006). Traditional healing practices sought by Muslim psychiatric patients in Lahore, Pakistan. *International Journal of Disability, Development and Education, 53*(4), 401–415.
Fatoye, F. O. (2003). Psychosocial correlates of substance use amongst secondary school students in south western Nigeria. *East African Medical Journal, 80*(3), 154–158.

Filazoglu, G., & Griva, K. (2008). Coping and social support and health related quality of life in women with breast cancer in Turkey. *Psychology, Health & Medicine, 13*(5), 559–573.

Friedman, M., & Saroglou, V. (2010). Religiosity, psychological acculturation to the host culture, self-esteem and depressive symptoms among stigmatized and nonstigmatized religious immigrant groups in Western Europe. *Basic and Applied Social Psychology, 32*, 185–195.

Gal, G., Goldberger, N., Kabaha, A., Haklai, Z., Gerasisy, N., Gross, R., & Levav, I. (2012). Suicidal behavior among Muslim Arabs in Israel. *Social Psychiatry and Psychiatric Epidemiology, 47*, 11–17.

Gencoz, F., Vatan, S., Walker, R. L., & Lester, D. (2007). Hopelessness and suicidality in Turkish and American respondents. *Omega: Journal of Death and Dying, 55*(4), 311–319.

Ghandour, L. A., Karam, E. G., & Maalouf, W. E. (2009). Lifetime alcohol use, abuse and dependence among university students in Lebanon: Exploring the role of religiosity in different religious faiths. *Addiction, 104*, 940–948.

Ghorbani, N., Watson, P., Ghramaleki, F. A., Morris, R. J., & Hood, R. W. (2000). Muslim attitudes towards religion scale: Factors, validity and complexity of relationships with mental health in Iran. *Mental Health, Religion and Culture, 3*(2), 125–132.

Hamdan, A., & Tamim, H. (2011). Psychosocial risk and protective factors for postpartum depression in the United Arab Emirates. *Archives of Women's Mental Health, 14*, 124–133.

Hestyanti, Y. R. (2006). Children survivors of the 2004 tsunami in Aceh, Indonesia: a study of resiliency. *Annals of the New York Academy of Sciences, 1094*, 303–307.

Hosseini, M., Salehi, A., Khoshknab, M. F., Rokofian, A., & Davidson, P. M. (2013). The effect of a preoperative spiritual/religious intervention on anxiety in Shia Muslim patients undergoing coronary artery bypass grant surgery: A randomized controlled trial. *Journal of Holistic Nursing*. doi:10.1177/0898010113488242.

Inelmen, E. M., Gazeroo, M., Inelmen, E., Sergi, G., & Manzato, E. (2010). Alcohol consumption and suicide: A country-level analysis. *Italian Journal of Public Health, 7*(3), 106–114.

Inozu, M., Clark, D. A., & Karanci, A. N. (2012). Scrupulosity in Islam: A comparison of highly religious Turkish and Canadian samples. *Behavior Therapy, 43*, 190–202.

Jahangir, F., Rehman, H., & Jan, T. (1998). Degree of religiosity and vulnerability to suicidal attempt/plans in depressive patients among Afghan refugees. *International Journal for the Psychology of Religion, 8*(4), 265–269.

Johnstone, J., & Tiliopoulos, N. (2008). Exploring the relationship between schizotypal personality traits and religious attitude in an international Muslim sample. *Archive for the Psychology of Religion, 30*, 241–253.

Kabiru, C. W., Beguy, D., Crichton, J., & Ezeh, A. C. (2010). Self-reported drunkenness among adolescents in four sub-Saharan African countries: association with adverse childhood experiences. *Child and Adolescent Psychiatry and Mental Health, 4*, 17.

Kagimu, M., Guwatudde, D., Rwabukwali, C., Kaye, S., Walakira, Y., & Ainomugisha, D. (2012). Religiosity for HIV prevention n Uganda: A case study among Muslim youth in Wakiso district. *African Health Sciences, 12*(3), 282–290.

Kamal, Z., & Loewenthal, K. M. (2002). Suicide beliefs and behavior among young Muslims and Hindus in the UK. *Mental Health, Religion and Culture, 5*(2), 111–118.

Khamis, V. (2012). Impact of war, religiosity and ideology on PTSD and psychiatric disorders in adolescents from Gaza Strip and South Lebanon. *Social Science & Medicine, 74*, 2005–2011.

Khan, M. M., Aklimunnessa, K., Kabir, M. A., Kabir, M., & Mori, M. (2006). Tobacco consumption and its association with illicit drug use among men in Bangladesh. *Addiction, 101*(8), 1178–1186.

Khan, Z. H., & Watson, P. (2006). Construction of the Pakistani Religious Coping Practices Scale: Correlations with religious coping, religious orientation, and reactions to stress among Muslim university students. *International Journal for the Psychology of Religion, 16*(2), 101–112.

Khoshtinat, V. (2012). The impact of adherence to Islamic beliefs via public health on university students' tendency to drug consumption. *International Research Journal of Applied and Basic Sciences, 3*(10), 2155–2164.

Kuyel, N., Cesur, S., & Ellison, C. G. (2012). Religious orientation and mental health: A study with Turkish university students. *Psychological Reports, 110*(2), 535–546.

Lester, D., & Abdel-Khalek, A. (2007). A Taoist orientation and mental health in Kuwaiti and American students. *Perceptual and Motor Skills, 105*(3, Pt. 1), 921–922.

Levav, I., & Aiesenberg, E. (1989). Suicide in Israel: Crossnational comparisons. *Acta Psychiatrica Scandinavica, 79*, 468–473.

Mirzamani, M., & Mohammadi, M. R. (2003). Religious values in a group of psychiatric outpatients. *Psychological Reports, 92*(3 Pt 1), 787–790.

Ndetei, D. M., Muriungi, S. K., Owoso, A., Mutiso, V. N., Mbwayo, A. W., Khasakhala, L. I., Barch, D. M., & Mamah, D. (2012). Prevalence and characteristics of psychotic-like experiences in Kenyan youth. *Psychiatry Research, 196*, 235–242.

Ndom, R. J. E., & Adelekan, M. L. (1996). Psychosocial correlates of substance use among undergraduates in Ilorin University, Nigeria. *East African Medical Journal, 73*, 541–547.

Noon, H. M., Haneef, M. A. M., Yusof, S. A., & Amin, R. M. (2003). Religiosity and social problems in Malaysia. *Intellectual Discourse, 11*, 77–87.

Nuraskikin, M. S., Aini, A., Aida Syarinaz, A. A., Ng, C. G. (2010). Validity and reliability of the Malay version of Duke University Religion Index (DUREL-M) among a group of nursing students. *Malaysian Journal of Psychiatry 19*(2). MJP Online Early.

Nurasikin, M. S., Khatijah, L. A., Aini, A., Ramil, M., Aida, S. A., Zainal, N. Z., & Ng, C. G. (2013). Religiousness, religious coping methods and distress level among psychiatric patients in Malaysia. *International Journal of Social Psychiatry, 59*(4), 332–338.

Ozbay, O. (2008). Does social capital deter youth from cheating, alcohol use, and violence in Turkey?: Bringing torpil in. *Journal of Criminal Justice, 36*(5), 403–415.

Pedersen, W., & Kolstad, A. (2000). Adolescent alcohol abstainers: Traditional patterns in new groups. *Acta Sociologica, 43*, 219–233.

Pritchard, C., & Amanullah, S. (2007). An analysis of suicide and undetermined deaths in 17 predominantly Islamic countries contrasted with the UK. *Psychological Medicine, 37*(3), 421–430.

Razali, S. M., Aminah, K., & Khan, U. A. (2002). Religious-cultural psychotherapy in the management of anxiety patients. *Transcultural Psychiatry, 39*(1), 130–136.

Razali, S. M., Hasanah, C. I., Aminah, K., & Subramaniam, M. (1998). Religious–sociocultural psychotherapy in patients with anxiety and depression. *Australian and New Zealand Journal of Psychiatry, 32*, 867–872.

Rezaeian, M. (2010). Suicide among young Middle Eastern Muslim females: The perspective of an Iranian epidemiologist. *Crisis, 31*(1), 36–42.

Rodek, J., Sekulic, D., & Pasalic, E. (2009). Can we consider religiousness as a protective factor against doping behavior in sport? *Journal of Religion and Health, 48*(4), 445–453.

Saffari, M., Pakpour, A. H., Naderi, M. K., Koenig, H. G., Baldacchino, D. R., & Piper, C. N. (2013). Spiritual coping, religiosity and quality of life: a stud on Muslim patients undergoing haemodialysis. *Nephrology, 18*, 269–275.

Salib, E., & Youakim, S. (2001). Spiritual healing in elderly psychiatric patients: A case-control study in an Egyptian psychiatric hospital. *Aging & Mental Health, 5*(4), 366–370.

Scholte, W. F., Olff, M., Ventevogel, P., de Vries, G.-J., Jansveld, E., Lopes Cardozo, B., et al. (2004). Mental Health Symptoms Following War and Repression in Eastern Afghanistan. *Journal of the American Medical Association, 292*(5), 585–593.

Shah, A., & Chandia, M. (2010). The relationship between suicide and Islam: a cross-national study. *Journal of Injury and Violence Research, 2*(2), 93–97.

Sisask, M., Varnik, A., Kolves, K., Bertolote, J. M., Bolhari, J., Botega, N. J., Fleischmann, A., Vijayakumar, L., & Wasserman, D. (2010). Is religiosity a protective factor against attempted suicide: A cross-cultural case-control study. *Archives of Suicide Research, 14*, 44–55.

Suhail, K. (2001). Death anxiety in a Pakistani sample. *Journal of the Indian Academy of Applied Psychology, 27*(1–2), 19–27.

Suhail, K., & Akram, S. (2002). Correlates of death anxiety in Pakistan. *Death Studies, 26*(1), 39–50.

Suhail, K., & Ghauri, S. (2010). Phenomenology of delusions and hallucinations in schizophrenia by religious convictions. *Mental Health, Religion and Culture, 13*(3), 245–259.

Taleghani, F., Yekta, Z. P., & Nasrabadi, A. N. (2006). Coping with breast cancer in newly diagnosed Iranian women. *Journal of Advanced Nursing, 54*(3), 265–272.

Tavabi, A. A., & Iran-Pour, E. (2011). The association between religious beliefs and mental health amongst medical students. *Journal of the Pakistan Medical Association, 61*, 135–138.

Tek, C., & Ulug, B. (2001). Religiosity and religious obsessions in obsessive-compulsive disorder. *Psychiatry Research, 104*(2), 99–108.

Templer, D. I. (1972). Death anxiety: Extraversion, neuroticism, and cigarette smoking. *Omega, 3*, 53–56.

Tomas-Sabado, J., & Gomez-Benito, J. (2004). Note on death anxiety in Spain and five Arab countries. *Psychological Reports, 95*(3 Pt 2), 1239–1240.

Tuncay, T., Musabak, I., Gok, D. E., & Kutlu, M. (2008). The relationship between anxiety, coping strategies, and characteristics of patients with diabetes. *Health and Quality of Life Outcomes, 6*, 79.

Uddin, E. (2007–2008). Religious attitude, religiosity, and arrack drinking patterns among Muslim, Hindu, Santa, and Oaraon communities in Rasulpur Union, Bangladesh. *International Quarterly of Community Health Education, 28*, 351–370.

Van den Branden, S., & Broeckaert, B. (2011). Living in the hands of god. English Sunni e-fatwas on (non-) voluntary euthanasia and assisted suicide. Medicine. *Healthcare and Philosophy, 14*, 29–41.

Vasegh, S., & Mohammadi, M. R. (2007). Religiosity, anxiety, and depression among a sample of Iranian medical students. *International Journal of Psychiatry in Medicine, 37*(2), 213–227.

Wahass, S., & Kent, G. (1997). Coping with auditory hallucinations: A cross-cultural comparison between Western (British) and non-Western (Saudi Arabian) patients. *Journal of Nervous and Mental Disease, 185*, 664–668.

Watson, P., Ghorbani, N., Davison, H., Bing, M. N., Hood, R. W., Jr., & Ghramaleki, A. F. (2002). Negatively reinforcing personal extrinsic motivations: Religious orientation, inner awareness, and mental health in Iran and the United States. *International Journal for the Psychology of Religion, 12*(4), 255–276.

Yorulmaz, O., Gencoz, T., & Woody, S. (2009). OCD cognitions and symptoms in different religious contexts. *Journal of Anxiety Disorders, 23*, 401–406.

Yuniarti, K. W., Dewi, C., Ningrum, R. P., Widiastuti, M., & Asril, N. M. (2013). Illness perception, stress, religiosity, depression, social support, and self management of diabetes in Indonesia. *International Journal of Research Studies in Psychology, 2*(1), 25–41.

Zarghami, M., Valaie, N., Sartakhti, A. A., Mehraban, M., Mahmoudi, R., & Monesi, F. S. (2010). Attitudes of Iranian interns and residents towards euthanasia. *World Applied Sciences Journal, 8*(4), 486–489.

Zuraida, N. Z., & Ahmad, H. S. (2007). Religiosity and suicide ideation in clinically depressed patients. *Malaysian Journal of Psychiatry, 16*, 12–15.

Chapter 8
Religion and Positive Emotions in Muslims

The psychological benefits of religious faith have been emphasized in Islam since early times. According to Al-Dhahabi (1961) in *Prophetic Medicine*, a treatise written in the fourteenth century, "Prayers often produce happiness and contentment in the mind; they suppress anxiety and extinguish the fire of anger. They increase love for truth and humility before people; they soften the heart, create love and forgiveness and dislike of the vice of vengeance. Besides, often sound judgment occurs to the mind [due to concentration about difficult matters] and one finds correct answers [to problems]. One also remembers forgotten things .... One can discover the ways to solve matters worldly and spiritual. And one can effectively examine oneself—particularly when one strenuously exercises oneself in prayers" (p. 140).

Religious involvement not only appears to help neutralize negative emotions and prevent addictive behaviors but also has the potential to increase the experience of positive emotions. By positive emotions we mean feelings and experiences such as happiness, life satisfaction, well-being, hope, and optimism, as well as improvement of meaning and purpose, self-esteem, sense of control, and a wide range of positive character traits. But, let us look now at what the research has found.

Well-Being

Eight studies have examined relationships between religiosity and well-being, happiness, or life satisfaction in Muslim-majority countries, including five from Kuwait and one each from Pakistan, Malaysia, and Algeria. A number of studies have also compared Muslims and non-Muslims on well-being.

Religiosity. Suhail and Chaudhry (2004) surveyed a random sample of 973 Pakistanis ages 16–80 living in Lahore (50 % women), examining relationships between religiosity and well-being. An 18-item religiosity scale was used to assess Islamic beliefs and practices. Work satisfaction was measured using a 3-item scale, marital satisfaction by a 2-item scale, and personal subjective well-being by two

H.G. Koenig and S. Al Shohaib, *Health and Well-Being in Islamic Societies: Background, Research, and Applications*, DOI 10.1007/978-3-319-05873-3_8,

items (one assessing life satisfaction and the other personal happiness). Uncontrolled correlations revealed significant positive associations between religiosity and marital satisfaction ($r = +0.08$, $p \leq 0.05$), work satisfaction ($r = +0.09$, $p \leq 0.01$), personal happiness ($r = +0.12$, $p \leq 0.001$), and overall life satisfaction ($r = +0.10$, $p \leq 0.01$). In a regression model that controlled for other predictors, religiosity was positively related to happiness ($B = +0.10$, $p = 0.001$) independent of work satisfaction, social support, income, and marital satisfaction. Religiosity also predicted higher overall life satisfaction ($B = +0.07$, $p = 0.05$) independent of work and marital satisfaction, income, and social support.

Baroun (2006) examined relationships between religiosity and happiness in 941 Kuwaiti adolescents in grades 6–12 (mean age 17). Religiosity was assessed using the 10-item Hoge Intrinsic Religious Motivation scale and by a single question on self-rated religiosity. Happiness and life satisfaction were measured using single questions with responses ranging from 0 (very low) to 10 (very high). Intrinsic religiosity was positively related to both happiness ($r = +0.12$) and life satisfaction ($r = +0.26$), as was self-rated religiosity ($r = +0.28$ and $r = +0.29$, respectively) (all $p < 0.001$, uncontrolled).

Abdel-Khalek from Kuwait University has published a series of reports examining religiosity and happiness in Kuwait. In his first study, Abdel-Khalek (2006) surveyed 2,210 Muslim college students at Kuwait University (mean age 21, 52 % women), examining relations between religiosity and happiness. Both were assessed using single questions with responses ranging from 0 to 10. Men were happier than women, but not by much (7.1 vs. 6.6, respectively). Happiness was positively correlated with religiosity in both men ($r = +0.33$) and women ($r = +0.31$). Controlling for measures of mental and physical health, religiosity remained significantly related to happiness in both men ($B = +0.16$) and women ($B = +0.15$) (both $p < 0.0001$).

In a second study, Abdel-Khalek (2007) analyzed data on 6,339 Muslim Kuwaiti adolescents ages 15–18 (50 % female). Religiosity and happiness were measured in the same manner as in the 2006 study. Again, religiosity was slightly higher in boys than girls (7.9 vs. 7.5) and was positively correlated with happiness in boys ($r = +0.26$) and girls ($r = +0.27$). Controlling for mental health, physical health, anxiety, and depression, religiosity remained correlated with happiness in both boys ($B = +0.16$) and girls ($B = +0.13$) (both $p < 0.001$). In a third study, Abdel-Khalek (2008) surveyed 424 adult Kuwaiti personnel working for the Kuwait State in government ministries, institutions, and the private sector. The same methodology as above was used, except that happiness was also assessed using the Oxford Happiness Inventory (OHI) and life satisfaction by the Satisfaction with Life Scale. Again, self-rated religiosity in men was positively correlated with happiness ($r = +0.39$, self-rating of happiness; $r = +0.30$, Oxford happiness scale) and life satisfaction (+0.28). Similar relationships were found in women ($r = +0.43$, self-rating of happiness; $r = +0.31$, Oxford happiness scale; $r = +0.30$, life satisfaction) (all $p < 0.01$, uncontrolled).

A study by Noor (2008) surveyed 389 employed married Malaysian women (average age 36) with one or more children living at home, examining relationships between religiosity and life satisfaction (given the high stress these women were experiencing given their multiple roles). Religiosity was measured using the 14-item Muslim Attitude toward Religion Scale (MARS; Wilde). Life satisfaction was assessed using a standard 5-item scale (Diener). The uncontrolled correlation between religiosity and life satisfaction was positive ($r = +0.25$, $p < 0.01$). Hierarchical regression controlling for age, education, negative affect, and work experience revealed that the relationship with life satisfaction persisted ($p < 0.001$). Religiosity also interacted with age and work experience ($p < 0.05$). For younger women, high religiosity moderated the adverse effects of low work experience on life satisfaction. For the older women, high work experience was correlated with high life satisfaction only in women with high religiosity.

Tiliouine and colleagues (2009) analyzed the relationship between religiosity and subjective well-being in a convenience sample of 2,909 adults age 18 or older in Algeria (40 % with a university education and 62 % single). Researchers assessed religiosity by administering a 16-item Islamic Religiosity Scale made up of religious practices and religious altruism subscales. Well-being was assessed using a 7-item Personal Well-Being Index. Both religious practices and religious altruism were positively related to well-being ($r = +0.20$ and +0.22, respectively, $p < 0.005$). After controlling for pain, anxiety, and sleep quality, religiosity remained significantly and positively correlated with personal well-being in both those who were healthy and those who were sick. This was especially true for religious altruism, which involved advising others to do good and avoiding sin, considering charity as a religious duty, praising God at beginning and end of work, tolerating others for God's sake, and seeking relief from God when anxious/sad.

Finally, Ashkanani (2009) surveyed 266 patients and family members of those severely injured in a car accident (65 %) or related to those who died as a result of a car accident (35 %). All participants were recruited from the orthopedic hospital Al Razi Hospital in Kaifan, Kuwait (56 % male). Religiosity was measured using 10 items from the Al Kandari religiosity scale. Subjective well-being was assessed using the 84-item Ryff Inventory. After controlling for income and age, religiosity was positively related to well-being ($B = 0.36$, $p < 0.001$). In women, 30 % of the total variance in well-being was accounted for by religiosity compared to 27 % in men.

We also identified one study that compared Muslims and non-Muslims on well-being. Kazarian (2005) examined differences in psychological well-being between 182 Christian and Muslim students (mean age 19) at the American University of Beirut, finding no differences in well-being between the two religious groups. Only poor family functioning predicted lower levels of well-being.

Missed Studies. Our 2010 systematic review did not likely uncover all studies in Muslims on religiosity and well-being, given the large volume of studies published on this topic. We did not search for missed studies, since relationships between religiosity and well-being appeared to be quite consistent based on our review above.

Recent Research. At least 12 additional studies in Muslims have been published since 2010. Abdel-Khalek and Lester (2010) surveyed 235 Kuwaiti college students using the Oxford Happiness Index (OHI) and single-item self-ratings of happiness, health, social support, and religiosity, along with a number of other established multi-item scales assessing life satisfaction, optimism and pessimism, hope, self-esteem, and emotional affect. Religiosity was positively correlated with happiness scores on the OHI, self-rating of happiness, and self-rating of life satisfaction (*r*s ranging from +0.19 to +0.33, all $ps<0.01$, uncontrolled). A second study by Abdel-Khalek (2011a) examined religiosity, happiness, and life satisfaction using the same measures above in a sample of 224 Egyptian college students. Again, he found a positive relationship between religiosity and happiness (OHI) ($r=+0.25$), life satisfaction (Life Satisfaction Index) ($r=+0.31$), self-rated life satisfaction ($r=+0.48$), and self-rated happiness ($r=+0.27$) (all $p<0.01$, uncontrolled). Besides these two studies, seven additional recent reports by Abdel-Khalek indicated similar findings in adolescents, young, and middle-age Kuwaitis (Abdel-Khalek 2012a), Kuwaiti adolescents (Abdel-Khalek 2011b), younger adults from Qatar (Abdel-Khalek 2013a), Lebanese adolescents (Abdel-Khalek 2012b), Kuwaiti and Egyptian college students (Abdel-Khalek 2012c), Kuwaiti and Palestinian children and adolescents (Abdel-Khalek and Eid 2011), and Saudi children and adolescents (Abdel-Khalek 2009).

In one of the few studies in older adults, Momtaz and colleagues (2010) surveyed 1,367 widowed and married elderly Muslims from Malaysia, examining relationships between intrinsic–extrinsic religiosity (modified 11-item Gorsuch I-E scale) and well-being (WHO-5 index). The objective was to determine if the religiosity might buffer (reduce) the negative emotional effects of widowhood. Religiosity was divided into personal religiosity (intrinsic) and social religiosity (extrinsic). Results indicated that widowhood was related to lower well-being. Both personal and social religiosity were related to greater well-being in the overall sample ($p<0.01$, after controlling for multiple demographic and health variables). Personal (intrinsic), but not social religiosity, mediated the relationship between widowhood and well-being.

In a second report, Momtaz and colleagues (2011a) examined the effect of religiosity on the relationship between social isolation and well-being in 1,415 community-dwelling Muslim older adults in Malaysia. The same measures of well-being and religiosity were used in this as in the previous study, along with a standard measure of social isolation. Religiosity (combined personal and social) was positively related to greater well-being ($r=+0.27$, $p<0.01$, uncontrolled), an association that persisted in hierarchical regression models that controlled for multiple demographic factors ($B=+0.80$, $p<0.01$). Furthermore, there was a significant interaction between religiosity and social isolation such that among older adults with greater religiosity, the negative relationship between social isolation and well-being was much weaker than in those with low religiosity. A third study by Momtaz and colleagues (2011b) in the same sample using the same measures found that religiosity moderated the negative impact of chronic medical illness on well-being, such that this relationship was weaker in those with high religiosity (suggesting a buffering effect, as it had for social isolation).

Finally, Ismail and Desmukh (2012) examined religiosity and well-being in 150 persons ages 18–60 in Pakistan. Religiosity was assessed using frequency of religious attendance, prayer, and importance of belief. Life satisfaction was assessed with the 5-item Satisfaction with Life Scale (Diener). Religiosity and life satisfaction were strongly related ($r = +0.76$), especially frequency of prayer ($r = +0.79$) (uncontrolled). This correlation is extremely high, much higher than any previously reported correlation between religiosity and well-being (or for that matter, any indicator of mental health).

One last study deserves mention, given the impact that "social norms" regarding religiosity may have on the relationship between religiosity and well-being (since religious social norms are very strong in Muslim populations). Stavrova and colleagues (2013) from the University of Cologne (Germany) examined relationship between religiosity and well-being using data from the World and European Values Studies that have data on 101,682 persons in 64 countries. They found that among countries where religiosity is the social "norm," there was a strong relationship between personal religiosity (attendance, subjective religiosity, importance of God) and both happiness and life satisfaction, whereas in countries where fewer people are religious, the relationship was much weaker or nonexistent. Among countries with the highest religious social norms were Indonesia, Ghana, and Iraq (two Muslim countries out of three), and those with the lowest religious norms were Norway, Sweden, and France.

Summary. In our systematic review, we identified eight studies examining relationships between religiosity and well-being in Muslim-majority countries (Table 8.1). Since 2010, at least 12 additional studies have been published. All 20 studies (100 %) found significant positive relationships between religiosity and well-being, regardless of Muslim country or age of participants. Furthermore, studies indicate that religiosity buffers (reduces) the negative effects of social isolation and chronic medical illnesses on well-being in older adults. Only one study compared Christians and Muslims with regard to well-being and no differences were found.

Hope

Our 2010 systematic review uncovered no studies that examined relationships between religiosity/spirituality (R/S) and hope in Muslim-majority countries. However, it did identify a study by Ai and colleagues (2003) of 138 refugees (93 % Muslim) from Kosovo and Bosnia in the USA that examined relationships between religiosity (measured using self-rated religiosity and multi-item scales of negative and positive religious coping) and hope (assessed using the 12-item Hope Scale, developed by Snyder). No relationships were found between hope and religiosity or positive religious coping, although there was a significant inverse relationship between hope and negative religious coping ($r = -0.22$, $p < 0.01$, uncontrolled).

Missed Studies. In the present systematic review, we could find no other studies besides the one above that examined hope in Muslim populations prior to 2010.

Recent Research. Since our 2010 review we identified an additional two studies, one conducted in Egypt and the other examining Somali refugees in Hungary. A study by Rabie and colleagues (2011) focused on religiosity and hope among 80

Table 8.1 Religiosity and well-being in Muslims

Authors (year)	Method	Sample size	Participants	Location	Controls	Findings
Suhail and Chaudhry (2004)	CS	973	Adults ages 16–80	Pakistan	MC	P
Baroun (2006)	CS	941	Adolescents	Kuwait	None	P
Abdel-Khalek (2006)	CS	2,210	University students	Kuwait	MC	P
Abdel-Khalek (2007)	CS	6,339	Adolescents	Kuwait	MC	P
Abdel-Khalek (2008)	CS	424	Adult workers	Kuwait	None	P
Noor (2008)	CS	389	Married adult women	Malaysia	MC	P
Tiliouine et al. (2009)	CS	2,909	Adults ages 18 or over	Algeria	MC	P
Ashkanani (2009)	CS	266	Injured patients and family	Kuwait	SC	P
Momtaz et al. (2010)	CS	1,367	Older widowed/married	Malaysia	MC	P
Momtaz et al. (2011a)	CS	1,415	Older adults, community	Malaysia	MC	P
Abdel-Khalek (2009)	CS	7,211	Children and adolescents	Saudi Arabia	SC	P
Abdel-Khalek and Lester (2010)	CS	235	University students	Kuwait	None	P
Abdel-Khalek (2011a)	CS	224	University students	Egypt	None	P
Abdel-Khalek (2011b)	CS	499	Adolescents	Kuwait	None	P
Abdel-Khalek and Eid (2011)	CS	1,937/1,009	Children and adolescents	Kuwait/Pales	SC	P
Abdel-Khalek (2012a)	CS	1,420	Adolescents, students, adults	Kuwait	None (?)	P
Abdel-Khalek (2012b)	CS	239	Adolescents	Lebanese	None (?)	P
Abdel-Khalek (2012c)	CS	577/674	University students	Egypt/Kuwait	SC	P
Ismail and Desmukh (2012)	CS	150	Adults ages 18–60	Pakistan	None	P
Abdel-Khalek (2013a)	CS	244	University students	Qatar	None (?)	P

CS cross-sectional, *NA* no association, *P* significant positive association, *NG* significant negative association, *C* complex association, *MC* multiple controls, *SC* some controls patients suffering from cancer in Egypt. Religiosity was measured using the 14-item Religious Orientation Scale-Revised (Gorsuch). Hope was assessed using the Beck Hopelessness Scale (lower scores indicating more hope). Results indicated an indirect positive relationship between hopelessness scores and external religiosity scores, although the relationship was not statistically significant (only abstract available, so study details lacking).

The second study was by Kroo and Nagy (2011) who examined 53 traumatized Muslim Somali refugees at reception centers in Hungary (83 % men, 83 % ages 18–29). Hope was measured using the 12-item Adult Trait Hope Scale (Snyder). Posttraumatic growth (PTG) was assessed using the 21-item Post-Traumatic Growth Scale. Religiosity was assessed using three measures: (1) a 5-item scale that included one question on self-rated religiosity and four questions assessing the spirituality of trauma survivors; (2) a question that asked about religious change ("Has your relationship with God or your beliefs changed since your experience?"); and (3) the 14-item brief RCOPE. Religiosity (5-item scale) was related to greater PTG ($r=+0.30$) and PTG scores were related to greater hope ($r=+0.48$), but the relationship between religiosity and hope was not examined. Among those who indicated a significant change in their religious beliefs (23 %), all indicated that their beliefs had strengthened.

Summary. Two studies have examined religiosity and hope in Muslim-majority populations, and neither found a significant relationship (in contrast to studies on religiosity and well-being) (Table 8.2).

Optimism

Whereas hope concentrates on the personal attainment of specific goals (i.e., belief that there is light at the end of the tunnel in a specific difficult circumstance), optimism focuses more broadly on the possibility of achieving positive future outcomes (i.e., belief in good outcomes more generally across circumstances). Our 2010 systematic review uncovered only one study that examined the relationship between religiosity and optimism in a Muslim sample. Abdel-Khalek and Maltby (2008) surveyed 271 college students from Kuwait University and 205 college students from the UK. As usual, religiosity was assessed with a single self-rated item ranging from 0 to 10. Optimism was assessed using the Arabic Scale of Optimism and Pessimism. Optimism was significantly higher in Kuwaiti students (likely Muslim) than in UK students (likely Christian) (54.2 vs. 46.5, $p<0.001$). Religiosity and optimism, however, were not related in either Kuwaiti students or in students from the UK.

Missed Studies. In the present review, we identified five additional studies in Muslim-majority populations prior to 2010 that we missed in our 2010 systematic review. In the first of these, Ai and colleagues (2003) examined religiosity and optimism in a predominantly Muslim sample of 138 adult refugees from Kosovo and

Table 8.2 Religiosity and hope, optimism, meaning, self-esteem, and control in Muslims

Authors (year)	Method	Sample size	Participants	Location	Controls	Findings
Hope						
Ai et al. (2003)	CS	138	Kosovo/Bosnia refugees	USA	None	NA
Rabie et al. (2011)	CS	80	Cancer patients	Egypt	None	NA
Optimism						
Ai et al. (2003)	CS	138	Kosovo/Bosnia refugees	USA	None	P
Abdel-Khalek and Lester (2007)	CS	460	University students	Kuwait	None	P
Abdel-Khalek and Naceur (2007)	CS	244	University students	Algeria	None	P (female)
Abdel-Khalek and Maltby (2008)	CS	271	University students	Kuwait	None	NA
Ahmed (2009)	CS	174	Muslim youth	USA	None	P
Tiliouine et al. (2009)	CS	2,909	Adults ages 18 or over	Algeria	None	P
Khalad (2010)	CS	260	University students	Jordan	None	NA
Meaning and purpose						
Tiliouine and Belgoumidi (2009)	CS	495	University students	Algeria	SC (?)	P
Aflakseir (2012)	CS	60	University students (Muslim)	England	None	P
Lazenby et al. (2013)	CS	205	Cancer patients	Jordan	None	P
Self-esteem						
Watson et al. (2002)	CS	227	University students	Iran	None	P
Suhail and Chaudhry (2004)	CS	973	Adults ages 18–80	Pakistan	None	NA
Carlton-Ford et al. (2008)	CS	1,000	Adolescents ages 12–17	Iraq	MC	P
Khan and Watson (2004)	CS	121	Adults, mean age 28	Pakistan	None	P
French et al. (2008)	CS	183	Adolescents	Indonesia	MC	P
Fanni Asl et al. (2008)	CS	202	University students	Iran	None	P
Sirin et al. (2008)	CS	97	Adults ages 18–28 (Muslim)	USA	None	P
Abu-Rayya and Abu-Rayya (2009)	CS	520	Palestinian university students	Israel	None	P
Imam et al. (2009)	CS	358	University students	Malaysia	SC	P
Azaiza et al. (2010)	CS	145	Older Arab adults (>60)	Israel	None	NG

Ghaffari and Ciftci (2010)	CS	174	Muslim immigrants	USA	None	M
Friedman and Saroglou (2010)	CS	273	Muslim immigrants	Belgium	None	NG (indirect)
Sallquist et al. (2010)	P	136	Adolescents	Indonesia	None	P
Abdel-Khalek (2011b)	CS	499	Adolescents	Kuwait	None	P
Abdel-Khalek (2012c)	CS	577/674	University students	Egypt/Kuwait	MC	P
Locus of control (LOC)						
Mohammadi and Honarmand (2007)	CS	179	University students	Iran	(?)	P (females)
Cohen and Azaiza (2007)	CS	162	Older Muslim Arabs	Israel	MC	NA
Khan et al. (2011)	CC	159/163	Medical patients/controls	Pakistan	None	NG
Cirhinlioglu and Ozdikmenli-Demir (2012)	CS	430	University students	Turkey	MC	M

CS cross-sectional, *P* prospective, *NA* no association, *P* significant positive association with self-esteem or with internal LOC, *NG* significant negative association with self-esteem or positive association with external LOC, *MC* multiple controls, *SC* some controls, *M* mixed (for self-esteem, significant positive and negative associations based on interaction; for LOC, positive associations with both internal and external LOC)

Bosnia, finding a significant relationship between positive religious coping and higher optimism (measured by the Life Orientation Test, developed by Scheier and Carver) ($r = +0.26$, $p < 0.01$, uncontrolled).

Two studies by Abdel-Khalek and colleagues also examined this relationship. In the first, Abdel-Khalek and Lester (2007) examined religiosity and optimism in 460 Kuwaiti and 275 American college students. Religiosity was measured with the usual single self-rated question with responses ranging from 0 to 10. Optimism was assessed using the Arabic Scale of Optimism and Pessimism. Optimism was higher in American students compared to Kuwaiti college students (56.5 vs. 52.0, $p = 0.001$). Religiosity was significantly and positively related to optimism in both Kuwaiti ($r = +0.25$, $p < 0.001$, uncontrolled) and American ($r = +0.22$, $p < 0.001$) students. In the second study, Abdel-Khalek and Naceur (2007) examined religiosity and optimism in 244 Algerian Muslim college students, using the same measures as above, finding that religiosity was related to optimism in women ($r = +0.25$, $p < 0.05$, uncontrolled), but not in men.

In a fourth study, Ahmed (2009) examined religiosity and character strengths (including hope/optimism) among 174 Muslim youth ages 18–25 in America. Religiosity (assessed with the 10-item Religious Commitment Inventory) was positively related to hope/optimism (r [phi] = +0.54) in a subset of highly religious Muslim youth (over three-quarters of the sample). Finally, as reviewed earlier, Tiliouine and colleagues (2009) examined religiosity and optimism in 2,909 adults from Algeria (about 50 % ages 18–25), administering a 16-item Islamic Religiosity Scale with religious practice and religious altruism subscales. A single question assessed optimism. Religious practice and religious altruism were both related to greater optimism ($r = +0.17$ and $r = +0.22$, respectively, $p < 0.005$, uncontrolled).

Recent Research. Since 2010, at least one additional study has addressed this topic. Khalad (2010) compared the optimism of Jordanian and American college students, also examining the relationship with religiosity. Participants were 260 Jordanians and 167 Americans (both mean age 20) enrolled in introductory psychology classes. Americans attended a public university in northwestern USA. A single question assessed religiosity, with responses ranging from "not religious at all" (1) to "highly religious" (4). Optimism was measured using the standard 10-item Life Orientation Test. Results indicated no difference in religiosity between Jordanians and Americans, although American students were more optimistic (15.8 vs. 14.0, $p < 0.01$). Further analyses revealed that although Americans expected fewer negative outcomes than Jordanians, both groups were equal in their expectations of positive outcome. Religiosity was not related to optimism in either Jordanians or Americans.

Summary. We found seven studies that examined the religiosity–optimism relationship in Muslim populations (Table 8.2). Of those, five (71 %) reported significantly greater optimism among those who were more religious. Three studies also compared optimism in Muslim and Christian populations (the US and UK), finding that American students were more optimistic than either Kuwaiti or Jordanian students, although Kuwaiti students were more optimistic than students in the UK.

Meaning and Purpose

In our 2010 systematic review we could find no studies in Muslim-majority countries that had examined the relationship between R/S and meaning/purpose.

Missed Studies. In our current review, we identified one study missed in the systematic review. Unfortunately, only the abstract was retrievable. In that study, Tiliouine and Belgoumidi (2009) surveyed 495 Muslim college students from Algeria (mean age 21). Researchers administered the 60-item Comprehensive Measure of Islamic Religiosity, and a measure of meaning in life. Although statistics of association were not given in the abstract, the authors indicated that religious belief and religious altruism were both significantly related to meaning in life. In fact, they indicated that the relationship between religiosity and personal well-being was almost entirely due to the relationship between religiosity and meaning in life.

Recent Research. At least two other studies since 2010 have now examined relationships with meaning and purpose in life. Aflakseir (2012) surveyed 60 Muslim students at the University of Southampton and Birmingham in England. Purpose in life was assessed using the Life Attitude Profile-Revised scale (Reker). Religiosity was assessed using the 6-item Strength of Spiritual Belief Scale and a single item assessing importance of religious beliefs in life. Purpose in life was associated with both spirituality ($r=+0.32$) and importance of religiosity ($r=+0.35$) (both $p<0.05$, uncontrolled). Personal meaning was also associated with both spirituality ($r=+0.35$) and religiosity ($r=+0.37$) (both $p<0.05$). In the second study, Lazenby and colleagues (2013) surveyed 205 cancer patients from Amman, Jordan (average age 48), administering the Arabic Functional Assessment of Chronic Illness Therapy-Spiritual Well-Being scale to assess mental health, meaning, and religious faith. This scale contains a peace subscale (mental health), a meaning/purpose in life subscale, and a faith subscale (religiosity). Meaning/purpose in life was significantly and positively correlated with religious faith ($r=+0.42$, $p=0.01$).

Summary. All three studies that have examined the relationship between religiosity and purpose/meaning in life in Muslims have found significant positive relationships (Table 8.2). The role that Islamic beliefs and practices play in giving those with medical illness a sense of meaning and purpose was underscored in a recent qualitative study of 19 Jordanian men with coronary artery disease. This study described how men's religious beliefs gave their illness meaning and purpose. First, religious beliefs helped them to see that the illness was a test of their obedience to God's will. Second, if they carried their burden of illness faithfully without complaint, the illness could help to compensate for sins and help purify their lives.

Self-Esteem

Self-esteem is important for Muslims just as it was for the Bedouin Arabs who existed before the emergence of Islam. A sense of pride and defense of one's honor, family, and tribe has long been highly valued in Arabic culture. For Muslims, self-esteem is a consequence of belief in and connection with God. Believing that God is on a person's side as long as he or she does good gives a person power to accomplish things in life. Self-esteem comes from practices such as prayer, helping the poor, and believing in the equality of all persons. Self-esteem is critical for mental health, and could help to explain the impact that Islamic beliefs and practice have on the well-being of Muslims.

Our systematic review identified three studies in Muslim-majority countries that examined relationships between R/S and self-esteem. First, Watson and colleagues (2002) surveyed 227 college students from Tehran, Iran (all Muslim) and 220 from the University of Tennessee (the majority Baptists and Methodists). The purpose was to examine relationships between religiosity, self-esteem, and other sociodemographic and health characteristics in each religious group. Religiosity was assessed using the Religious Orientation Scale (Allport), a measure of intrinsic and extrinsic religiosity. Self-esteem was measured using the standard scale in the field (Rosenberg). Intrinsic religiosity was significantly and positively related to self-esteem in the Iranian sample ($r = +0.35$, $p < 0.001$, uncontrolled) and in the American sample ($r = +0.34$, $p < 0.001$).

In a study reviewed earlier, Suhail and Chaudhry (2004) surveyed a random sample of 973 community-dwelling Pakistanis ages 16–80 (50 % female), assessing factors related to well-being, including religiosity and self-esteem. Religiosity was measured using an 18-item Islamic beliefs and practices scale, whereas self-esteem was assessed using the 10-item Rosenberg scale. Religiosity was not related to self-esteem ($r = +0.02$, $p = \text{ns}$) in that study.

Carlton-Ford and associates (2008) examined a random sample of 1,000 adolescents (ages 12–17) living in Baghdad following the U.S.-Iraq war of 2003, examining factors related to self-image and self-esteem. Religiosity was assessed using a single question that asked about whether faith was important on a 1–4 scale. Self-esteem was assessed using a 6-item version of the Rosenberg scale, which was divided into positive questions ("regard" or high esteem) and negative questions ("derogation" or low esteem). Religiosity was positively related to high self-esteem ($r = +0.16$, $p \leq 0.001$, uncontrolled) and inversely related to low self-esteem ($r = -0.10$, $p \leq 0.001$). In a multiple regression model that controlled for multiple other predictors, of all characteristics measured, religiosity (importance of faith) was the strongest predictor of high self-esteem ($B = +0.34$, $p < 0.001$).

Missed Studies. In the present review, we identified six additional studies missed by our 2010 review. First, Khan and Watson (2004) surveyed 121 Pakistani Muslims examining religiosity and self-esteem (mean age 28; 51 % female). Religious interest was assessed using a single item rated from 0 to 9, and religious motivation was measured using a 3-item intrinsic–extrinsic scale (Gorsuch). Self-esteem was assessed, as usual, with the 10-item Rosenberg scale. Intrinsic religiosity was positively associated with self-esteem ($r = +0.33$, $p < 0.001$) overall, but the association was primarily found in women ($r = +0.47$, $p < 0.001$, uncontrolled) and weakened in men ($r = +0.15$, $p = \text{ns}$).

French and colleagues (2008) examined religious involvement and self-esteem in 183 eighth and ninth grade Muslim adolescents in Indonesia (mean age 13).

Spirituality was assessed using a 19-item Daily Spiritual Experiences scale adapted from the standard 16-item scale of Underwood, and was administered to both adolescents and parents (who rated the adolescents on the scale). Religiosity of adolescents and parents was also assessed using a checklist of religious practices. Self-esteem, in turn, was measured using a set of adolescent self-competence scales (Harter). The results of a structural equation model indicated that religious involvement (based on reports by both adolescents and parents) was significantly and positively correlated with adolescent self-esteem.

Fanni Asl and colleagues (2008) analyzed data from 202 college students at Mohaghegh Ardabilli University in Iran, examining relationships between religiosity and self-esteem (only abstract available). Religiosity was assessed with the Nelson religious beliefs practice test, and self-esteem by the Rosenberg scale. Results again indicated a significant positive relationship between religious beliefs and practices and self-esteem ($p<0.05$, uncontrolled).

In a mixed methods study, Sirin and colleagues (2008) examined how Muslim Americans' identifications were correlated with religious practices and cultural adaptation. The sample was made up of 97 young adults ages 18–28, with a slight majority being female. Religiosity was assessed with a 6-item scale developed for the study that focused on religious activities and beliefs. Self-esteem was assessed using two religion-specific versions of the Collective Self-Esteem Scale (Luhtanen). Results indicated that religiosity was positively related to Muslim aspects of self-esteem ($r=+0.40$, $p<0.001$, uncontrolled), but not to American aspects of self-esteem.

Abu-Rayya and Abu-Rayya (2009) examined factors related to psychological well-being in 520 Muslim and 334 Christian Palestinian college students in Israel (mean age 24). Religious identity was assessed using the Multi-Religion Identity Measure, a scale developed by the authors. Self-esteem was again measured using the 10-item Rosenberg scale. Religious identification was positively related to self-esteem in both Muslim ($r=+0.52$, $p<0.001$, uncontrolled) and Christian ($r=+0.46$, $p<0.001$) students. In both groups, religious identification was even more strongly related to self-esteem than was ethnic identification.

Finally, Imam and colleagues (2009) surveyed 358 students at the International Islamic University of Malaysia (mean age 22, 87 % female), examining relationships between spiritual and psychological health. The 20-item Spiritual Well-Being (SWB) Scale (Palouzian), adapted for use in Muslims, was administered along with the 10-item Rosenberg self-esteem scale and other measures of well-being. The SWB scale consists of two 10-item subscales, a religious and an existential well-being subscale. Overall spiritual well-being and self-esteem did not differ between men and women. Controlling for age, gender, and education, religious well-being was positively associated with self-esteem (partial $r=+0.37$, $p<0.001$).

Recent Research. Several studies have examined relationships with self-esteem since our 2010 review. Azaiza and colleagues (2010) examined death and dying in 145 Arab Muslims age 60 or over living in Israel (two-thirds women). The sample was divided between community-dwelling adults (55 %) and nursing home patients (45 %). Religiosity was assessed using a single item that asked participants to categorize themselves as secular, traditional, religious, or very religious. Self-esteem was again measured using the 10-item Rosenberg scale. Although there was no relationship between religiosity and self-esteem in the overall sample, among nursing home patients religiosity was *inversely* related to self-esteem ($r = -0.22$, $p < 0.05$, uncontrolled). No explanation was given for this finding, although nursing home patients with low self-esteem may have been more likely to turn to religion for comfort.

Next, Ghaffari and Ciftci (2010) surveyed 174 Muslim immigrants to the USA (ages 18–61), examining religious behaviors and attitudes, perceived discrimination, and self-esteem. Religious practices were assessed using a 3-item scale (prayer, service attendance, self-rated religiosity), and religious attitudes were measured using the 14-item MARS. Self-esteem was assessed using the standard Rosenberg scale. In this study, self-esteem was not related to either religious attitudes or behavior. However, *perceived discrimination* appeared to moderate the relationship between religiosity and self-esteem. For both religious behaviors and attitudes, the relationship with self-esteem was positive among those with low perceived discrimination and negative for those with high perceived discrimination.

In another related study, Friedman and Saroglou (2010) surveyed 273 Muslims in Belgium (mean age 22; 81 % second-generation immigrants; 53 % women), examining religiosity, acculturation, religious intolerance, and self-esteem. For comparison, a group of 155 Christian immigrants (mean age 22; 60 % second-generation immigrants; 61 % women) was also examined. Religiosity was assessed using an 8-item intrinsic religiosity scale (Gorsuch). Self-esteem was again assessed using the Rosenberg scale. Results indicated that intrinsic religiosity was significantly higher in Muslims compared to Christians (41.3 vs. 30.5, $p < 0.001$, uncontrolled), and self-esteem was also significantly higher in Muslims (33.4 vs. 32.1, $p < 0.01$). Intrinsic religiosity, however, was not related to self-esteem in either Muslims or non-Muslims. A bootstrapping method was used to examine indirect effects. When this was done, religiosity had a significant *negative* total indirect effect on self-esteem in Muslims acting through perceived religious tolerance and feelings of anger toward the host society ($M = -0.03$, 95 % CI −0.05 to −0.02).

To our knowledge, only one longitudinal study has examined religiosity and self-esteem in Muslims. Sallquist and colleagues (2010) assessed a group of 136 Muslim adolescents (mean age 14, 44 % female) in Indonesia at T1 (baseline), T2 (7 months later), and T3 (16 months after T2). At T2, religiosity was assessed by having both parents and adolescents rate the consistency of adolescents' religious behaviors in eight areas. Spirituality was also assessed by having parents and adolescents complete a 19-item revised version of the Daily Spiritual Experiences scale (Underwood). Self-esteem (cognitive and global) was assessed at T3 using standard measures. Results indicated that adolescent religiosity at T2 predicted greater cognitive self-esteem ($r = +0.31$, $p < 0.01$, uncontrolled) and marginally greater global self-esteem ($r = +0.10$, $p = \text{ns}$) at T3. Likewise, T2 adolescent spirituality predicted cognitive self-esteem ($r = +0.19$, $p < 0.05$) and global self-esteem

($r = +0.15$, $0.05 < p < 0.10$) at T3. Structural equation modeling found that T2 religiosity/spirituality (R/S) was positively related to T1 self-esteem (baseline) but not to T3 self-esteem on follow-up.

Abdel-Khalek has conducted two studies examining religiosity and self-esteem. In the first, Abdel-Khalek (2011b) explored relationships between religiosity, well-being, and self-esteem in 499 Muslim adolescents in Kuwait (50 % female, average age 17). Religiosity and religious belief were assessed using single items that were self-rated from 0 to 10. Self-esteem was again measured using the Rosenberg scale. Religiosity and strength of religious belief were both positively associated with self-esteem ($r = +0.49$ and $r = +0.50$, respectively, $p < 0.01$, uncontrolled). In the second study, Abdel-Khalek (2012c) analyzed data from two samples of college students, one from Egypt ($n = 577$) and one from Kuwait ($n = 674$). Religiosity was assessed using a single self-rated item ranging from 0 to 10, and self-esteem by the Rosenberg scale. Again, a stepwise regression model demonstrated that religiosity was independently related to greater self-esteem.

Summary. Although our systematic review only identified three studies, two of which found greater self-esteem in Muslims who were more religious, the present review identified six additional studies published prior to 2010 and six more studies published since 2010. Thus, a total of 15 studies were identified. Of those, 11 (73 %) found significant positive relationships between religiosity and self-esteem, two found significant negative relationships, one reported mixed results, and one reported no association (Table 8.2). In the study that found mixed results (Muslim immigrants to USA) the relationship between religiosity and self-esteem was moderated by perceived discrimination. In the study that examined Muslim immigrants to Belgium, the inverse relationship between religiosity and self-esteem was indirect, acting through perceived religious intolerance and feelings of anger toward the host society.

Sense of Control

Locus of control (LOC) is a concept that has to do with a person's sense of control in life. LOC is divided into two types: internal (where the individual feels in control of his or her life) and external (where the individual feels life is controlled by external agents, such as the government or powerful other people). As noted in Chap. 6, an internal LOC is known to be associated with better mental health (and external LOC with worse mental health). Our 2010 systematic review uncovered two studies that examined R/S and LOC in Muslims, one in a Muslim country (Iran) and one in Israel.

In the first study, Mohammadi and Honarmand (2007) surveyed 179 Muslim college students in Tehran, Iran (54 % male). Only the abstract was available, which limits our description. LOC was measured using Rotter's Locus of Control Scale (the standard measure of LOC in the field). The authors reported a significant positive relationship between religiosity and internal LOC in women, but not in men. Women were more religious than men, but men scored higher on internal LOC than did women.

In the second study, Cohen and Azaiza (2007) surveyed a random sample of 358 Jews and 162 Muslim Arabs ages 50–75 living in Israel, examining factors related to health LOC in these two populations. Arab respondents were younger, had more children, and had less education and lower financial status than Jews. The 11-item Health Locus of Control Scale (Wallston) was used to assess participants' sense of control over their health (5 questions assessing internal control and six questions assessing external control). Religiosity was measured using a single question that had respondents self-categorize themselves into one of four groups ranging from secular to very religious. In the combined group of Arabs and Jews, there was no relationship between religiosity and internal LOC, but religiosity was related to a higher external LOC ($r = +0.10$, $p < 0.05$, uncontrolled). Arabs scored significantly higher than Jews on external LOC. When analyses were controlled for gender, age, education, and economic status, however, the relationship between religiosity and external LOC disappeared (i.e., was explained largely by education level).

Missed Studies. We also identified several additional studies missed in our 2010 review. Although none examined relationships between LOC and religiosity, they did compare LOC between Muslims and non-Muslims.

In the first study, Lester and colleagues (1991) compared LOC (Rotter scale), depression, and suicidal ideation between American (Christian), Philippine (Christian), and Turkish (Muslim) college students. External LOC was significantly higher in American and Turkish students compared to Philippine students ($F = 15.8$, $p < 0.0001$), meaning that students from the Philippines demonstrated greater internal LOC than students in either of the two other groups. In addition, consistent with previous research, having a higher external LOC was associated with a greater likelihood of considering suicide in the Turkish students.

Next, Khayyer (2000) surveyed 210 Muslim and 2010 Jewish school students ages 11–14 living in Iran. Students were matched on gender, education, age, and father's education. LOC was measured using the Nowicki-Strickland Scale for Children. Researchers found no difference in internal or external LOC between Muslim and Jewish students.

In a third study, Arslan (2001) interviewed 277 business managers concerning the Protestant Work Ethic (PWE), one component of which was an internal LOC (based on agreement with the two statements "Most people who do not succeed in life are just plain lazy" and "People who fail at a job have usually not tried hard"). Religious affiliations of the managers were 100 Protestants (from Great Britain), 103 Catholics (Ireland), and 74 Muslims (Turkey). LOC was compared between religious groups. Results indicated that Muslim managers scored significantly higher on internal LOC than either Protestant or Catholic managers ($p < 0.001$).

In a fourth study, Ghorbani and colleagues (2004) compared LOC and other psychological factors between 325 university students from Tehran, Iran (Muslim), and 401 university students from Chattanooga, Tennessee (Christian). LOC was measured using three Multidimensional Locus of Control Scales (MLCS; Levenson), which included internal control, chance control, and powerful others control. Results indicated that scores on internal control, chance control, and powerful others control were all significantly higher in Iranians than in Americans, especially chance control ($F=13.3$, $p<0.001$, uncontrolled). Cultural interpretation of the questions on this scale, however, may have influenced responses.

Finally, Srnka and colleagues (2007) examined the impact that moral reasoning had on ethically problematic business situations among 60 students enrolled in marketing and accounting classes in Austria (Christian) and 60 students in Turkey (Muslim) (most age 20–25). One category of arguments in moral reasoning involved an internal LOC (defined as "considering whether a person has the free choice of acting morally or immorally"). An internal LOC was less likely to be used by students in Turkey (0.7 %) than among students in Austria (1.7 %), and mean scores of LOC were significantly lower in students from Turkey compared to those from Austria (0.10 vs. 0.25, $p<0.05$, uncontrolled).

Recent Research. Our current review identified three additional studies on this topic published since 2010, two examining religiosity and LOC in Muslims and one comparing LOC in Muslims and non-Muslims.

The first study was complex and hard to follow, but we attempt to describe it here. Khan and colleagues (2011) surveyed 159 hospitalized Pakistani patients (mean age 48) with diabetes, cancer, or heart disease, and a healthy control group of 163 persons (mean age 28) selected from the university and broader community. Religious interest was assessed using a single question with responses ranging from 0 to 6, and religious orientation by a 3-item intrinsic–extrinsic religiosity scale (Gorsuch). Religious coping was measured using a 14-item scale (Islamic Positive Religious Coping and Identification Scale) made up of three dimensions (positive Islamic coping, Islamic identification, and extra-prayer commitment). In addition, negative religious coping was assessed using a 3-item Punishing Allah Reappraisal scale. The MLCS (Levenson) was used to assess internal, chance, and powerful others control. The General Health Questionnaire (GHQ) and a 5-item life satisfaction scale (LSS) assessed emotional functioning. A factor analysis of responses on the MLCS, GHQ, and LSS identified three factors: poor psychological functioning, external LOC, and life satisfaction/internal LOC (which we will call internal LOC).

Uncontrolled analyses using the combined sample of cases and controls ($n=322$) indicated no relationship between positive Islamic coping, Islamic identification, or intrinsic religiosity and either an external or internal LOC. However, extra-prayer commitment and religious interest were both positively associated with an external LOC, as was the Punishing Allah Reappraisal subscale ($r=+0.20$, $p<0.001$, uncontrolled). No religious measures were associated with an internal LOC, except Punishing Allah Reappraisal, which was inversely related to it ($r=-0.18$, $p<0.001$). Separate analyses in patients and in controls that adjusted for age and employment found that in neither group was positive Islamic coping related to internal or external LOC. Punishing God Reappraisal, while unrelated to either internal or external LOC in patients, was positively related to external LOC ($B = +0.23$, $p < 0.01$) and inversely related to internal LOC ($B = -0.28$, $p < 0.001$) in healthy controls.

In the second study, Cirhinlioglu and Ozdikmenli-Demi (2012) examined relationships between religious orientation, LOC, and depressive symptom in 430 Muslim college students from Turkey. Details are minimal given that only the study abstract was available to us. Researchers reported results based on hierarchical regression analyses stratified by gender. In both men and women, intrinsic religiosity was positively related to belief in fate, but negatively related to belief in chance. In women, intrinsic religiosity was inversely related to belief in "the meaningless effort," which was interpreted as indicating that intrinsically religious women were more likely to feel that individual effort was meaningful, suggesting an internal LOC. Extrinsic religiosity, in turn, was positively related to belief in fate among both men and women, but not to other LOC measures.

In the final study, Zulfikar (2012) compared internal LOC in Muslims and Christians who were working in the USA. Muslims ($n = 96$) were recruited from various national Turkish organizations. Christians (313 Protestants, 86 Catholic, 128 other, and 180 "none") were recruited from the faculty and staff of the University of North Carolina at Chapel Hill. Internal LOC, assessed by a 5-item subscale, was one of five factors that made up a Protestant Work Ethic (PWE) scale. In comparing scores on each of the five internal LOC items between those with no affiliation, Catholics, Protestants, and Muslims, Muslims scored the highest on all five internal LOC items (with the difference being statistically significant on most of them). In fact, Muslims scored the highest on the PWE overall, even higher than Protestants.

Summary. More work is needed in Muslim populations on the relationship between religiosity and LOC. So far, the research shows a range of findings with little consistency. In the four studies of religiosity and LOC in Muslims, each reported a different finding: one found a positive relationship with internal LOC, one with external LOC, one reported mixed findings, and one found no association (Table 8.2). When comparing Muslims with other religious groups, the results depend on how LOC was measured. When internal LOC was measured as a component of the PWE, Muslims scored higher on internal LOC than Christians (and even higher than Protestants). When measured using more traditional LOC scales, Muslims tended to score higher on external LOC or there was no difference between Muslims and other religious groups. However, bear in mind that positive correlations between religiosity and an external LOC in Muslims or higher scores by Muslims (vs. non-Muslims) on external LOC may result from how questions on external LOC scales are interpreted. Belief that God is in control of events or belief in destiny (fate), strong teachings in Islam, may be used as indicators of an external LOC in some scales. We would argue that positive responses to questions like these do not necessarily reflect an external LOC as understood in the West. In the West, external LOC is the view that powerful other people control a person's future and that the individual is helpless to do anything about it, which is known to be associated with poor mental health and maladjustment.

Personality Traits

Personality traits are enduring, long-standing patterns of relating to self and others. "Character" traits are sometimes used synonymously with "personality" traits. We will use the term personality traits here. As noted in the last chapter, the most common way that personality traits are measured today is by the NEO Personality Inventory. The NEO assesses the "Big Five" personality traits: extraversion, neuroticism, conscientiousness, agreeableness, and openness. Personality traits may also be measured using the Eysenck Personality Inventory (especially in Europe) that assesses personality extremes along a continuum of introversion vs. extroversion, neuroticism vs. stability, and psychoticism vs. socialization. Other personality measures are also used, and these vary depending on how personality is defined. We focus here on the traits measured using the NEO and Eysenck personality inventories, and on qualitative reports when they are available.

Extraversion

Extraverted people tend to be more outgoing, talkative, and energetic in social situations. Our 2010 systematic review uncovered two studies that examined relationships between R/S and extraversion in Muslim-majority populations.

In the first study, Nielsen and Stevens (2001) surveyed 62 Malaysian Muslim college students (mean age 21). Half of the sample were asked to identify the most important religious experience they had ever had and the other half were asked to identify the most important spiritual experience. Participants were then asked to describe how they felt during these experiences by having them choose from a list of 80 seven-point semantic differentials (adjectives) based on Costa and McCrae's "Big Five" personality traits. There were significant differences on personality traits experienced during religious experiences compared to how they felt during spiritual experiences. Respondents indicated that they felt more extraverted, more stable (less neurotic), and more open during religious experiences compared to how respondents felt during spiritual experiences (all statistically significant, uncontrolled). There was also a trend for respondents to feel more agreeable during religious (vs. spiritual) experiences ($p=0.08$). Although this study did not examine the relationship between religiosity and these personality traits per se, the findings give some indication on how religiosity might affect these traits.

In the second study, one that was reviewed earlier, Suhail and Chaudhry (2004) surveyed 973 persons aged 16–80 living in Lahore, Pakistan. Religiosity was assessed using an 18-item measure of Islamic beliefs and practices. Personality was assessed using the extraversion subscale of the Eysenck Personality Inventory. Religiosity was unrelated to scores on the extraversion subscale.

Missed Studies. Our current review also uncovered two studies missed in our 2010 systematic review. In the first study, Wilde and Joseph (1997) examined relationships between scores on the MARS and extraversion as measured by the Eysenck Personality Inventory in 50 Muslim college students at the University of Essex in England. After controlling for gender and age, no association was found between religiosity and extraversion. In the second study, Aguilar-Vafaie and Moghanloo (2008) examined personality traits and religiosity in 359 Iranian college students at Tarbiat Modarres University in Tehran. Religiosity was assessed using the Islamic Religious Orientation Scale (IROS) made up of Creeds/Rituals and Morals subscales. The Revised NEO Personality Inventory assessed personality traits. Both IROS subscales (Creeds/Rituals and Morals) were significantly and positively associated with extraversion ($r=+0.25$ and $r=+0.24$, respectively, $p<0.001$, uncontrolled).

Recent Research. Since our 2010 review, several other studies have examined relationships between extraversion and religiosity. Salmanpour and Issazadegan (2012) surveyed 484 university students at AZAD University of Naqadeh in Iran (mean age 25, equally divided by gender). Relationships between personality, religious involvement, and other psychological characteristics were examined. The 21-item intrinsic–extrinsic religiosity scale (Allport & Ross) was administered along with the 60-item NEO Personality Inventory. Intrinsic religiosity (in this study, low scores indicated high intrinsic religiosity) was inversely correlated with extraversion ($r=-0.23$, $p<0.01$, uncontrolled), meaning that greater intrinsic religiosity was associated with greater extraversion. Extrinsic religiosity (high scores indicating high extrinsic religiosity) had a weak positive relationship with extraversion ($r=+0.09$, $p<0.05$), such that higher extrinsic religiosity was associated with higher extraversion.

Aghababaei (2012) examined religiousness and two personality scales, a 50-item NEO Personality Inventory and the 60-item HEXACO Personality Inventory, in 190 students at the University of Tehran, Iran (67 % female, average age 21). Religious interest (single self-rated scale 0–9) and religious orientation (3-item measure, Gorsuch) were both assessed. Correlational analyses (uncontrolled) revealed no relationship between either religious interest or religious orientation and extraversion on the NEO or HEXACO inventories. In a second report from a larger sample of 1,000 Iranian college students (four different samples combined), Aghababaei (2013) examined the same relationships, except focused on the NEO Personality Inventory. Religious measures included a 14-item measure of religious orientation (Gorsuch), a single-item measure of religious orientation, a single item measure of religious interest, and a 4-item Gratitude to God scale. Again, no religious measures were associated with extraversion.

Finally, Abdel-Khalek (2013b) administered the Eysenck Personality Inventory and the 14-item MARS to 227 Kuwaiti Muslim college students (mean age 20, equally divided by gender). Islamic religiosity was positively correlated with extraversion in women ($r=+0.24$, $p<0.001$, uncontrolled), but not in men.

Summary. Thus, seven studies have examined relationships between religiosity and extraversion, six out of those in college students. Three of seven studies reported positive relationships between religiosity and greater extraversion (similar to the 39 % of studies in Christians that reported positive associations). One additional study reported that Muslim college students felt more extraverted during religious experiences than during spiritual experiences (Table 8.3).

Table 8.3 Religiosity and personality traits in Muslims

Authors (year)	Method	Sample size	Participants	Location	Controls	Findings
Extraversion						
Wilde and Joseph (1997)	CS	50	University students (Muslim)	England	SC	NA
Nielsen and Stevens (2001)	CS	62	University students	Malaysia	None (?)	P (?)
Suhail and Chaudhry (2004)	CS	973	Adults ages 18–80	Pakistan	None	NA
Aguilar-Vafaie and Moghanloo (2008)	CS	359	University students	Iran	None	P
Salmanpour and Issazadegan (2012)	CS	484	University students	Iran	None	P
Aghababaei (2012)	CS	190	University students	Iran	None	NA
Aghababaei (2013)	CS	1,000	University students	Iran	None	NA
Abdel-Khalek (2013a)	CS	227	University students	Kuwait	None	P (females)
Neuroticism						
Wilde and Joseph (1997)	CS	50	University students (Muslim)	England	SC	NA
Nielsen and Stevens (2001)	CS	62	University students	Malaysia	None (?)	P (?)
Aguilar-Vafaie and Moghanloo (2008)	CS	359	University students	Iran	None	P
Abdel-Khalek (2010)	CS	487	University students	Kuwait	None	P
Salmanpour and Issazadegan (2012)	CS	484	University students	Iran	None	NA
Aghababaei (2012)	CS	190	University students	Iran	None	NA
Aghababaei (2013)	CS	1,000	University students	Iran	None	P
Abdel-Khalek (2013a)	CS	227	University students	Kuwait	None	P (females)
Conscientiousness						
Nielsen and Stevens (2001)	CS	62	University students	Malaysia	None (?)	NA (?)
Aguilar-Vafaie and Moghanloo (2008)	CS	359	University students	Iran	None	P
Salmanpour and Issazadegan (2012)	CS	484	University students	Iran	None	P
Aghababaei (2012)	CS	190	University students	Iran	None	P
Aghababaei (2013)	CS	1,000	University students	Iran	None	P

(continued)

Table 8.3 (continued)

Authors (year)	Method	Sample size	Participants	Location	Controls	Findings
Agreeableness						
Nielsen and Stevens (2001)	CS	62	University students	Malaysia	None (?)	P (?)
Aguilar-Vafaie and Moghanloo (2008)	CS	359	University students	Iran	None	P
Aghababaei (2012)	CS	190	University students	Iran	None	P
Aghababaei (2013)	CS	1,000	University students	Iran	None	P
Salmanpour and Issazadegan (2012)	CS	484	University students	Iran	None	P
Openness to new experiences						
Nielsen and Stevens (2001)	CS	62	University students	Malaysia	None (?)	P (?)
Aguilar-Vafaie and Moghanloo (2008)	CS	359	University students	Iran	None	P
Salmanpour and Issazadegan (2012)	CS	484	University students	Iran	None	NA
Aghababaei (2012)	CS	190	University students	Iran	None	NA
Aghababaei (2013)	CS	1,000	University students	Iran	None	P

CS cross-sectional, *P* prospective, *NA* no association, *P* significant positive association with extraversion, agreeableness, conscientiousness, or openness to experiences, or significant negative correlation with neuroticism, *MC* multiple controls, *SC* some controls

Neuroticism

Neurotic persons tend to be characterized by a long-standing pattern of anxiety, moodiness, worry, and shyness, and respond poorly to stress. Our 2010 systematic review uncovered only one study that touched on the relationship between religiosity and neuroticism in Muslims. As noted earlier, Malaysian college students who were more religious reported being more stable (less neurotic) during religious experiences compared to how they felt during spiritual experiences (Nielsen and Stevens 2001).

Missed Studies. In our current review, however, two additional studies were found. These were both reviewed under extraversion. Wilde and Joseph (1997) found no associations between religiosity (assessed using the MARS) and neuroticism as measured using the Eysenck Personality Inventory in Muslim college students in England. The second study by Aguilar-Vafaie and Moghanloo (2008) in 359 Iranian college students found that neuroticism measured by the NEO Personality Inventory was inversely related to Islamic Creeds/Rituals ($r=-0.18$, $p<0.001$, uncontrolled) and even more strongly inversely related to Islamic Morals ($r=-0.42$, $p<0.001$).

Recent Research. With regard to research conducted since 2010, the same four studies that assessed religiosity and extraversion cited above also examined relationships with neuroticism. One additional study examined neuroticism only (Abdel-Khalek 2010).

Abdel-Khalek (2010) assessed religiosity and personality in 487 Kuwaiti college students using both the NEO Personality Inventory and the Factorial Arabic Neuroticism Scale (FANS). Religiosity was assessed using two questions, a self-rated religiosity item ranging from 0 to10 and a self-rated strength of religious belief item ranging from 0 to 10. Results indicated that both religiosity and strength of religious belief were inversely related to neuroticism on the NEO ($r=-0.13$, $p<0.005$ and $r=-0.22$, $p<0.0001$) and on the FANS ($r=-0.14$, $p<0.005$ and $r=-0.25$, $p<0.0001$, uncontrolled).

In their study of 484 Iranian college students, Salmanpour and Issazadegan (2012) reported that intrinsic and extrinsic religiosity were both unrelated to neuroticism assessed using the NEO. Likewise, Aghababaei (2012), in his study of 190 Iranian college students, found no relationship between neuroticism (assessed by the NEO) and religious interest, intrinsic religiosity, or extrinsic religiosity, but did find a significant positive relationship between neuroticism/emotionality (assessed using the HEXACO) and extrinsic religiosity-personal type ($r=+0.24$, $p<0.01$, uncontrolled). In the second report by Aghababaei (2013) involving four samples of Iranian students, he reported an inverse relationship between intrinsic religiosity and neuroticism ($r=-0.15$, $p<0.01$, uncontrolled) in Sample 1 ($n=300$), no relationship in Sample 2 ($n=181$), and inverse relationships in Sample 3 ($n=197$) and in Sample 4 ($n=322$) between Gratitude to God and neuroticism ($r=-0.23$ and $r=-0.16$, both $p<0.01$). Finally, Abdel-Khalek (2013b) reported an inverse relationship between religiosity and neuroticism in women Kuwaiti college students ($r=-0.31$, $p<0.05$, uncontrolled), but not in men.

Summary. Thus, four of seven studies (all in college students) found lower neuroticism in Muslims who were more religious, and three found no association (Table 8.3). One additional study reported that Muslim college students felt more stable (less neurotic) during religious experiences than during spiritual experiences. The percentage of studies in Muslims reporting an inverse relationship (57 %) with neuroticism is higher than that in studies reported among Christians (24 %).

Conscientiousness

Conscientious individuals tend to be efficient, goal oriented, well organized, careful, and self-disciplined. Only one study identified in our 2010 systematic review examined religiosity and conscientiousness in Muslims (Nielsen and Stevens 2001). However, while this study in Malaysian college students likely examined the relationship (i.e., how students felt during religious compared to spiritual experiences), they did not discuss the results in the paper, probably because there was no difference.

Missed Studies. Our current review identified one study missed in our 2010 review. In a study reviewed above, Aguilar-Vafaie and Moghanloo (2008) examined religiosity (IROS) and personality (NEO) in 359 Iranian college students. They reported a strong positive correlation between conscientiousness and Islamic Creeds/Rituals ($r=+0.32$, $p<0.001$) and Islamic Morals ($r=+0.50$, $p<0.001$).

Recent Research. Since our 2010 systematic review, at least three additional studies have now examined relationships between religiosity and conscientiousness in Muslims. We already described those studies when discussing other personality traits above. In the first one, Aghababaei (2012) examined personality (assessed with NEO and HEXACO) and religiosity (3-item I-E scale of Gorsuch and religious interest question) in 190 Iranian college students, finding that conscientiousness measured by the NEO was positively related to religious interest ($r=+0.22$, $p<0.01$, uncontrolled), intrinsic religiosity ($r=+0.21$, $p<0.01$), and extrinsic religiosity-P (personal type) ($r=+0.14$, $p<0.05$). When conscientiousness was measured using the HEXACO inventory, however, the only relationship present was found with extrinsic religiosity-S (social type) ($r=-0.14$, $p<0.05$, uncontrolled).

In Aghababaei's (2013) second report involving four subsamples of Iranian college students, where personality was measured only with the NEO, conscientiousness was again positively associated with intrinsic religiosity ($r=+0.24$, $p<0.01$) and extrinsic religiosity-P ($r=+0.26$, $p<0.01$) in Sample 1 ($n=300$). These relationships with conscientiousness were also present in Sample 2 ($n=181$) ($r=+0.21$, $p<0.01$, and $r=+0.14$, $p<0.05$, respectively), plus there was a positive association with religious interest ($r=+0.22$, $p<0.01$). Conscientiousness was also positively associated with Gratitude to God scores in Sample 3 ($n=197$) ($r=+0.27$, $p<0.01$) and in Sample 4 ($n=322$) ($r=+0.30$, $p<0.01$).

Finally, Salmanpour and Issazadegan (2012), in their study of 484 Iranian college students, also reported a strong negative relationship between intrinsic religiosity ($r = -0.34$, $p < 0.01$, uncontrolled) and conscientiousness (meaning greater IR was associated with greater conscientiousness) and no relationship was found between conscientiousness and extrinsic religiosity.

Summary. We identified five studies that have examined relationship between religiosity and conscientiousness in Muslims, again all conducted in college students and none controlling for other influential variables (Table 8.3). Four of the five reported significant positive relationships between religiosity and conscientiousness (similar to the two-thirds of studies that found positive relationships in Christian populations).

Agreeableness

Individuals characterized by agreeableness tend to be cooperative, kind, sympathetic, warm, and considerate toward others. Our 2010 systematic review uncovered no studies that examined the relationship with religiosity and agreeableness, except that Nielsen and Stevens (2001) found that Muslims tended to report feeling more agreeable during religious experiences compared to how they felt during spiritual experiences.

Missed Studies. We missed one study, and that was Aguilar-Vafaie and Moghanloo's (2008) study of Iranian college students. These researchers found robust positive correlations between agreeableness and both Islamic Creed/Rituals ($r = +0.25$) and Islamic Morals ($r = +0.53$) ($p < 0.001$, uncontrolled).

Recent Research. Since 2010 at least three studies (all described above) have examined relationships with agreeableness. Salmanpour and Issazadegan (2012) study in Iranian college students found that intrinsic religiosity was inversely related to agreeableness ($r = -0.16$, $p < 0.01$) (meaning that intrinsic religiosity was positively correlated with agreeableness), whereas no relationship was found with extrinsic religiosity. Aghababaei's (2012) study of 190 Iranian college students found no association between intrinsic religiosity and agreeableness, but did find a positive relationship between agreeableness and religious interest ($r = +0.25$, $p < 0.01$) and extrinsic religiosity-P ($r = +0.19$, $p < 0.01$). In Aghababaei's second report (2013) involving Iranian college students in four separate samples, intrinsic religiosity and extrinsic religiosity-P were both positively related to agreeableness in Sample 1 ($r = +0.24$ and $r = +0.19$, $p < 0.01$); religious interest and extrinsic religiosity-P were both positively related to agreeableness in Sample 2 ($r = +0.26$ and $r = +0.18$, respectively, both $p < 0.01$); and Gratitude to God was positively related to agreeableness in both Sample 3 and Sample 4 ($r = +0.44$ and $r = +0.23$, respectively, $p < 0.01$).

Summary. At least five studies have examined relationships between religiosity and agreeableness, all in college students. All five reported significant positive relationships, although none controlled for possible confounders (Table 8.3). Again, these findings are similar to those in Christians where 86 % of studies found positive relationships.

Openness to Experience

Those who score high on this trait tend to have active imaginations, prefer variety, are more curious, and prefer new experiences to familiar routines or traditional ways of life. In Christian populations, there is a slight tendency for this trait to characterize the "spiritual but not religious" group, i.e., those who reject traditional religion in favor of a more self-defined, individualized spirituality.

The only study identified in our 2010 systematic review was the Nielsen and Stevens (2001) study, which found (interestingly) that Malaysian Muslim college students felt more open to new experiences during religious experiences than during spiritual experiences.

Missed Studies. One additional study, as noted above, examined this relationship in 359 Iranian college students (Aguilar-Vafaie and Moghanloo 2008). Investigators found that openness to experience was unrelated to Islamic Creeds/Rituals but was positively related to Islamic Morals ($r = +0.12$, $p < 0.05$).

Recent Research. Since our 2010 systematic review, at least three additional studies (as described above) have examined relationships with openness. Salmanpour and Issazadegan's (2012) study of 484 Iranian college students found that intrinsic religiosity was unrelated to openness and extrinsic religiosity was negatively related to it ($r = -0.18$, $p < 0.01$). In his study of 190 Iranian college students, Aghababaei (2012) also found that interest in religion and intrinsic religiosity were unrelated to openness whether it was measured by the NEO or by the HEXACO Personality Inventory. Likewise, extrinsic religiosity-P was not related to openness on either the NEO or the HEXACO, although extrinsic religiosity-S was weakly inversely related to openness on the NEO ($r = -0.14$, $p < 0.05$) and on the HEXACO ($r = -0.16$, $p < 0.05$). In Aghababaei's (2013) second report on Iranian students, again extrinsic religiosity-S was inversely related to openness ($r = -0.11$, $p < 0.05$) in Sample 1; interest in religion (but no other religious characteristics) was positively related to openness in Sample 2 ($r = +0.17$, $p < 0.05$); and Gratitude to God was positively related to openness in Sample 3 ($n = 197$, $r = +0.16$, $p < 0.05$) but not Sample 4.

Summary. Thus, five studies have examined relationships between religiosity and openness to experience in Muslims. Excluding relationships with extrinsic religiosity, two of the four studies found significant positive relationships with religiosity (although weak) and two found no association (Table 8.3). One additional study reported that Muslim college students in Malaysia felt more open during religious experiences than during spiritual experiences. Again, these findings are not greatly different than reported in Christian populations where 42 % of studies found positive relationships between religiosity and openness.

Other Personality Traits

Other personality traits include schizotypal (difficulty establishing and maintaining close interpersonal relationships), authoritarianism (showing respect for authority and social conventions), and certain positive personality traits (self-regulation, kindness, warmth, prudence, etc.). Studies in Muslims have shown that religiosity is positively associated with a right-wing authoritarian personality (Ji and Ibrahaim 2007) (as is in Christian populations), with personality traits such as kindness, self-regulation, and prudence (Ahmed 2009), and with lower scores on schizotypal personality (Johnstone and Tiliopoulos 2008).

Summary and Conclusions

Just as religiosity is related to fewer negative emotions and less emotional disorder in Muslims, it is also associated with more positive emotions and healthier psychological traits. This means greater well-being and happiness, greater optimism, more of a sense of meaning and purpose in life, higher self-esteem, and more positive personality traits such as lower neuroticism, greater conscientiousness, more agreeableness, and more openness to new experiences. These associations are similar to those found in Christian populations. In Muslim populations, however, there is less research and less consensus on findings with regard to hope and sense of personal control. Most of these studies are cross-sectional in design, few control for important confounding variables, and few prospectively examine how religiosity influences the experience of positive emotions over time. Furthermore, no randomized clinical trials have yet examined whether religious interventions might actually increase psychological well-being and other positive emotions in Muslims. Much further research, then, is needed. We now turn to the question of whether deeply religious Muslims also experience better social and community health.

References

Abdel-Khalek, A. M. (2006). Happiness, health, and religiosity: Significant relations. *Mental Health, Religion and Culture, 9*(1), 85–97.

Abdel-Khalek, A. M. (2007). Religiosity, happiness, health, and psychopathology in a probability sample of Muslim adolescents. *Mental Health, Religion and Culture, 10*(6), 571–583.

Abdel-Khalek, A. M. (2008). Religiosity, health, and well-being among Kuwaiti personnel. *Psychological Reports, 102*(1), 181–184.

Abdel-Khalek, A. M. (2009). Religiosity, subjective well-being, and depression in Saudi children and adolescents. *Mental Health, Religion and Culture, 12*, 803–815.

Abdel-Khalek, A. M. (2010). Religiosity, subjective well-being, and neuroticism. *Mental Health, Religion and Culture, 13*, 67–79.

Abdel-Khalek, A. M. (2011a). Subjective well-being and religiosity in Egyptian college students. *Psychological Reports, 108*, 54–58.
Abdel-Khalek, A. M. (2011b). Religiosity, subjective well-being, self-esteem, anxiety among Kuwaiti Muslim adolescents. *Mental Health, Religion and Culture, 14*, 129–140.
Abdel-Khalek, A. M. (2012a). Subjective well-being and religiosity: A cross-sectional study with adolescents, young and middle-age adults. *Mental Health, Religion and Culture, 15*(1), 39–52.
Abdel-Khalek, A. M. (2012b). Happiness, health, and religiosity: significant association among Lebanese adolescents. *Mental Health, Religion and Culture.* E-pub ahead of print.
Abdel-Khalek, A. M. (2012c). Associations between religiosity, mental health, and subjective well-being among Arabic samples from Egypt and Kuwait. *Mental Health, Religion and Culture, 15*(8), 741–758.
Abdel-Khalek, A. M. (2013a). The relationships between subjective well-being, health, and religiosity among young adults from Qatar. *Mental Health, Religion and Culture, 16*(3), 306–318.
Abdel-Khalek, A. M. (2013b). Personality dimensions and religiosity among Kuwait Muslim college students. *Personality and Individual Differences, 54*, 149–152.
Abdel-Khalek, A. M., & Eid, G. K. (2011). Religiosity and its association with subjective well-being and depression among Kuwaiti and Palestinian Muslim children and adolescents. *Mental Health, Religion and Culture, 14*(2), 117–127.
Abdel-Khalek, A. M., & Lester, D. (2007). Religiosity, health, and psychopathology in two cultures: Kuwait and USA. *Mental Health, Religion and Culture, 10*(5), 537–550.
Abdel-Khalek, A. M., & Lester, D. (2010). Personal and psychological correlates of happiness among a sample of Kuwaiti Muslim students. *Journal of Muslim Mental Health, 5*, 194–209.
Abdel-Khalek, A. M., & Maltby, J. (2008). The comparison of predictors of death obsession within two cultures. *Death Studies, 32*(4), 366–377.
Abdel-Khalek, A. M., & Naceur, F. (2007). Religiosity and its association with positive and negative emotions among college students from Algeria. *Mental Health, Religion and Culture, 10*(2), 159–170.
Abu-Rayya, M. H., & Abu-Rayya, H. M. (2009). Ethnic identification, religious identity, and psychological well-being among Muslim and Christian Palestinians in Israel. *Mental Health, Religion and Culture, 12*(2), 147–155.
Aflakseir, A. (2012). Religiosity, personal meaning, and psychological well-being: A study among Muslim students in England. *Pakistan Journal of Social and Clinical Psychology, 9*(2), 27–31.
Aghababaei, N. (2012). Religious, honest and humble: Looking for the religious person within the HEXACO model of personality structure. *Personality and Individual Differences, 53*, 880–883.
Aghababaei, N. (2013). Between you and God, where is the general factor of personality? Exploring personality-religion relationships in a Muslim context. *Personality and Individual Differences, 55*, 196–198.
Aguilar-Vafaie, M. E., & Moghanloo, M. (2008). Domain and facet personality correlates of religiosity among Iranian college students. *Mental Health, Religion and Culture, 11*, 461–483.
Ahmed, S. (2009). Religiosity and presence of character strengths in American Muslim youth. *Journal of Muslim Mental Health, 4*, 104–123.
Ai, A. L., Peterson, C., & Huang, B. (2003). The effect of religious-spiritual coping on positive attitudes of adult Muslim refugees from Kosovo and Bosnia. *International Journal for the Psychology of Religion, 13*, 29–47.
Al-Dhahabi, M. I. (1961). *Al-Tibb al-Nabawi (Prophetic Medicine).* Cairo, Egypt: Mutafā al-Halabī [cited in Rahman F (1998). Health and Medicine in the Islamic Tradition (pp. 44–45). Chicago, IL: ABC International Group].
Ashkanani, H. R. (2009). The relationship between religiosity and subjective well-being: A case of Kuwaiti car accident victims. *Traumatology, 15*, 23–28.
Arslan, M. (2001). The work ethic values of Protestant British, Catholic Irish and Muslim Turkish managers. *Journal of Business Ethics, 31*, 321–339.
Azaiza, F., Ron, P., Shoham, M., & Gigini, I. (2010). Death and dying anxiety among elderly Arab Muslims in Israel. *Death Studies, 34*, 351–364.

Baroun, K. A. (2006). Relations among religiosity, health, happiness, and anxiety for Kuwaiti adolescents. *Psychological Reports, 99*(3), 717–722.

Carlton-Ford, S., Ender, M. G., & Tabatabai, A. (2008). Iraqi adolescents: Self-regard, self-derogation, and perceived threat in war. *Journal of Adolescence, 31*(1), 53–75.

Cirhinlioglu, F. G., & Ozdikmenli-Demir, G. (2012). Religious orientation and its relation to locus of control and depression. *Archive for the Psychology of Religion, 34*, 341–362.

Cohen, M., & Azaiza, F. (2007). Health-promoting behaviors and health locus of control from a multicultural perspective. *Ethnicity & Disease, 17*(4), 636–642.

Fanni Asl, A., Narimani, M., & Ghaffari, M. (2008). A survey of relationship between religious beliefs practice, self-esteem and mental health and scholar performance of collegians. *The Social Sciences, 3*(5), 359–363.

French, D. C., Eisenberg, N., Vaughan, J., Purwono, U., & Suryanti, T. A. (2008). Religious involvement and the social competence and adjustment of Indonesian Muslim adolescents. *Developmental Psychology, 44*, 597–611.

Friedman, M., & Saroglou, V. (2010). Religiosity, psychological acculturation to the host culture, self-esteem and depressive symptoms among stigmatized and non-stigmatized religious immigrant groups in Western Europe. *Basic and Applied Social Psychology, 32*, 185–195.

Ghaffari, A., & Ciftci, A. (2010). Religiosity and self-esteem of Muslim immigrants to the United States: The moderating role of perceived discrimination. *International Journal for the Psychology of Religion, 20*, 14–25.

Ghorbani, N., Watson, P. J., Krauss, S. W., Davison, H. K., & Bing, M. N. (2004). Private self-consciousness factors: Relationships with need for cognition, locus of control, and obsessive thinking in Iran and the United States. *Journal of Social Psychology, 144*, 359–372.

Imam, S. S., Nurullah, A. S., Makol-Abdul, P. R., Rahman, S. A., & Noon, H. M. (2009). Spiritual and psychological health of Malaysian youths. *Research in the Social Scientific Study of Religion, 20*, 85–101.

Ismail, Z., & Desmukh, S. (2012). Religiosity and psychological well-being. *International Journal of Business and Social Science, 3*(11), 20–28.

Ji, C. H., & Ibrahaim, Y. (2007). Islamic religiosity in right-wing authoritarian personality: The case of Indonesian Muslims. *Review of Religious Research, 49*, 28–146.

Johnstone, J., & Tiliopoulos, N. (2008). Exploring the relationship between schizotypal personality traits and religious attitude in an international Muslim sample. *Archive for the Psychology of Religion, 30*, 241–253.

Khan, Z. H., & Watson, P. J. (2004). Religious orientation and the experience of Eid-ul-Azha among Pakistani Muslims. *Journal for the Scientific Study of Religion, 43*, 537–545.

Kazarian, S. S. (2005). Family functioning, cultural orientation, and psychological well-being Among University Students in Lebanon. *Journal of Social Psychology, 145*(2), 141–152.

Khalad, Y. (2010). Dispositional optimism among American and Jordanian college students: Are Westerners really more upbeat than Easterners? *International Journal of Psychology, 45*, 56–63.

Khan, Z. H., Watson, P. J., & Chen, Z. (2011). Differentiating religious coping from Islamic identification in patient and non-patient Pakistani Muslims. *Mental Health, Religion and Culture, 14*, 1049–1062.

Khayyer, M. (2000). Comparison of locus of control among Muslim and Jewish school students in Iran. *Psychological Reports, 87*, 183–187.

Kroo, A., & Nagy, H. (2011). Posttraumatic growth among traumatized Somali refugees in Hungary. *Journal of Loss and Trauma, 16*, 440–458.

Lazenby, M., Khatib, J., Al-Khair, F., & Neamat, M. (2013). Psychometric properties of the functional assessment of chronic illness therapy-spiritual well-being (FACIT-Sp) in an Arabic-speaking, predominantly Muslim population. *Psycho-Oncology, 22*, 220–227.

Lester, D., Castromayor, I. J., & Icli, T. (1991). Locus of control, depression, and suicidal ideation among American, Philippine, and Turkish students. *Journal of Social Psychology, 131*, 447–449.

Mohammadi, S. D., & Honarmand, M. M. (2007). Relationship between religiousness and locus of control and the role of gender differences. *Psychological Research, 9*(3–4), 47–64.

Momtaz, Y. A., Haimid, T. A., Ibrahim, R., Yahaya, N., & Abdullah, S. S. (2011a). Moderating effect of Islamic religiosity on the relationship between chronic medical conditions and psychological well-being among elderly Malays. *Psychogeriatrics, 12*, 43–53.

Momtaz, Y. A., Hamid, T. A., Ibrahim, R., Yahaya, N., & Chai, S. T. (2011b). Moderating effect of religiosity on the relationship between social isolation and psychological well-being. *Mental Health, Religion and Culture, 14*(2), 141–156.

Momtaz, Y. A., Ibrahim, R., Hamid, T. A., & Yahaya, N. (2010). Mediating effects of social and personal religiosity on the psychological well-being of widowed elderly people. *Omega, 61*, 145–162.

Nielsen, M. E., & Stevens, R. (2001). Descriptions of religious experience among U.S. Christians and Malaysian Muslims. *North American Journal of Psychology, 3*(1), 77–90.

Noor, N. M. (2008). Work and women's well-being: Religion and age as moderators. *Journal of Religion and Health, 47*(4), 476–490.

Rabie, M. A., Meguid, M. A., Nivert, Z., & Moussa, M. (2011). Depressive symptoms and hopelessness among patients with cancer: Role of religiosity. *Middle East Current Psychiatry, 18*(3), 157–164.

Sallquist, J., Eisenberg, N., French, D. C., Purwono, U., & Suryanti, T. A. (2010). Indonesian adolescents' spiritual and religious experiences and their longitudinal relations with socioemotional functioning. *Developmental Psychology, 46*, 699–716.

Salmanpour, H., & Issazadegan, A. (2012). Religiosity orientations and personality traits with death obsession. *International Journal of Psychological Studies, 4*(1), 150–157.

Sirin, S. R., Bikmen, N., Mir, M., Fine, M., Zaal, M., & Katsiaficas, D. (2008). Exploring dual identification among Muslim-American emerging adults: A mixed methods study. *Journal of Adolescence, 31*, 259–279.

Srnka, K. J., Gegez, A. E., & Arzova, S. B. (2007). Why is it (un-)ethical? Comparing potential European partners: A Western Christian and an Eastern Islamic country—On arguments used in explaining ethical judgments. *Journal of Business Ethics, 74*, 101–118.

Stavrova, O., Fetchenhauer, D., & Schlosser, T. (2013). Why are religious people happy? The effect of the social norm of religiosity across countries. *Social Science Research, 42*, 90–105.

Suhail, K., & Chaudhry, H. R. (2004). Predictors of subjective well-being in an Eastern Muslim culture. *Journal of Social and Clinical Psychology, 23*(3), 359–376.

Tiliouine, H., & Belgoumidi, A. (2009). An exploratory study of religiosity, meaning in life and subjective wellbeing in Muslim students from Algeria. *Applied Research in Quality of Life, 4*(1), 109–127.

Tiliouine, H., Cummins, R. A., & Davern, M. (2009). Islamic religiosity, subjective well-being, and health. *Mental Health, Religion and Culture, 12*(1), 55–74.

Watson, P., Ghorbani, N., Davison, H., Bing, M. N., Hood, R. W., Jr., & Ghramaleki, A. F. (2002). Negatively reinforcing personal extrinsic motivations: Religious orientation, inner awareness, and mental health in Iran and the United States. *International Journal for the Psychology of Religion, 12*(4), 255–276.

Wilde, A., & Joseph, S. (1997). Religiosity and personality in a Moslem context. *Personality and Individual Differences, 23*, 899–900.

Zulfikar, Y. F. (2012). Do Muslims believe more in Protestant work ethic than Christians? Comparison of people with different religious background living in the U.S. *Journal of Business Ethics, 105*, 489–502.

Chapter 9
Religion and Social Health in Muslims

Social health involves a number of domains, including social support (number and quality of social connections), marital stability (satisfaction and harmony within marriage), the absence of antisocial behaviors, and high social capital (social trust and community engagement). All have been related to the mental and physical health of individuals and populations, and are key to thriving families and communities (House et al. 1988; Uchino 2006). One might even argue that they are essential for the economic health of nations and the ability of those nations to compete in the world marketplace (Kawachi 1999).

Social Support

Social support is a strong predictor of positive health outcomes, and social isolation is known to have the opposite effect. In fact, social isolation has recently been found to predict mortality to a similar degree as traditional risk factors such as smoking, obesity, hypertension, and high cholesterol (Pantell et al. 2013). Our 2010 systematic review uncovered only two studies that examined relationships between R/S and social support in Muslims, one study in Kuwait and one in Pakistan. In the first study, Al-Kandari (2003) surveyed 223 Kuwaitis (80 % Sunni, 20 % Shiite; age range 18–75; half women), examining relationships between religiosity and various aspects of health including social support. Religious commitment was assessed using a 15-item Muslim religiosity scale. Social support was assessed by asking about the number of close friends and relatives (two questions). Results indicated that religiosity was strongly and positively related to number of close relatives ($r=+0.46$, $p<0.01$, uncontrolled) and close friends ($r=+0.36$, $p<0.01$).

In the second study, described earlier in this chapter, Suhail and Chaudhry (2004) analyzed data from 973 community-dwelling persons ages 16–80 living in Lahore, Pakistan. Religiosity was assessed by an 18-item Islamic beliefs and practices scale. Social support was measured by a 2-item scale that asked about amount of help

H.G. Koenig and S. Al Shohaib, *Health and Well-Being in Islamic Societies: Background, Research, and Applications*, DOI 10.1007/978-3-319-05873-3_9,

provided by close relatives and number of close friends. In that study, religiosity was unrelated to social support.

Missed Studies. Our current review also uncovered two additional studies missed in our 2010 review. Levav and colleagues (2008) surveyed 695 residents of the Gaza and West Bank (mostly Sunni Muslim) prior to the Israeli government's removal of settlers in 2005. Religiosity was measured by a single question asking respondents to categorize themselves as secular, traditional, national religious, and national ultra-religious. Social support was assessed using a 5-item index that asked about family and friends. Results indicated that those who described themselves as "secular" were significantly more likely to have no family and report lower social support compared to those who were religious ($F=9.9$, $p<0.0001$).

The second study by Aflakseir and Coleman (2009) examined relationships between religious coping and mental health in 78 disabled Iranian veterans of the war between Iraq and Iran between 1980 and 1988. Average age of respondents was 44 at the time of the survey, all were men, and 99 % were married. Religious coping was measured using a 22-item scale adapted from the RCOPE (Pargament), including 6-item religious practice, 6-item benevolent reappraisal, 4-item negative religious coping, 3-item passive religious coping, and 3-item active religious coping subscales. Social support was assessed using an established 19-item measure from the Medical Outcomes Study. Correlational analysis revealed that religious coping was strongly and positively related to social support ($r=+0.48$, $p<0.01$). In fact, religious coping was the strongest correlate of social support among all characteristics measured.

Muslims vs. Non-Muslims. We also found two studies comparing Muslim Arabs living in Israel and Israeli Jews, both reporting that social support was higher in Muslims than in Jews, one examining perceived levels of support (Ben-Ari and Gil 2004) and the other examining availability of support (Pines and Zaidman 2003).

Recent Research. Since our 2010 review, at least two additional studies have examined religiosity and social support in Muslims. Rambod and Rafii (2010) analyzed relationships between social support and quality of life in 202 Iranian hemodialysis patients (mean age 55.6, 53 % women). The Quality of Life Index (Ferrans) used in the study included a section on "psychological–spiritual" satisfaction and importance. Social support was measured using a 25-item subscale of the Personal Resources Questionnaire (Weinert). Results indicated a positive correlation between scores on the psychological–spiritual subscale and perceived social support ($r=+0.63$, $p\leq 0.05$). The second study by Momtaz and colleagues (2011) from Malaysia examined relationships between religiosity, social isolation, and well-being in a national random sample of 1,415 community-dwelling Muslim adults ages 60 or over (mean age 70, 51 % female). Religiosity was assessed using the 14-item intrinsic–extrinsic religiosity scale (Gorsuch), and social isolation (the inverse of social support) by the 6-item Lubben social network scale. Uncontrolled analyses indicated that religiosity was inversely related to social isolation (–0.11, $p<0.01$). In addition, religiosity moderated the inverse relationship between social isolation and psychological well-being, such that the inverse relationship between social isolation and well-being was much stronger in those with low religiosity.

Summary. Of the six studies that have examined religiosity–social support relationships, 5 (83 %) reported significant positive relationships (Table 9.1). Again, these findings are identical to those found in Christian populations during our 2010 systematic review, where 83 % of studies found great religiosity associated with greater social support.

Marital Stability

Surprisingly, there are only a few studies examining religiosity and marital stability or marital satisfaction in Muslim populations. Although it is commonly accepted that divorce rates are high in Western countries, rates are also pretty high in several Muslim countries (see Table 9.2). Our systematic review identified two studies that examined relationships between religiosity and marital stability in Muslim-majority countries (Pakistan and Turkey), and both reported significant positive relationships. A third study from Syria examined rates of physical abuse by religious group, finding higher rates of abuse in Muslim marriages. We review these studies now below.

In a study already reviewed several times, Suhail and Chaudhry (2004) examined religiosity and marital satisfaction in a community sample of 973 adults in Lahore, Pakistan. Marital satisfaction was assessed by respondent agreement to the following 2 items: "My life partner is my best friend" and "If re-born, I will marry the same person." Religiosity was assessed using an 18-item scale that assessed Islamic beliefs and practices. Correlational analysis revealed a positive relationship between religiosity and marital satisfaction ($r = +0.08$, $p < 0.05$, uncontrolled).

In the second study, Hunler and Gencoz (2005) examined 92 married couples ($n = 184$ individuals) in Turkey to determine relationships between religiosity and marital satisfaction. Average age of participants was 50 and average marriage duration was 25 years. Religiousness was measured using a 31-item scale that assessed religious beliefs and behaviors. Marital satisfaction was measured using the standard 32-item Dyadic Adjustment Scale (DAS). Also administered were a 9-item Marital Problem Solving Scale (MPSS), a 16-item Submissive Acts Scale (SAS), and a 20-item Hopelessness Scale (HS). Correlational analysis revealed no relationship between religiosity and the DAS, MPSS, or HS, although there was a positive correlation with the SAS ($r = +0.20$, $p < 0.01$). Regression analysis was used to predict marital satisfaction (DAS), controlling for SAS, HS, MPSS, duration of marriage, marital style, and education. Results indicated that religiosity was significantly and positively associated with marital satisfaction in that analysis ($B = +0.27$, $p < 0.05$).

In the third study, Maziak and Asfar (2003) from the Syrian Center for Tobacco Studies in Aleppo surveyed 411 women randomly selected from primary care centers in Aleppo, with the goal of determining rates and predictors of physical abuse among low-income women (mean age 28, 88 % married, 91 % Muslim). Abuse was assessed using the WHO 20-item Self-Reporting Questionnaire. Current physical abuse was reported by 23.1 % of the overall sample and by 26.2 % of married women (with regular physical abuse reported by 3.3 % of married women). In 87 %

Table 9.1 Religiosity and social health in Muslims

Authors (year)	Method	Sample size	Participants	Location	Controls	Findings
Social support						
Al-Kandari (2003)	CS	223	Adults ages 18–75	Kuwait	None	P
Suhail and Chaudhry (2004)	CS	973	Adults ages 16–80	Pakistan	None	NA
Levav et al. (2008)	CS	695	Adults, average age 42	Israel	None	P
Aflakseir and Coleman (2009)	CS	78	Disabled war veterans	Iran	None	P
Rambod and Rafii (2010)	CS	202	Hemodialysis patients	Iran	None	P
Momtaz et al. (2011)	CS	1,415	Adults age 60 or over	Malaysia	None	P
Marital stability						
Ilyas (1991)	CS	600	300 married couples	Bangladesh	MC	P
Suhail and Chaudhry (2004)	CS	973	Adults ages 16–80	Pakistan	None	P
Hunler and Gencoz (2005)	CS	184	Couples average age 50	Turkey	MC	P
Asamarai et al. (2008)	CS	173	Married men and women	USA	None	P
Ahmadi and Hossein-Abadi (2009)	CS	1,320	600 couples	Iran	None	P
Chapman and Cattaneo (2013)	CS	296	Adult Muslims	USA	None	P
Delinquency/crime						
Al-Thakeb and Scott (1981)	CS	599	College students	Kuwait	(?)	P
Barber (2001)	CS	6,000	Youth age 14	Palestine	MC	P
Herzog (2003)	CS	198	Muslim adults	Israel	MC	M
Noon et al. (2003)	CS	2,869	High school students	Malaysia	None	P
French et al. (2008)	CS	182	Adolescents, mean age 14	Indonesia	MC	P
Ozbay (2008)	CS	974	College students	Turkey	MC	NG
Serajzadeh (2008)	CS	1,522	College students	Iran	MC	P
Koster et al. (2009)	CS	20,155	Adults in 70 countries	–	MC	P
French et al. (2011)	P	1,010	Adolescents ages 13–15	Indonesia	SC	P
Mirzamani (2011)	CC	137 vs. 40	Prisoners vs. controls	Iran	None	P
Krause et al. (2012)	CS	895	High school students	Malaysia	MC	P

Social capital						
Barber (2001)	CS	6,000	Youth age 14	Palestine	None	P
Brigaitis (2005)	CS	12,604	Adult Muslims	Muslim countries	MC	M
Inoguchi and Hotta (2006)	CS	14,000	Adults age 20–69	Central/South Asia	None	P
Jamal (2007)	CS	2,742	Adult Muslims	Arab countries	MC	(P)
Ozbay (2008)	CS	974	College students	Turkey	None	NA
Berggren and Bjornskov (2011)	CS	109	Countries	Worldwide	SC	NG
Asadollahi et al. (2012)	CS	201	Muslims over 60	Iran	None	NG
Sarkissian (2012)	CS	18,000 (?)	Adult Muslims	Nine Muslim countries	None	M
Krause et al. (2012)	CS	895	High school students	Malaysia	SC	P
Krause et al. (2013)	CS	596	High school students	Malaysia	MC	P

CS cross-sectional, *P* prospective, *CC* case control, *NA* no association, *P* significant positive association, (*P*) trend positive association ($0.05 < p < 0.10$), *NG* significant negative association, *M* mixed (both significant positive and negative findings), *C* complex association, *MC* multiple controls, *SC* some controls

Table 9.2 Divorce rates per 1,000 by country[a]

	Divorce rate
Western countries	
Russia	4.7
United States	3.6
Germany	2.3
Canada	2.1
France	2.1
United Kingdom	2
Brazil	1.4
Italy	0.9
Mexico	0.8
Ireland	0.7
Islamic countries	
Jordan	2.6
Kuwait	2.2
Egypt	1.9
Iran	1.7
Turkey	1.6
Qatar	1.1
Saudi Arabia	1.1
Syria	1
Libya	0.3

[a]Divorce demography. Wikipedia (http://en.wikipedia.org/wiki/Divorce_demography) (last accessed 8 October 2013)

of cases, abuse was by the husband. Physical abuse among Muslims was 25.3 % vs. 0 % among non-Muslims ($p<0.001$). Factors related to abuse based on regression analysis were age, education, marital status, rural vs. urban residence, economic status, mental distress, and smoking. Religion could not be examined since all abused women were Muslim.

Missed Studies. Our recent research review identified a few additional studies missed by our 2010 review. Ilyas (1991) surveyed a random community sample of 300 Muslim couples in Dhaka, Bangladesh (mean age 35, married an average of 10 years). Religiosity was measured using a 4-item scale of Islamic practices. Marital satisfaction was assessed using the 29-item Marital Adjustment Scale (developed by the author). Correlational analyses revealed a significant relationship between marital satisfaction and religiosity of husband and religiosity of wife, although the relationship was stronger with husband religiosity. In stepwise regression models that controlled for other predictors, the husband's religious practices were significantly related to both the husband's marital satisfaction ($B=+0.16$, $p<0.001$) and the wife's marital satisfaction ($B=+0.15$, $p=0.001$). When husband's religiosity was controlled for in the model, however, wife's religiosity no longer predicted her marital satisfaction.

Abu-Rayya (2007) examined marital well-being and religiosity in 156 Christian European women (mean age 39) married to Israeli Muslim Arabs. Marital satisfaction was assessed with the 32-item Spanier DAS and the 36-item Personal Assessment of Intimacy in Relationships (PAIR) Scale. Since all women were Christian, a 7-item Christian religiosity scale was used to measure religiosity (Francis Scale of Attitude toward Christianity). Interestingly, while religiosity was associated with greater self-esteem ($r=+0.42$, $p<0.001$), positive affect ($r=+0.51$, $p<0.001$), and less negative affect ($r=-0.54$, $p<0.001$), it was inversely related to marital satisfaction ($r=-0.35$, $p=0.01$) and marital intimacy ($r=-0.47$, $p<0.001$). Having different religious belief systems, particularly among those with strong beliefs, may have adversely affected marital quality. Although these results do not apply to religiosity and marital satisfaction among Muslim couples, they are relevant to satisfaction in mixed Muslim–Christian marriages.

Asamarai and colleagues (2008) examined importance of religiosity in spouse selection and marital satisfaction among 173 married Muslim men and women attending an Islamic cultural community center (mosque) in Minneapolis, Minnesota (USA). A 10-item scale was used to assess the importance of religiosity in choice of spouse (religiosity itself was not measured, but rather importance of religiosity in spouse selection). Marital satisfaction was assessed using the Assessment of Muslim Marital Satisfaction scale developed specifically for this study. Among women, correlations between importance of religiosity in choosing a spouse and all six dimensions of marital satisfaction and total marital satisfaction were positive and significant (intimacy, communication, mutual respect, conflict resolution, child-rearing agreement), with correlations ranging from +0.13 (for child rearing) to +0.34 (for conflict resolution). In men, however, there were no significant correlations between importance of religiosity in spouse selection and overall marital satisfaction or any of its dimensions.

Finally, Ahmadi and Hossein-Abadi (2009) surveyed a random sample of 660 couples (1,320 individual participants) from Tehran, Iran, studying relationships between religiosity, marital satisfaction, and child rearing. Religiosity was assessed using the Revised Religious Fundamentalist Scale (RRFS), by which participants were divided into four groups (a little religiosity, average, much, and too much religiosity). Marital satisfaction was assessed using the PAIRS (above) and a 47-item version of the ENRICH scale (a standard measure of marital satisfaction). In addition, a 10-item measure of child rearing was developed specifically for this study. Results indicated that across the four religious groups above, overall marital satisfaction increased in a linear fashion ($F=37.8$, $p<0.0001$, uncontrolled), as did each of the subscales of marital satisfaction (general satisfaction, communication, conflict resolution, financial management, sexual relationship, parenting, etc.). Likewise, amount of supervision and control of children increased in a stepwise fashion across the religious groups from low to high religiosity ($p<0.00001$, uncontrolled).

Few studies have compared Muslims and non-Muslims with regard to marital stability. We could find only one report based on national divorce statistics in Israel, finding that Muslim Arabs had a considerably lower divorce rate than Jews (Central Bureau of Statistics 1998).

Recent Research. Since our 2010 review we could find no studies that examined the relationship between religiosity and marital stability in Muslim-majority countries or populations. This is remarkable given the 3.5-year period that this latest review covered (2010–2013). However, we did find a study on marital quality in American Muslims. Chapman and Cattaneo (2013) conducted an online survey sent out to members of several Muslim community organizations, including those who were currently married, age 18 or older, Muslim, and living in the USA. A total of 296 persons responded. Participants were 49 % women, 57 % under age 35, 56 % within first 10 years of marriage, and nearly half with a graduate college degree. Standard measures of marital quality were assessed by the questionnaire, including marital satisfaction, confidence in the marriage, marital instability, negative interactions, positive interactions, problems in marriage, discord with in-laws, and domestic violence. Religiosity was measured using a 3-item scale with scores ranging from 3 to 18. Uncontrolled analyses indicated that religiosity was positively related to marital satisfaction ($\rho = +0.15$, $p < 0.05$) and marital confidence ($\rho = +0.16$, $p < 0.05$), inversely related to discord with mother-in-law ($\rho = -0.21$, $p < 0.01$) and abuse from mother-in-law ($\rho = -0.17$, $p < 0.05$), and was unrelated to abuse from spouse. Researchers only briefly discussed these positive findings (acknowledging that religiosity was associated with greater marital satisfaction); they did not explain why this might be so.

Summary. Of six studies that have examined the religiosity–marital stability relationship in Muslim populations, all six reported significant positive relationships with marital satisfaction or marital adjustment (Table 9.1). However, one study reported that physical abuse is more common among Muslim marriages in Syria (before the revolutionary war there), and one study found that religiosity in European Christian women married to Muslim men, while related to better mental health, was significantly and inversely related to marital satisfaction and marital intimacy. We could not find many studies comparing marital stability in Muslims vs. non-Muslims. However, one study reported a lower divorce rate in Muslims than Jews in Israel. More research is needed in Muslim countries to explore the role that religion plays in fostering marital satisfaction and stability.

Delinquency and Crime

Our 2010 systematic review identified three studies that examined relationships between religiosity and delinquency or crime, including one each in Palestine, Indonesia, and Turkey. Two of the three found significant inverse relationships, and one study reported greater political violence associated with greater religiosity in Turkey.

Barber (2001) analyzed data on a sample of 6,000 Palestinian youth (age 14) in 1994–1995, examining relationships between political violence, individual functioning (including antisocial behavior), and social contexts (including religion). Youth came from the West Bank, Gaza Strip, and East Jerusalem. Religiosity was measured using a 5-item index of self-rated religiosity, religious behavior, and importance of religion. Antisocial behavior was assessed by yes/no responses to four questions regarding use of alcohol beverages, use of tobacco, stealing, and running away from home. Correlational analyses revealed that religiosity was inversely related to antisocial behavior in males ($r = -0.20, p < 0.001$) and in females ($r = -0.11, p < 0.001$). Structural equation modeling with all variables in the model confirmed the inverse relationship with religiosity.

Next, French and colleagues (2008) surveyed 183 Indonesian Muslim adolescents (mean age 13), examining relationships between spirituality/religiosity and social competence, including antisocial and problem behavior. Participants came from public schools segregated by religion. Spirituality was assessed using a 19-item daily spiritual experiences scale, and religion was assessed by frequency of behaviors (fasting, reading Qur'an in Malaysian and Arabic, attending mosque, performing daily prayers). Religiosity was self-assessed by the adolescent and by the parent regarding the adolescent. Antisocial behaviors examined were lying to parents, fighting, skipping school, taking money without permission, sneaking out of house, associating with deviant peers, viewing pornographic materials, and taking money (again, as reported by adolescent and by parent). Religiosity self-ratings by adolescent and adolescent ratings by parent were both inversely related to antisocial behavior (five of eight relationships were statistically significant). A structural equation model confirmed these inverse relationships.

Ozbay (2008) surveyed 974 college students in Turkey (50 % male, mean age 21) assessing religiosity and antisocial acts, including political violence. Religiosity was measured by three questions asking about whether the youth talked with friends about religion, whether youth's mother talked with their friends or neighbors on religious topics, and whether youth's father talked to friends and neighbors about religion. The latter two questions regarding youths' mothers and fathers were combined into a 2-item index as a measure of religious environment. Antisocial behavior was assessed with a 4-item index that asked about cheating on exams, alcohol use, fighting for the purpose of gaining political power on campus (political violence), and fighting for other reasons. Regression analysis indicated that mother/father's talking with friends/neighbors about religion was positively related to political violence by youth ($B = +2.91, p \leq 0.01, n = 409$).

Missed Studies. We missed several additional studies in our 2010 systematic review. In a study of 599 college students in Kuwait, Al-Thakeb and Scott (1981) found that the perceived severity of moral crimes (adultery, distribution of pornography, etc.) was similar (and in need of punishment) to that reported for violent crime. The strongest predictor of participants' perception of the seriousness reported for crime was religiosity, which was assessed by a scale measuring Islamic fundamentalism (details lacking due to availability of abstract only).

Groves and colleagues (1987) used cross-national data from the United Nations to examine offender and offense rates for crimes and their relationship to religion. The purpose was to test the hypothesis that "The Islamic religion preserves a 'sense of community'." Data used in this analysis were based on crimes reported by member countries in the United Nations between 1970 and 1975. The power of this study was weak because analyses were conducted at the country level and there were only 47 countries (33 non-Islamic and 14 Islamic[1]). Researchers found that female adult offenses per 100,000 tended to be lower in Islamic countries (41.6 vs. 111.1, $p=0.09$), and were significantly lower for male juvenile offenses (12.0 vs. 106.2, $p<0.05$). Furthermore, specific kinds of offenses were significantly less frequent in Islamic countries, including theft (142.2 vs. 1,147.2, $p<0.01$) and fraud (12.3 vs. 114.6, $p=0.01$). However, when controlling for "per capita gross domestic product," all differences between Islamic and non-Islamic countries lost significance. Researchers concluded that the economic factor was the primary reason for the differences in crime rates between Islamic and non-Islamic countries, and that the Islamic factor (religion) was secondary.

Serajzadeh (2001–2002) from the University of Tehran also compared crime statistics in developed and developing (Islamic and non-Islamic) nations based on data from the United Nations in 1980. Islamic countries included Bangladesh, Kuwait, Pakistan, Qatar, and the United Arab Emirates. Crime rates per 100,000 were lower in Islamic countries than in non-Islamic developing countries and were lower than in non-Islamic developed countries (Canada, the USA, the UK, etc.) for crimes such as assault, homicide, rape, robbery, fraud, and theft. Overall, rate of crime in developing Islamic countries was only two-thirds that of developing non-Islamic countries (694.2 vs. 1,028.5 per 100,000) and only about one-tenth as common as in developed non-Islamic countries (694.2 vs. 5,968.5 per 100,000). Lower crime rates were attributed to racial and religious uniformity, cohesiveness of the family network, the religious worldview of Islam, the lower tolerance of criminal behavior in terms of public opinion, and the severity of punishment. For a more detailed discussion of the role of Islamic religious belief in crime prevention, see Al-Khalifah (1994).

More recently, Serajzadeh (2008) examined social determinants of perceived seriousness of crime in a random national sample of 1,522 college students in Iran. Participants were 57 % male, 87 % single, nearly 90 % between ages of 17 and 28, and 95 % Shi'ite Muslim. Religiosity was measured using a 21-item scale assessing religious beliefs, practices, feelings, consequences, and knowledge. Students noted the seriousness of 24 criminal acts on a scale from 1 to 20 (minor to serious), and then an index of seriousness was developed based on responses. The offenses rated the highest in seriousness after intentional homicide were those of a sexual nature (rape, pedophilia, married woman's adultery, married man's adultery). Religiosity was positively related to total score on the seriousness of crime index ($r=+0.46$, $p<0.01$) and, in fact, was the strongest of all predictors. Regression analysis controlling for other factors confirmed religiosity as the strongest predictor of crime

[1] Islamic: Algeria, Bahrain, Cyprus, Egypt, Indonesia, Iran, Iraq, Kuwait, Morocco, Oman, Pakistan, Qatar, Syria, and Turkey. Non-Islamic: Argentina, Australia, Austria, Bahamas, Barbados, Chile, Costa Rica, Denmark, Ecuador, El Salvador, Finland, France, Germany, Greece, Guiana, Ireland, Italy, Jamaica, Japan, Malaysia, Maldives, San Marino, Singapore, Spain, Sweden, Switzerland, Trinidad and Tobago, the UK, the USA, Yugoslavia, Norway, Canada, and Mauritius.

seriousness (explaining 21 % of the variance, and replicating the 1981 report initially described above).

Religiosity and attitudes toward the seriousness of crime were also examined by Herzog (2003) among a representative sample of 987 adults in Israel, comparing Muslims ($n=198$) and Jews ($n=633$). Religiosity was assessed by the self-rated categories of secular, religious, and very religious. A total of 14 crime scenarios were presented to respondents, who were asked to rank the seriousness of the crime from 1 (not serious at all) to 11 (very serious). After controlling for age, education, gender, and income, religiosity for Muslim respondents was significantly and positively related to seriousness of crime for girl rape, apartment burglary, false testimony, inflating bills, clerk bribery, and watch theft, but was inversely related to seriousness of crime for wife assault. When Muslims and Jews were compared, Muslim respondents rated significantly higher crime seriousness for drug selling, illegal sexual relations, and abortions, but significantly lower crime seriousness than Jews for wife murder, wife assault, and rape.

Noon and colleagues (2003) examined the relationship between religiosity and social problems in a random sample of 2,869 Muslim secondary school students in Malaysia, near Singapore. Participants were 69 % Muslim and equally divided between male and female. Religiosity was measured using a multi-item scale that assessed ideological, ritualistic, experiential, consequential, and intellectual aspects of religion. Participant involvement in a wide variety of social problems was assessed, including stealing, running away from home, illegal motorbike racing, truancy, vandalism, gangsterism, and watching pornographic videos. Religiosity in the Muslim subsample was inversely related to every single one of the social problems above, with correlations ranging from $r=-0.09$ for running away from home to $r=-0.16$ for truancy, all at $p<0.01$ level (uncontrolled).

Finally, Koster and associates (2009) examined whether religious affiliation or religiosity was related to victimless crimes across 70 different countries. They analyzed data on 128,243 participants collected during the World Values Surveys (WVSs) that took place between 1981 and 2004. Religious affiliation [none ($n=32{,}048$), Christian ($n=74{,}934$), Muslim ($n=20{,}155$), and other ($n=10{,}106$)] was recorded. Level of religiosity was assessed by the question “How important is God in your life?” (response options 1–10). Justifiability of victimless crimes was assessed on a 1–10 scale (never to always justifiable) for (1) claiming government benefits not entitled, (2) accepting a bribe concerning professional duties, (3) cheating on taxes, and (4) not paying the fare while riding on public transportation. Responses to individual items were combined to form a “justifiability” scale (range 4–40). Results indicated that scores on justifiability of crime were highest in those indicating “none” for religious affiliation (10.2), lowest for Muslims (7.4), and in-between for Christians (9.3) ($p<0.01$). Regression analyses controlling for religion, gender, age, level of education, and importance of family in life revealed that religiosity was significantly and inversely related to justifiability of victimless crimes ($B=-0.43$, $p<0.01$). In that model both Muslim ($B=-0.19$, $p<0.01$) and Christian ($B=-0.13$, $p<0.01$) affiliation predicted less justifiability of crimes, compared to no religious affiliation.

Recent Research. Not much research has been done in this area since 2010. However, we did locate three additional studies. In the first, French and colleagues (2011) surveyed 1,010 Muslim adolescents ages 13–15 in Indonesia and followed them up a year later ($n=891$). The purpose was to determine the effect that adolescents' friends had on their level of religiosity and level of problem behavior. Religiosity was measured using a 22-item scale that assessed religious practices, and was administered at baseline (Y1) and in Year 2 (Y2). Problem behavior was assessed using a list of 20 behaviors that adolescents may have been involved in during the past month (stealing, lying to parents, fighting, skipping school, taking money, sneaking out of house, viewing pornographic materials, etc.). Religiosity and problem behavior of friends were also assessed directly from the friends themselves. Results were stratified by gender. Among boys, Y1 religiosity was inversely related to problem behaviors in Y1 ($r=-0.33$, $p<0.01$) and in Y2 ($r=-0.28$, $p<0.01$). Among girls, Y1 religiosity was also inversely related to problem behavior in Y1 ($r=-0.16$, $p<0.01$) and in Y2 ($r=-0.15$, $p<0.01$). Among boys, Y1 friend religiosity also predicted fewer adolescent problem behavior in Y1 ($r=-0.34$, $p<0.01$) and in Y2 ($r=-0.22$, $p<0.01$). Among girls, Y1 friend religiosity also predicted adolescent problem behavior in Y1 ($r=-0.10$, $p<0.05$), but surprisingly, predicted worse problem behavior in Y2 ($r=+0.11$, $p<0.05$, uncontrolled). Regression models controlling for gender and grade indicated that Y2 religiosity was inversely related to Y2 problem behavior in the overall group ($r=-0.10$, $p<0.05$). Thus, especially in boys, the adolescents' own religiosity and their friends' religiosity both predicted less problem behavior over time.

A second study by Mirzamani (2011) compared the characteristics of 137 prisoners at a military prison in Iran with 40 matched military personnel controls who had never been in prison. The purpose was to determine if religious values were associated with being in prison. Religious values were measured using a subscale of the Allport, Vernon, and Lindzey's Study of Values Test. Controls were matched with prisoners on marital status, age, and education. Results indicated that religious values were significantly lower in prisoners compared to non-prisoner controls (41.8 vs. 52.9, $p<0.001$, uncontrolled). Although not particularly surprising, these results confirm expectations.

The final study conducted by Krause and colleagues (2012) examined relationships between religiosity, spiritual strivings, at-risk behaviors, and pro-social behaviors in 895 third-year Muslim high school students (mean age 16, evenly divided by gender) in Malaysia, near Kuala Lumpur. Religiosity was measured using the 20-item Islamic Worldview Scale, the 8-item Spiritual Striving Scale, and frequency of mosque attendance. At-risk behaviors were assessed using a 9-item scale that measured loitering, smoking, gambling, drinking alcohol, viewing pornographic movies/books, drug use, kissing and premarital sex (not all necessarily indicating delinquent activities, but activities that place adolescents at risk for delinquency). Pro-social behavior was assessed using a 14-item Mu'amalat scale that measured engagement in positive relations with family, friends, and society. Results indicated that all three religious measures were associated with significantly lower at-risk behaviors and significantly higher pro-social and thriving behaviors ($p<0.01$ for all correlations).

Regression models that controlled for multiple other demographic, social, parental, and school predictors, and other religious predictors, confirmed that religious worldview predicted lower at-risk behaviors ($B = -0.12$, $p < 0.01$), and both religious worldview and spiritual strivings predicted pro-social behavior ($r = +0.16$ and $r = +0.38$, $p < 0.01$, respectively).

Summary. Thus, of 11 studies, 9 found significant inverse relationships between religiosity and delinquent or criminal behavior in Muslims (Table 9.1). One study found that the more the youths' parents talked to friends/neighbors about religion the greater the likelihood that youths would be engaged in political violence. One study also found that Muslims who were more religious (compared to those who were less religious) believed that assaulting a wife was a less serious criminal behavior. Finally, several studies have found that rates of crime are lower in Islamic countries compared to non-Islamic countries (including the USA and Europe). However, one of those studies (using 1977 data) found that controlling for gross domestic product per capita (i.e., income) explained the lower crime rates in Islamic countries (not religion).

Social Capital

Social capital, an indicator of community health, is defined as degree of civic involvement by members of a community, trust between members of the community, frequency of volunteering, and involvement in other community activities that strengthen the community. Stated another way, social capital emphasizes the importance of service to others, time spent with community groups, and trust between neighbors. Our systematic review in 2010 identified only one study that examined religiosity and social capital in Muslims, and that study found no consistent association. A second study in Israel compared Jews and Muslims on indicators of social capital, finding greater social capital in Jews than in Muslims in four of six areas.

In the study by Ozbay (2008) cited earlier, which examined 974 college students in Turkey, little relationship was found between "youth religion" (undefined) and a wide range of adolescent and parent social capital variables. Among two-dozen correlations in this study, significant associations were found only between youth religion and (1) parent control over youth's network, (2) family talking with friends/neighbors about religion, and (3) youth talking with friends about religion (the latter two representing autocorrelations with youth religion). No relationships were found with indicators of social capital such as mother or father being members in a community organization, youth civic tolerance, youth social capital deprivation, youth membership in organizations, youth trust, or youth voting.

The second study by Baron-Epel and colleagues (2008) compared Israeli Muslim Arabs and Jews on social capital. Interviews were conducted with a representative national sample of 3,365 adult Jews and 985 adult Arabs. Social capital was assessed with six indicators: a 2-item social trust scale, a single item on neighborhood safety, a single item on perceived helpfulness of people, a 2-item scale on trust in local and national authorities, a 2-item social support scale, and a single item on frequency of social contacts. Jews were more likely than Arabs to have high social trust (63.1 % vs. 38.8 %, $p<0.0001$), find people helpful (43.4 % vs. 19.4 %, $p<0.0001$), have trust in national and local authorities (32.6 % vs. 16.8 %, $p<0.0001$), and have high social support (49.7 % vs. 37.2 %, $p<0.0001$). There was no difference between Jews and Arabs on feeling safe in their neighborhood, and Arabs had more social contacts than Jews (61.0 % vs. 49.1 %, $p<0.0001$). These associations remained strong after controlling for gender, age, income, education, employment, marital status, and religiosity. Religiosity was not examined in relationship to social capital variables.

Missed Studies. We also uncovered several studies missed in our 2010 systematic review. In a study cited earlier of 6,000 Palestinian 14-year-olds, Barber (2001) examined associations between a 5-item measure of religious beliefs/behaviors and a 5-item measure of neighborhood social disorganization (a proxy of low social capital). Social disorganization was assessed by frequency of fights in which a weapon was used, violent arguments between neighbors, youth gang conflicts, people being hit by police, and overall bad feelings about the neighborhood. Religiosity was significantly and inversely associated with neighborhood social disorganization in boys ($r=-0.09$, $p<0.001$) and weakly inversely associated in girls ($r=-0.03$).

As part of his master's thesis at the University of North Texas, Brigaitis (2005) analyzed data from the 2000–2001 World Values Survey (WVS) that included responses from 12,604 Muslims from seven Muslim-majority countries and from seven countries with significant Muslim minorities ranging from 10 to 50 %.[2] The WVS included a range of religious variables that when factor analyzed resulted in three factors: internal religiosity (personal belief), belief in mosque, and religious participation (actual physical involvement in religious institutions). The three social capital indicators in the WVS were (1) importance of service to others, (2) time spent with sport, cultural, or communal groups, and (3) level of trust. Analyses were controlled for gender, age, marital status, and socioeconomic index. In Muslim participants, a significant positive correlation was found between personal religious belief and importance of service to others ($B=+0.17$, $p<0.001$). However, there was no relationship with trust, and personal religious belief was inversely related to time spent in group activities ($B=-0.07$, $p<0.001$). Belief in mosque was positively related to importance of service to others ($B=+0.11$, $p<0.001$) and social trust ($B=+0.05$, $p<0.001$), but was unrelated to time spent in group activities. Finally, religious participation (in mosque activities) was inversely related to importance of service to others ($B=-0.03$, $p=0.002$), positively related to time spent in group activities ($B=+0.27$, $p<0.001$), and unrelated to social trust. The author concluded that religiosity had little ability to generate interpersonal trust, although it did influence belief in the importance of social services and in actually engaging in social group activity.

Inoguchi and Hotta (2006) analyzed data collected by the AsiaBarometer 2005 survey of approximately 14,000 community-dwelling adults in 14 Central and South

[2] Bangladesh, Bosnia and Herzegovina, India, Indonesia, Iran, Jordan, Morocco, Nigeria, Pakistan, Uganda, Macedonia, Egypt, Tanzania, and Montenegro.

Asian countries, examining relationships between social capital, religious affiliation, and importance of God. Social capital was measured by several questions including those assessing community trust and engagement with institutions. Responses to the questions regarding community trust were examined by religious affiliation. Results indicated that Muslims, Hindus, Catholics, and Mahayana Buddhists had higher percentages of respondents who were generally trusting of people, compared to Hinayana Buddhists, Protestants, and other religions (atheists had the lowest trust, and Muslims had the highest trust). Higher importance of God was also related to greater trust ($p<0.001$). Another question asked if respondents thought people were generally helpful or were mostly looking out for themselves. Again, those who indicated greater importance of God were more likely to feel that people generally try to be helpful ($p<0.001$), with Muslims being the religious group most likely to indicate this. By country, general trust was highest in Maldives and Pakistan (both Muslim countries), whereas institutional engagement was highest in Kyrgyzstan (74 % Muslim), Mongolia (4 % Muslim), and Kazakhstan (70 % Muslim). Muslim countries, then, were among those with the highest levels of social capital.

Finally, Jamal (2007) at Princeton University examined relationships between religious attitudes and social trust in 2,742 Muslims in Arab countries using a multivariable logit model that controlled for many demographic, political, and gender attitudes. Results indicated that individuals who believed that religious leaders should be in government positions (an indicator of religiosity) tended to have higher levels of trust ($B=+0.08$, $0.05<p<0.10$). However, mosque attendance was unrelated to social trust, making researchers conclude, "mosque networks per se are not sufficient in increasing or decreasing levels of interpersonal trust" (p. 1343).

Recent Research. Several new studies since our 2010 review have examined relations between religiosity and social trust in Muslim populations. Berggren and Bjornskov (2011) analyzed data from the Gallup World Poll of 109 countries, examining relationships between importance of religion in daily life and social trust. They report a significant *inverse* relationship between importance of religion and social trust across all countries ($B=-0.24$, $p<0.01$), a negative relationship which increased in size as religious diversity increased. The authors explained that there is lower social trust in countries where a large proportion of the population is Muslim, since those populations are more religious than others. Furthermore, they sarcastically quote a saying attributed to the Prophet Muhammad, "An Arab is superior to a non-Arab in nothing but devotion" (p. 467). Of course, the country with the highest social trust and the lowest importance of religion was Sweden, the authors' home.

Asadollahi and colleagues (2012) surveyed 201 Muslim adults aged 60 or over from Ahwaz, Iran, examining relationships between religiosity and civic engagement. Civic engagement was assessed using a 24-item Aged Civic Engagement Scale developed for the study. Religiosity was measured using a 3-item scale that was not described. Religiosity was inversely related to civic engagement ($r=-0.10$, $p=0.02$, uncontrolled), leading the author to conclude that religiosity was unrelated to civic engagement in older adults (although, in fact, religiosity was related to lower civic engagement).

In a study reviewed earlier, Krause and associates (2012) examined relationships between religiosity and indicators of social capital in 895 Muslim high school students from Malaysia. Religiosity was measured using the 45-item Muslim Religiosity-Personality Inventory (MRPI). Social capital variables included school engagement (6-item scale) and youth organization involvement (2-item scale). After controlling for social desirability, gender, and school type, partial correlations between religiosity and both social capital variables were positive: school engagement ($r=+0.38, p<0.001$) and youth organization involvement ($r=+0.17, p<0.001$). In a second report on Malaysian students from the same area ($n=596$), Krause and colleagues (2013) examined relations using the same indicators of social capital and religiosity, except dividing religiosity into Islamic Worldview and Religious Personality (the two scales that make up the MRPI). Regression analyses controlling for gender, family structure, social desirability, and parenting factors revealed a significant relationship between Islamic Worldview and school engagement ($B=+0.18$, $p<0.01$), although no relationship was found with youth organization involvement or peer attachment. Religious Personality, in turn, was positively related to both youth organization involvement ($B=+0.09$, $p<0.05$) and school engagement ($B=+0.18$, $p<0.001$). Researchers concluded that religious involvement was a significant predictor of greater community engagement.

Sarkissian (2012) examined relations between religion and civic engagement using data from nine Muslim countries[3] collected during two waves of the World Values Survey (1999–2004 and 2005–2007). Religious characteristics measured were frequency of religious service attendance, active membership in a religious association, and frequency of prayer. Four measures of civic engagement were assessed, including belonging to secular associations, signing petitions, attending demonstrations, and joining boycotts. After controlling for gender, education level, class, and tolerance of others, religious service attendance was unrelated to measures of civic engagement except for joining boycotts, which was 9.4 % higher in those attending weekly or more. Active religious association membership significantly increased the likelihood of belonging to secular associations (46.4 %), signing petitions (7.8 %), and attending demonstrations (10.6 %), although was unrelated to attending boycotts. Finally, daily prayer significantly reduced the likelihood of all measures of civic engagement, including belonging to secular organizations (−3.8 %), signing petitions (−9.1 %), attending demonstrations (−8.8 %), and joining boycotts (−11.3 %). Researchers hypothesized that the negative effect of prayer on civic engagement was due to the heavy demand that conservative religious organizations have on their participants, which discourages participation in civic activities.

Finally, Addai and colleagues (2013) examined relations between religion and trust in Ghana, Africa, using data from the 2008 Afro-barometer survey that included 1,200 participants. Two measures of social capital were examined: interpersonal trust and institutional trust. Religious affiliation (16 % Muslim) and religious importance [1 = important (93 %), 0 = not important] were also measured. Uncontrolled correlations in the overall sample revealed that religious importance was unrelated

[3] Albania, Bangladesh, Burkina Faso, Egypt, Indonesia, Jordan, Kyrgyzstan, Mali, and Turkey.

to either interpersonal or institutional trust, although Muslim religious affiliation was related to significantly greater institutional trust ($r = +0.18, p < 0.01$). Controlling for age, gender, education, ethnicity, geographical region, political affiliation, and mental health variables using regression analysis, investigators found that religious importance remained unrelated to either measure of trust. However, a significant positive relationship emerged between Muslim affiliation and interpersonal trust ($B = +0.18$, $p < 0.001$), while the relationship with institutional trust decreased to non-significance. Researchers concluded that the effect of religion on trust was weak and weaker for institutional trust.

Summary. Research on religiosity and social capital in Muslim populations is still in the very early stages, and most of this research has been done by Westerners, not Muslims themselves. At least ten studies have now examined relationships between religiosity and some aspect of social capital, and five of those studies (50 %) reported only positive relationships, one found no association, two reported mixed results (both positive and negative relationships), and two found inverse or negative relationships (Table 9.1). Two additional studies compared indicators of social capital in Muslim populations with other religious groups. One study conducted in Israel found lower social capital in Muslims compared to Jews on four of six indicators, whereas another study found that social trust and institutional engagement were higher in Muslim-majority countries than in non-Muslim countries. Among the ten studies examining religiosity and social capital, two also examined differences between Muslims and non-Muslims. One study in 14 Central and South Asian countries found that Muslims and Muslim-majority countries had the highest level of social capital (trust), whereas the other study of 109 countries around the world suggested that Muslim countries had lower social capital (social trust). Thus, research findings to date are inconsistent, whether they involve relationships between religiosity and social capital in Muslim populations or differences in social capital between Muslims and other religious groups.

Summary and Conclusions

Social and community health in general (with rare exceptions) is better among Muslims who are more religious. By social health we mean greater social support, greater marital satisfaction and stability, lower delinquency and crime, and in about half of studies, greater social capital. Again, more and better-designed research is needed in almost every one of these areas, providing a great opportunity for researchers in Muslim countries to provide new and important contributions. Future research is needed that controls for relevant covariates that could influence the relationship between religiosity and social health. Longitudinal studies and clinical trials are desperately needed to provide information on the causal nature of these relationships (i.e., does religiosity or religious interventions actually cause changes in social health?). Relationships between religiosity and social health in Muslims appear similar to those found in Christians, and the differences in social health between Muslims and Christians are not great. This is what we would expect given the similarities in social and moral values between these two religious traditions, particularly among those who are devoutly committed to their faith.

References

Abu-Rayya, H. M. (2007). Acculturation, Christian religiosity, and psychological and marital well-being among the European wives of Arabs in Israel. *Mental Health, Religion & Culture, 10*(2), 171–190.

Addai, I., Opoku-Agyeman, C., & Ghartey, H. T. (2013). An exploratory study of religion and trust in Ghana. *Social Indicators Research, 110*, 993–1012.

Aflakseir, A., & Coleman, P. G. (2009). The influence of religious coping on the mental health of disabled Iranian war veterans. *Mental Health, Religion & Culture, 12*, 175–190.

Ahmadi, K., & Hossein-Abadi, F. H. (2009). Religiosity, marital satisfaction and child rearing. *Pastoral Psychology, 57*, 211–221.

Al-Kandari, Y. Y. (2003). Religiosity and its relation to blood pressure among selected Kuwaitis. *Journal of Biosocial Science, 35*(3), 463–472.

Al-Khalifah, A. H. M. (1994). Religiosity in Islam as a protective mechanism against criminal temptation. *American Journal of Islamic Social Sciences, 11*(1), 1–12.

Al-Thakeb, F., & Scott, J. E. (1981). The perceived seriousness of crime in the Middle East. *International Journal of Comparative and Applied Criminal Justice, 5*(2), 129–143.

Asadollahi, A., Rezaei, P., Faraji, N., & Saberi, L. F. (2012). Does religiosity have unsuitable effect on civic engagement of older adults? A research within aged citizens in the Southwest of Iran. *Journal of American Science, 8*(7), 421–426.

Asamarai, L. A., Solberg, K. B., & Solon, P. C. (2008). The role of religiosity in Muslim spouse selection and its influence on marital satisfaction. *Journal of Muslim Mental Health, 3*, 37–52.

Barber, B. K. (2001). Political violence, social integration, and youth functioning: Palestinian youth from the Intifada. *Journal of Community Psychology, 29*(3), 259–280.

Baron-Epel, O., Weinstein, R., Hviv-Mesika, A., Garty-Sandalon, N., & Green, M. S. (2008). Individual-level analysis of social capital and health: A comparison of Arab and Jewish Israelis. *Social Science & Medicine, 66*, 900–910.

Ben-Ari, A., & Gil, S. (2004). Well-being among minority students: The role of perceived social support. *Journal of Social Work, 4*(2), 215–225.

Berggren, N., & Bjornskov, C. (2011). Is the importance of religion in daily life related to social trust? Cross-country and cross-state comparisons. *Journal of Economic Behavior & Organization, 80*, 459–480.

Brigaitis, P. (2005). *Religious engagement and social capital in the Islamic context*. Masters' Thesis, University of North Texas. Retrieved May 10, 2013, from http://digital.library.unt.edu/ark:/67531/metadc4788/

Central Bureau of Statistics. (1998). *Statistic Abstract of Israel*. Abstract No. 49 (cited in Cohen & Savaya, 2003).

Chapman, A. R., & Cattaneo, L. B. (2013). American Muslim marital quality: A preliminary investigation. *Journal of Muslim Mental Health, 7*(2), 1–24. Online ahead of print (Permalink: http://hdl.handle.net/2027/spo.10381607.0007.201).

French, D. C., Eisenberg, N., Vaughan, J., Purwono, U., & Suryanti, T. A. (2008). Religious involvement and the social competence and adjustment of Indonesian Muslim adolescents. *Developmental Psychology, 44*(2), 597–611.

French, D. C., Purwono, U., & Triwahyuni, A. (2011). Friendship and the religiosity of Indonesian Muslim adolescents. *Journal of Youth and Adolescence, 50*, 1623–1633.

Groves, W. B., Newman, G., & Corrado, C. (1987). Islam, modernization and crime: A test of the religious ecology thesis. *Journal of Criminal Justice, 15*, 495–503.

Herzog, S. (2003). Religiosity and perceptions of crime seriousness by Jewish and Muslim respondents in Israel. *Deviant Behavior, 24*, 153–174.

House, J. S., Landis, K. R., & Umberson, D. (1988). Social relationships and health. *Science, 241*, 540–545.

Hunler, O. S., & Gencoz, T. (2005). The effect of religiousness on marital satisfaction: Testing the mediator role of marital problem solving between religiousness and marital satisfaction relationship. *Contemporary Family Therapy: An International Journal, 27*(1), 123–136.

Ilyas, Q. S. M. (1991). Relationship of religious and role variables with marital adjustment among Muslim couples in Bangladesh. *Pakistan Journal of Psychological Research, 6*(1–2), 1–30.

Inoguchi, T., & Hotta, Z. L. (2006). Quantifying social capital in Central and South Asia: Are there democratic, developmental, and regionalizing potentials? *Japanese Journal of Political Science, 7*(2), 195–220.

Jamal, A. (2007). When is social trust a desirable outcome? Examining levels of trust in the Arab world. *Comparative Political Studies, 40*, 1328–1349.

Kawachi, I. (1999). Social capital and community effects on population and individual health. *Annals of the New York Academy of Sciences, 895*, 120–130.

Koster, F., Goudriaan, H., & van der Schans, C. (2009). Shame and punishment: An international comparative study on the effects of religious affiliation and religiosity on attitudes to offending. *European Journal of Criminology, 6*(6), 481–495.

Krause, S. E., Hamzah, A., Ismail, I. A., Suandi, T., Hamzah, S. R., Dahalan, D., et al. (2012). Religious socialization among Malaysian Muslim adolescents: A family structure comparison. *Review of Religious Research, 54*, 499–518.

Krause, S. E., Ismail, I. A., Suandi, T., Hamzah, A., Hamzah, S. R., Dahalan, D., et al. (2013). Parenting and community engagement factors as predictors of religiosity among Muslim adolescents from Malaysia. *International Journal for the Psychology of Religion, 23*, 87–102.

Krauss, S. E., Hamzah, A., Ismail, I. A., Suandi, T., Hamzah, S. R., Dahalan, D., et al. (2014). Parenting, community and religious predictors of positive and negative developmental outcomes among Muslim adolescents. *Youth & Society, 46*(2), 201–227.

Levav, I., Kohn, R., & Billig, M. (2008). The protective effect of religiosity under terrorism. *Psychiatry, 71*(1), 46–58.

Maziak, W., & Asfar, T. (2003). Physical abuse in low-income women in Aleppo, Syria. *Health Care for Women International, 24*(4), 313–326.

Mirzamani, S. M. (2011). Comparison of value system among a group of military prisoners with controls in Tehran. *Iranian Journal of Psychiatry, 6*, 121–124.

Momtaz, Y. A., Hamid, T. A., Ibrahim, R., Yahaya, N., & Chai, S. T. (2011). Moderating effect of religiosity on the relationship between social isolation and psychological well-being. *Mental Health, Religion & Culture, 14*, 141–156.

Noon, H. M., Haneef, M. A. M., Yusof, S. A., & Amin, R. M. (2003). Religiosity and social problems in Malaysia. *Intellectual Discourse, 11*(1), 77–87.

Ozbay, O. (2008). Does social capital deter youth from cheating, alcohol use, and violence in Turkey?: Bringing torpil in. *Journal of Criminal Justice, 36*(5), 403–415.

Pantell, M., Rehkopf, D., Jutte, D., Syme, S. L., Balmes, J., & Adler, N. (2013). Social isolation: A predictor of mortality comparable to traditional clinical risk factors. *American Journal of Public Health, 103*(11), 2056–2062.

Pines, A. M., & Zaidman, N. (2003). Israeli Jews and Arabs: Similarities and differences in the utilization of social support. *Journal of Cross-Cultural Psychology, 34*(4), 465–480.

Rambod, M., & Rafii, F. (2010). Perceived social support and quality of life in Iranian hemodialysis patients. *Journal of Nursing Scholarship, 42*(3), 242–249.

Sarkissian, A. (2012). Religion and civic engagement in Muslim countries. *Journal for the Scientific Study of Religion, 51*(4), 607–622.

Serajzadeh, S. H. (2001–2002). Islam and crime: The moral community of Muslims. *Journal of Arabic and Islamic Studies, 4*, 111–131.

Serajzadeh, S. H. (2008). Social determinants of the seriousness of crime: an examination of a Muslim sample. *Social Compass, 55*(4), 541–560.

Suhail, K., & Chaudhry, H. R. (2004). Predictors of subjective well-being in an Eastern Muslim culture. *Journal of Social and Clinical Psychology, 23*(3), 359–376.

Uchino, B. N. (2006). Social support and health: A review of physiological processes potentially underlying links to disease outcomes. *Journal of Behavioral Medicine, 29*, 377–387.

Chapter 10
Religiosity and Behavioral Health in Muslims

One of the most important factors that link religious involvement and physical health is health behavior. We know that certain behaviors, practices, and habits influence physical health in a major way. Most people underestimate the impact that these factors (many of which are under the individual's control) have on health and longevity. For example, three health behaviors—regular exercise, consuming a healthy diet and maintaining an ideal body weight, and avoiding cigarette smoking—have been shown to reduce mortality by over 50 % over 10 years, may add as many as 14 years to a person's life span, and could reduce chronic diseases by nearly 80 % (Knoops et al. 2004; Ford et al. 2009; Lee et al. 2009; Kvaavik et al. 2010). The cost of poor health behaviors is also a financial one. Indeed, increasing healthcare costs due to aging populations threatens to overwhelm the economic stability of both developed and developing nations (Zohrabian and Philipson 2010). We now examine research in Muslim populations on the role that religiosity plays in five health behaviors: cigarette smoking, physical activity, diet, weight, and sexual behavior.

Cigarette Smoking

For Muslims, a "fatwa" involves religious rulings that that are not specifically discussed in the Qur'an or Hadith, but are felt by religious scholars to be warranted based on what is contained in these texts. A relatively recent fatwa now places a ban on cigarette smoking for Muslims (Ghouri et al. 2006; Muhamad and Mizerski 2013). When such a fatwa is issued, it becomes an integral part of Islamic law (sharia). Despite this, however, cigarette smoking is relatively high in Muslim countries, especially among men (e.g., Saudi Arabia 19 %, Turkey 51 %, Indonesia 69 %) (Ghouri et al. 2006). Our 2010 systematic review identified five studies that examined relationships between cigarette smoking and religiosity in Muslim-majority populations, and one qualitative study asked participants reasons for their not smoking.

H.G. Koenig and S. Al Shohaib, *Health and Well-Being in Islamic Societies: Background, Research, and Applications*, DOI 10.1007/978-3-319-05873-3_10,

Of the five quantitative studies, three reported significantly less smoking among Muslims who were more religious. We review these qualitative and quantitative studies and then examine research that has compared smoking in Muslims compared to non-Muslims.

Religiosity. In a qualitative study, Naing and Ahmad (2001) examined factors related to cigarette smoking in 180 male teachers and trainee teachers at secondary schools in Malaysia. The most common reason given for not smoking among non-smokers was that smoking was against their religious beliefs. In the first quantitative study to examine the subject, Ozcan and Ozcan (2002) analyzed data on religiosity and cigarette smoking in 4,767 high school students in Ankara, Turkey. No significant association was found between family religiosity or school type (religious vs. other) and smoking. Al-Kandari (2003) conducted a quantitative study that examined smoking and religiosity in 223 Kuwaitis ages 18–75, finding that religious commitment was inversely related to smoking ($r = -0.17, p < 0.05$). A third quantitative study by Afifi Soweid and colleagues (2004) surveyed 954 first-year college students in Beirut, Lebanon, finding that religiosity (4-item measure) was inversely related to smoking in the overall sample ($p < 0.001$, uncontrolled) and in both men and women when analyzed separately. Similar findings were reported by Nakhaee and associates (2009) who examined these relationships in 833 Muslim college students in Iran, finding that each of four religious activities (prayers, Qur'an reading, mosque attendance, fasting) were inversely related to smoking (all $p < 0.001$, uncontrolled). Combining the religious activities into an index and dividing the sample into high, medium, and low religiosity, researchers constructed a regression model that controlled for multiple other covariates. They found that those with high religiosity were about one-half as likely to smoke as those with low religiosity (OR = 0.53, 95 % CI 0.33–0.84, $p < 0.01$).

Finally, Yong and colleagues (2009) conducted an 18-month prospective study of 693 Muslim Malaysian and 1,539 Buddhist Thai adult smokers, finding that Thai Buddhists were more likely than Muslim Malaysians to have made an attempt to quit smoking (74.2 % vs. 47.9 %, $p < 0.001$). However, Malaysian Muslims were more likely to quit successfully (23.2 % vs. 16.8 %, $p = 0.05$). Note that 79 % of Malaysian Muslims and 88 % of Thai Buddhists said that their religion discouraged smoking. Only 8.1 % of Malaysian Muslims said that a fatwa (Islamic ruling) exists that forbids smoking in Islam, whereas 14.9 % said that Ramadan motivated them to quit smoking. After age, gender, income, education, locality, and daily cigarette consumption were controlled for in a regression model, religiosity did not predict either attempts to quit smoking or successful quitting. Although those who said that their religion discourages smoking were more likely to attempt quitting (OR = 3.37, 95 % CI 1.77–6.40), they were not more likely to be successful at quitting. In a later report, Yong and associates (2013) found that religious norms were more important in discouraging cigarette smoking in Muslims than were societal norms (whereas the opposite was true in Thai Buddhists).

Muslims vs. Non-Muslims. We identified seven additional studies that compared Muslims with non-Muslims on cigarette smoking. Adelekan et al. (1993) compared current and lifetime cigarette smoking between 483 Christian and 137 Muslim students at a Nigerian university in 1988. Christians were no more likely than Muslims to either currently smoke (10 % vs. 10 %, respectively) or have a lifetime history of smoking (38 % vs. 42 %). Likewise, Fatoye (2003) examined cigarette smoking in 557 high school seniors in southwestern Nigeria, finding that current and lifetime tobacco use were acknowledged by 7 % and 13 % of 46 Muslim students compared to 3 % and 8 % of 511 Christian students (no significant differences). Similarly, Pampel (2005) analyzing data from a sample of 5,111 men and 20,809 women ages 15–59 in Malawi and Zambia found few differences in cigarette smoking between Catholics, Protestants, and Muslims, all of whom tended to smoke less than those affiliated with other religions. Khan and colleagues (2006), examining 4,297 males ages 15–54 from Bangladesh, also found no differences in Muslims and non-Muslims in likelihood of smoking cigarettes. When these researchers later (Khan et al. 2009) stratified their sample (increased now from 4,297 to 12,155) into those living in slum and non-slum areas, significant differences were found. While there was no difference in smoking between Muslims and Christians in slum areas, Muslims were less likely to smoke than were Christians in non-slum areas (44.1 % vs. 61.6 %, $p<0.01$).

Two additional studies have found differences in smoking behavior between Muslims and Christians. Chaturvedi and colleagues (2003) surveyed 1,831 Hindus, Muslims, and Christians in Northeast India, finding that Hindus and Muslims were less likely to use tobacco than Christians (25.9 % and 22.2 % vs. 42.85, respectively, $p<0.01$). Similar findings were reported by Bradby and associates (2006) who examined Christian, Muslim, and Hindu/Sikh high school students in Scotland asking them at ages 14–15 ($n=620$) and at 18–20 years old ($n=375$) whether they had ever smoked cigarettes. At ages 14–15, Christian boys were more likely (45 %) than Muslims (32 %) or Sikh/Hindu (24 %) to have ever smoked, although these differences disappeared by ages 18–20. Among girls, Christians at ages 14–15 were also more likely (59 %) than Muslims (31 %) and Sikh/Hindu (17 %) to have ever smoked, and this pattern continued when they were 18–20 years old (75 % Christian, 51 % Muslim, 9 % Sikh/Hindu).

Missed Studies. Our 2010 systematic review missed several studies that examined religiosity and smoking in Muslims or compared Muslims to non-Muslims. Islam and Johnson (2003) examined correlates of smoking behavior in 461 Muslim students in 7th to 12th grades attending school in Fairfax County, Virginia (50 % female, 42 % from Saudi Arabia). Students were asked "How effective do you think religious advice is in preventing youth from smoking?" with responses ranging from not effective whatsoever (1) to very effective (4) (called "religious influence"). Susceptibility to smoking, experimentation with cigarettes (ever smoked), and smoking behavior in the past 30 days were assessed. Religious influence was inversely related to susceptibility to smoking ($r=-0.23$, $p<0.05$) and to ever having smoked ($r=-0.16$, $p<0.05$). When other predictors were controlled in a regression model, high religious influence predicted a 28 % reduction in likelihood of ever having smoked (OR$=0.72$, 95 % CI 0.57–0.92, $p<0.05$), which was particularly strong in females (OR$=0.60$, 95 % CI 0.40–0.80).

Vucina and Becirevic (2007) surveyed 732 high school students from Mostar (Bosnia), where about 50 % of the population are Muslim and 50 % are Christian. They examined risk and protective factors regarding cigarette smoking and use of other drugs. Mean age was 16.8 and 51 % were female. Smoking was a common practice with 70 % having smoked cigarettes at least once and 42 % smoking within the last 30 days. Religiosity was assessed using a 19-item measure with two subscales, one measuring religious beliefs and the other religious practices. In addition, importance of religious faith was assessed with a single item ranging from 1 (not important at all) to 7 (extremely important). Religious affiliation was not reported. Religious beliefs ($r=-0.09$, $p<0.05$), religious practices ($r=-0.12$, $p<0.001$), and faith ($r=-0.09$, $p<0.05$) were all inversely correlated with cigarette smoking. However, after controlling for multiple sociodemographic, individual, family, and peer factors, no religious measure significantly predicted cigarette use (although it is likely that the effect of religiosity was explained by these other factors).

In a qualitative study, Khader and Alsadi (2008) examined factors related to smoking behavior among 712 college students in Jordan (52 % males, mean age 21). Current smoking was present in 56.9 % of men and 11.4 % of women. Reasons for not smoking were explored. The most common reason given was adverse effects on health (36 %). The second most common reason was religious belief (33 %).

One additional study examined differences in smoking by religious affiliation. Bachir and Chaaya (2008) identified determinants of smoking during pregnancy in 538 pregnant women hospitalized in Lebanon. Smoking included both narghile and cigarettes. Religious affiliation of participants was either Christian (19 %) or Muslim (81 %). Logistic regression was used to determine predictors of cigarette smoking during pregnancy, controlling for age, education, personal problems, financial problems, nervousness, and social support. Results indicated that Muslim women were nearly three times more likely than Christian women to smoke (OR=2.75, 95 % CI=1.32–5.70, $p<0.01$).

Recent Research. Since our 2010 systematic review, at least three additional studies have now examined relationships between religiosity and smoking. Divsalar and colleagues (2010) examined religiosity and other factors related to cigarette smoking in 1,065 students at Kerman University of Medical Sciences in Iran (77 % female, 23 % smoking). Religiosity was assessed using a 40-item religious attitude scale. Results indicated significantly lower religiosity ($p=0.01$) in smokers compared to nonsmokers, regardless of general health status. A second quantitative study by Kamal and associates (2011) surveyed 474 male college students in Bangladesh (91 % Muslim, mean age 23). A total of 35 % currently smoked (lower than the national average of 64 %) and an additional 25 % said they had quit within the past 30 days. Students in the department of religion were least likely to smoke (1.2 %), significantly different from students in other departments. The finding persisted after controlling for year in school, rural–urban residence, mother's education and occupation, financial status, and whether father or other family members smoked.

We are aware of only one randomized clinical trial that has examined the effects of a religious intervention to decrease smoking in Muslims. Tahlil and colleagues (2013) compared an Islamic-based intervention (IBP) to a health-based intervention (HBP), a combined intervention, and a non-treated control group in 477 seventh and eighth grade students in Aceh, Indonesia. Randomization was at the school level such that eight junior high schools were randomly assigned to a control group (two schools) or to one of the three smoking intervention groups (two schools each). As a result, 109 students were assigned to the IBP, 122 to the HBP, 109 to the combined program, and 128 to the no-intervention control group. Outcomes were Islamic knowledge about smoking, positive attitude toward smoking, intention to smoke, smoking in the past week, smoking in the past 30 days, and percent lifetime smoking. The HBP involved eight 2-h classroom lectures over 8 weeks on smoking prevention knowledge and skill development. The IBP consisted of eight 2-h sessions over 8 weeks that involved teaching and practicing smoking prevention skills based on Islamic teachings that included basic concepts of Islam, health concepts in Islam, expected smoking behavior in Islamic societies, and Islamic law regarding smoking. The combined intervention included components of the two other interventions (HBP and IBP) delivered in eight 2-h sessions over 8 weeks. Those in the control group received no smoking prevention education.

Groups were added together for analysis. Those receiving the IBP ($n=109$) were added with those receiving the combined program ($n=109$) to form the Islamic Group ($n=218$), and those receiving the HBP ($n=122$) were added to those in the control group ($n=128$) to form the Non-Islamic Group. Results indicated that compared to the Non-Islamic Group, those in the Islamic Group had a significantly greater increase in Islamic knowledge ($B=+3.5$, $p<0.001$) and decrease in positive attitudes toward smoking ($B=-7.1$, $p<0.001$), although there was no difference regarding intention to smoke in the future. Likewise, there was no difference between groups in smoking during past week, smoking during past 30 days, or lifetime smoking. Researchers concluded that while the Islamic-based program influenced knowledge and attitudes, it did not have much of an effect on smoking intention or behavior. However, the rate of smoking among students was low to begin with, i.e., 8 %, and this may have reduced the power of the study to detect differences between treatments.

Summary. Of nine studies that examined relationships between religiosity and smoking or smoking attitudes, six found significantly less smoking among Muslims who were more religious. In addition, a randomized clinical trial found that an Islamic intervention to influence attitudes toward smoking and smoking behaviors was effective in altering attitudes toward smoking, but had no influence on behavior (Table 10.1). Eight additional studies compared smoking behavior between Muslims and non-Muslims. Four found no difference in smoking between Muslims and Christians, three reported less smoking in Muslims than Christians, and one study in hospitalized pregnant women found more smoking in Muslims than Christians.

Table 10.1 Religiosity and health behaviors in Muslims

Authors (year)	Method	Sample size	Participants	Location	Controls	Findings
Cigarette smoking						
Ozcan and Ozcan (2002)	CS	4,767	High school students	Turkey	MC	NA
Al-Kandari (2003)	CS	223	Adults ages 18–75	Kuwait	None	P
Islam and Johnson (2003)	CS	461	Muslim high school students	USA	MC	P
Afifi Soweid et al. (2004)	CS	954	College students (1st year)	Lebanon	None	P
Vucina and Becirevic (2007)	CS	732	High school students	Bosnia	MC	NA
Nakhaee et al. (2009)	CS	833	College students	Iran	MC	P
Yong et al. (2009)	PC	693	Adult smokers	Malaysia	MC	NA
Divsalar et al. (2010)	CS	1,065	College students	Iran	None	P
Kamal et al. (2011)	CS	474	College students	Bangladesh	MC	P
Tahlil et al. (2013)	RCT	477	7th and 8th graders	Indonesia	–	P (attitudes)
Exercise						
Cohen and Azaiza (2007)	CS	162	Adult Arabs	Israel	MC	NA
Kahan (2009)	CS	214	Arab college students	USA	MC	NG
Merom et al. (2012)	CS	970	Palestinian adults	Israel	None	NA
Diet						
Cohen and Azaiza (2007)	CS	162	Adult Arabs	Israel	MC	NG
Weight						
Perk et al. (2001)	PC	17	Hypertensive men	Israel	None	P
Kahan (2007)	CS	215	Arab college students	USA	MC	NG
Woofenden (2012)	CS	291	Female college students	Jordan	None	NA
Bharmal et al. (2013)	CS	120	Asian Indians (Muslim)	USA	MC	NA
Sexual behavior						
Lagarde et al. (2000)	CS	858	Adults ages 15–59	Senegal	MC	NA
Herzog (2003)	CS	198	Arab adults	Israel	MC	NA
Trinitapoli and Regnerus (2006)	CS	978	Adult men	Malawi	MC	P

Mohammadi et al. (2006)	CS	1,385	High school students	Iran	MC	(P)
Gilbert (2008)	CS	231	College students	Senegal	SC	P
Yasan et al. (2009)	CS	638	College students	Turkey	MC	P
Shirazi and Morowatisharifabad (2009)	CS	200	College students	Iran	None	P
Kagimu et al. (2011)	CS	2,224	Muslim youth (15–24)	Uganda	None	P
Rahman et al. (2012)	CS	1,032	High school students	Malaysia	SC	P

CS cross-sectional, *PC* prospective, *CC* case control, *RCT* randomized clinical trial, *NA* no association, *P* significant positive association, (*P*) trend positive association ($0.05 < p < 0.10$), *NG* significant negative association, *M* mixed (both significant positive and negative findings), *C* complex association, *MC* multiple controls, *SC* some controls, *Q* qualitative report

Physical Activity/Exercise

Regular physical activity and exercise is known to influence mental and physical health in children, adolescents, and adults (Biddle and Asare 2011; Penedo and Dahn 2005). Within Muslim countries and immigrant populations, physical activity does not have the same priority it does in some Western nations. Involvement in regular exercise or sports may be seen as taking time away from work, from achieving educational or career goals, or possibly even from religious activity. Young Muslims who are increasingly influenced by Western culture may also prefer to hang out, watch TV, spend time on the Internet, etc., which tend to decrease physical activity (Kahan 2003). In general, however, Islam itself encourages physical activity and sport in both men and women, although some interpretations of Islam may discourage such activity (Walseth and Fasting 2003). This is especially true for women, where the use of the veil, gender segregation, issues related to "sexual excitement" with physical activity, and the power relationship between men and women may have an influence. For whatever reason, the general impression is that Muslim populations tend to be less physically active than other religious groups.

Our systematic review uncovered only one study among Muslims that examined the relationship between physical activity and religiosity. Cohen and Azaiza (2007) surveyed a random, population-based sample of 358 Jews and 162 Arabs ages 50–75 in Israel, examining factors related to health behaviors such as exercise. Degree of religiosity was assessed with a single question that asked respondents to categorize themselves as secular, mildly religious, moderately religious, or very religious. Physical exercise was assessed using the Health-Promoting Behaviors Questionnaire. Results indicated that among both men and women, Muslim Arabs scored significantly lower on physical exercise than Jews ($p<0.001$, controlled for gender, age, education, economic status, and other variables). Religiosity was unrelated to frequency of physical exercise in bivariate or multivariate analyses in the combined group.

Missed Studies. The present review uncovered one additional study prior to 2010 by Kahan (2009). He recruited 214 Arab college students in southern California to examine correlates of physical activity. Religious affiliation was determined (49 % Muslim, 51 % non-Muslim), and religiosity was measured using a 6-item scale with response options ranging from 1 to 7 (total score divided into low, medium, or high for analysis). Variables that measured physical activity were energy expenditure (kcal/kg), step count, and participation in 20 activities that required physical activity. Results indicated no difference between Muslims and non-Muslims on energy expenditure, overall step count/day, or likelihood of engaging in vigorous physical activities. While Muslims were less likely than non-Muslims to be among those averaging more than 10,000 steps per day (29.5 % vs. 42.2 %, $p=0.05$), they were more likely to engage in at least one vigorous physical activity (sport) per week (37.1 % vs. 24.8 %, $p=0.05$). Religiosity was unrelated to energy expenditure or vigorous physical activity participation. However, those with medium religiosity had a higher overall step count than those with high religiosity (9,916/day vs. 8,536, $p=0.02$) and were more likely to be among those averaging more than 10,000 steps per day (46.0 % vs. 23.7 %, $p = 0.01$). The association persisted after controlling for gender, body mass index, religion, and acculturation. Based on this study, it is unclear whether Muslims are more or less active than non-Muslims, and those who are highly religious appear to be less active (at least on steps taken per day) than those with medium religiosity.

Recent Research. At least four studies since our 2010 systematic review have examined relationships between religion and exercise/physical activity in Muslim populations. Williams and colleagues (2010) examined risk factors for coronary heart disease, including exercise, among 1,065 healthy South Asians living in West London, UK (vs. 818 white Europeans). Religious affiliation was recorded (15.8 % Muslim, $n = 179$), and religiosity was measured using a 4-item version of the Santa Clara Strength of Religious Faith scale. Strength of religious faith was highest among Muslims. However, compared to the other groups (Sikh, Hindus, white Europeans), Muslims were significantly more likely to be engaged in sedentary behavior (55 % more than 3 h/day vs. 43–48 % for other groups, $p < 0.01$). Muslims were also less likely to engage in moderate or vigorous physical activity during the week (63 % vs. 74–79 %, $p < 0.01$). The relationship between physical activity and religiosity in Muslims was not examined.

Lerner-Geva and colleagues (2010) studied differences in lifestyle among women in midlife (ages 45–64) from three different religious groups in Israel: long-term Jewish residents ($n = 540$), Jewish immigrants from Russia ($n = 151$), and Arabs ($n = 123$). "Healthy lifestyle" was defined as currently not smoking, physically active during the past year, and healthy dietary habits. Results indicated that healthy lifestyle was significantly less common among Arab women (9.7 % for Arabs vs. 15.5 % for Russian immigrant Jews and 39.5 % for long-term Jewish residents, $p < 0.0001$).

Kalter-Leibovici and associates (2011) examined risk factors for adult-onset diabetes in a random national sample of 544 Arabs and 548 Jews in Israel. A physical activity score was calculated based on the frequency and duration of leisure and non-leisure physical activity. Results were stratified by diabetic status. Among non-diabetics, 36.3 % of Arabs scored in the lower third on the physical activity score compared to 21.1 % of Jews. Likewise, 30.7 % of Arabs scored in the upper third of physical activity compared to 39.5 % of Jews. The differences were even more pronounced among diabetics, where 65.8 % of Arabs scored in the lower one-third on physical activity compared to 32.3 % of Jews, and 11.4 % of Arab diabetics scored in the upper one-third on physical activity compared to 41.5 % of Jewish diabetics. Although these differences were not compared statistically, given the sample size they are almost certainly significant.

Finally, Merom and colleagues (2012) compared physical activity levels between 970 Palestinians and 712 Israelis ages 24–74 living in East and West Jerusalem. Concerning religiosity, respondents categorized themselves as orthodox, traditional, or secular. A scale was used to assess 28 specific physical activities of different effort levels during a typical week in the past month. Minutes of each activity were multiplied by its frequency to come up with energy expenditure during a typical week (MET/min/wk). Results indicated no relationship between physical activity and religiosity in Palestinian men or women. However, Palestinian men expended nearly twice as much MET/min/wk in energy compared to Israeli men (7,161 vs. 3,638, $p < 0.0001$). Among women, however, there was no difference.

Summary. Of three studies that have examined religiosity and exercise in Muslims, two found no association and the third found less physical activity among the more religious. Additional research is clearly needed, although it appears that greater religious involvement among Muslims is either unrelated to physical activity or inversely related to it, perhaps for the reasons noted earlier. The general impression that Muslims tend to be less physically active than other religious groups appears to be confirmed by the research. Of six studies that compared Muslims with other faith traditions (Jews, Sikh, Hindu), Muslims exercised less or were less physically active in four studies (three from Israel and one from the UK). One study reported mixed findings among Muslims in the USA, and one found that Palestinian Muslims were more physically active than Jews in Jerusalem. No studies, however, have compared exercise or physical activity between Muslims and non-Muslims in Muslim-majority countries.

Diet

Eating patterns and food intake is important to Muslims. Based on the Qur'an and Sunna, certain foods are considered forbidden (haram), whereas others are lawful and permitted (hallal). Forbidden foods include pork, blood, and meat that have not been prepared according to Islamic rulings (Regenstein et al. 2003). Furthermore, fasting is an important practice, not only during the month of Ramadan but at other times as well (see Chap. 2). Although no food or liquid is to be consumed from sunrise (Sahur) to sunset (Iftar), Muslims eat a greater variety of foods during Ramadan than during the rest of the year and increase their intake of sugary foods and drinks (Dima-Cozma and Cozma 2012). On average, however, Muslims tend to experience a mild drop in average blood sugar levels and lose about 3–8 lb during Ramadan. Despite the importance of food and fasting in Islam, our 2010 systematic review identified no research that examined the relationship between religiosity and diet or quality of nutritional intake in Muslim-majority countries.

Missed Studies. However, during the current review, we uncovered several studies relevant to this topic. First, Bonne and colleagues (2007) examined characteristics associated with eating halal meat among 576 adults (mean age 31) attending a national conference of Muslims in France. Identity as a Muslim was assessed using a single statement, "I consider myself a Muslim," with a 5-point response range from totally disagree to totally agree. The outcome, halal meat consumption, was assessed with the question, "How many times do you intend to eat halal meat in the next 7 days, today included?" Interestingly, results indicated no relationship between identity as a Muslim and intention to eat halal meat. However, among those with strong identity as Muslims, the decision of whether or not to eat halal meat was determined by the opinion of other important persons and institutions, i.e., the norms and rules prescribed by their religion. Thus, it appears that religion does influence the type of food consumed, at least among those with strong Muslim identity.

In a study described earlier, Cohen and Azaiza (2007) compared a random population-based sample of 358 Jews and 162 Arabs ages 50–75 in Israel, examining health-promoting behaviors and religiosity. Among those behaviors was eating a balanced diet, assessed with a single question with responses ranging from 1 (strongly disagree) to 5 (strongly agree). Results from a multivariate regression model, adjusting for gender, age, education, economic status, religiosity, and locus of health control, indicated that Arabs were significantly less likely to say they ate a balanced diet compared to Jews ($B = -0.12$, $p < 0.01$). Likewise, religiosity (assessed on a 4-point scale from secular to very religious) was also significantly and inversely related to eating a balanced diet in that same statistical model ($B = -0.12$, $p < 0.01$).

The last study involves breastfeeding. This practice is associated with better childhood and adult health and both the World Health Organization and the American Academy of Pediatrics recommend that babies be breastfed exclusively for the first 4–6 months of life. Al-Sahab and colleagues (2008) analyzed data from a prospective study of 1,320 healthy newborn infants from Beirut, Lebanon, who were followed for their first year of life. Muslims were 3.5 times more likely than Christians to exclusively breastfeed their infants for the first 4 months after birth (OR = 3.5, 95 % CI 2.5–4.8). After controlling for gender of pediatrician, parity, early discharge, maternal age, and maternal employment status using stepwise regression, Muslims were still nearly twice as likely as Christians to breastfeed for at least 4 months. As stated in the Qur'an, "We have commanded people to be good to their parents: their mothers carried them, with strain upon strain, and it takes 2 years to wean them" (31:14).

Recent Research. Although we could find no studies since our 2010 review that examined the relationship between religiosity and diet or nutritional intake in Muslims, two studies (both cited earlier) compared Muslims with non-Muslims on dietary habits and food consumption. First, Williams and associates (2010) compared the dietary practices of 1,065 healthy South Asians (including 179 Muslims) and 818 white Europeans living in London, UK. Age- and gender-adjusted analyses revealed that Muslims had the lowest fruit/vegetable intake (one serving or more per day) when compared to Sikhs, Hindus, and white Europeans (19.6 % vs. 26.7 %, 28.1 % and 42.0 %, respectively, $p < 0.05$). However, Muslims were more likely to eat low-fat products than the other groups (73.3 % vs. 58.6 %, 61.7 % and 52.5 %, respectively, $p < 0.05$). Muslims were also less likely to eat full-fat products (12.1 % vs. 16.1 % for Sikhs and 18.0 % for Hindus), but were more likely to do so than white Europeans (8.7 %).

Finally, Kalter-Leibovici and colleagues (2011) compared diabetic risk factors in a population-based sample of 544 Arabs and 548 Jews in Israel. They found that the average dietary energy density of food eaten (kcal/g) was higher in Arabs than in Jews among nondiabetics (29.5 % high density in Arabs vs. 19.7 % density in Jews) and even more so among diabetics (35.4 % vs. 17.5 %). Thus, according to this study, Arabs in Israel are more likely than Jews to eat high-calorie foods.

Summary. There is not enough evidence yet to conclude that religiosity is related to a better or worse diet or that Muslims are more or less likely to consume a better diet than members of other religious groups. Only one study examined the effects of religiosity on diet, and it found that great religiosity was associated with a lower likelihood of eating a balanced diet. Four studies compared Muslims with other religious groups. Two of these reported that Muslims in Israel ate a less balanced diet or a higher calorie diet than Jews. One found that while Muslims were less likely to eat fruits and vegetables than Sikhs, Hindus, or white Europeans in the UK, they were more likely to eat a low-fat diet than the other religious groups. In the last study, and only one conducted in a Muslim-majority country (Lebanon), researchers found that Muslims were more likely to breastfeed their infants for the recommended time. More research is clearly needed in Muslim-majority countries on the relationship between religiosity and dietary behavior.

Weight

The Qur'an says, "Eat from the good things We have provided for you, but do not overstep the bounds, or My wrath will descend on you. Anyone on whom my wrath descends has truly fallen" (20:81). Furthermore, extravagance is discouraged: "eat and drink [as We have permitted] but do not be extravagant: God does not like extravagant people" (7:31). Nevertheless, a large female body is venerated in Muslim Arab society, and in some Muslim countries, over 90 % of women say that they currently want to gain weight or did in the past (Rguibi and Belahsen 2006). There may also be Islamic beliefs regarding Allah's will concerning one's body size that may discourage attempts to lose weight or seek a healthy body weight (Batnizky 2011). Furthermore, religious rituals and social events often encourage elaborate and excessive food preparation to demonstrate hospitality, and guests may overeat as a show of appreciation and to avoid insulting their hostess.

Consequently, of the eight countries in the world with the highest average body mass index (BMI) per person, three of these are Muslim-majority countries: Kuwait (#1), Egypt (#6), and United Arab Emirates (#8) (however, note that the USA is #2 on this list) (Bond 2013). Unfortunately, not much research has examined the relationship between religiosity and weight or BMI in Muslim countries. Our 2010 systematic review located only one such study, which examined the effect of the Ramadan fast on weight among hypertensive Muslims living in Israel. Perk and colleagues (2001) studied 17 hypertensive Muslim adults living in Israel (mean age 57, 88 % men). Blood pressure and weight were determined before and during the last week of Ramadan. During Ramadan, although there was no change in blood pressure, participants lost an average of 3.1 lb ($p<0.002$).

Missed Studies. In a previously cited study of 214 Arab American college students in the USA (49 % Muslim, 54 % female), Kahan (2007) reported relationships between religion, religiosity, and physical activity. One-third of the sample (33.2 %) was overweight or obese. Those who were overweight were more likely to be Muslim (39.1 % vs. 27.5 % for non-Muslim, $p=0.05$) and were more likely to be high on religiosity (40.2 % vs. 26.7 % for non-overweight individuals, $p<0.05$). After controlling for other factors in a regression model (gender, socio-economic status, acculturation, and physical activity), Muslims were 3.6 times more likely to be overweight (OR = 3.62, 95 % CI 1.51–8.72), and those who were high on religiosity were 2.5 times more likely to be overweight (OR = 2.46, 95 % CI 1.17–5.18).

Latzer and associates (2009) examined differences in BMI between 926 Muslim, 128 Christian, and 87 Druze girls ages 12–18 year living in Israel. Participants were systematically sampled throughout Israel from schools randomly selected from urban and rural settings. Girls affiliated with the Druze religion were more likely to be currently dieting (44.5 % vs. 29.9 % of Christians and 28.3 % of Muslims, $p<0.05$), and also had lower BMI scores (18.9 vs. 20.8 for Christians and 20.9 for Muslims, $p<0.0001$). Religiosity was not examined.

Recent Research: Several studies since 2010 have compared Muslims with non-Muslims on body weight or BMI. In the previously cited study by Lerner-Geva and colleagues (2010), researchers compared BMI between female long-term Jewish residents ($n=540$), Jewish immigrants from Russia ($n=151$), and Arabs ($n=123$). Obesity was more common among Arab women than other groups (49.1 % obese vs. 34.4 % of Russian immigrants and 21.4 % of Jewish long-term residents ($p<0.0001$, uncontrolled).

Dunkel and associates (2010) surveyed 95 Muslim women and 106 non-Muslim women (88 % Christian) in middle to upper-middle class neighborhoods of Illinois and Iowa, in order to determine relationships between body satisfaction, BMI, and Muslim dress preferences. The sample was stratified into younger (ages 18–26) and older (ages 40–74) women. Participants were divided into five groups: non-Muslims, Muslims wearing Western dress alone, Muslims wearing Western dress with veil, Muslims wearing Muslim dress but without veil, and Muslims wearing Muslim dress with veil. The last group was considered to be the most religious (or at least, most compliant with Muslim religious cultural practice). Among younger women, Muslims who wore Muslim dress with veil ($n=28$) had the lowest BMI and non-Muslim women ($n=54$) had the highest BMI (20.25 vs. 23.17, respectively, $p<0.05$). Among older women, Muslims who wore Muslim dress with veil ($n=28$) also had lower BMI than non-Muslim women ($n=51$) (24.61 vs. 28.15, respectively, $p<0.05$).

In the previously described study by Kalter-Leibovici and associates (2011), which examined a population-based sample of 544 Arabs and 548 Jews from an urban area of Israel, researchers measured BMI in diabetics and nondiabetics in each group. The prevalence of obesity ($BMI \geq 26.0$) was lower in Arabs than in Jews for both nondiabetics (24.2 % vs. 33.0 %, respectively) and diabetics (47.2 % vs. 65.6 %, respectively). This is despite the fact that both nondiabetic and diabetic Arabs exercised less and consumed higher calorie foods than Jews.

In a study that focused on religiosity and body image, Woofenden (2012) measured BMI in 291 female college students in Jordanian and 189 female students in America. Jordanian women (97 % Muslim) ranged in age from 18 to 43 (mean age 21), with BMI ranging from 13.7 to 58.1. American women (75 % Christian) ranged in age from 18 to 63 (mean age 20.0), with BMI ranging from 16.3 to 50. Religious faith was assessed using the 10-item Santa Clara Strength of Religious Faith Scale. Results indicated that average BMI was significantly higher in American compared to Jordanian students (23.6 vs. 21.7, $t=4.7$, $p<0.001$). Strength of religious faith was unrelated to BMI in either Americans or Jordanians.

Hossain and colleagues (2012) analyzed data on 10,115 married, currently non-pregnant women ages 15–49 in Bangladesh (90 % Muslim). Adjusting for age, education, number of families, wealth, number of children, age at first childbirth, age when married, and husband's education using regression analysis, results revealed that average BMI was significantly higher among Muslim women compared to non-Muslims ($B=+0.51$, $p<0.001$).

Finally, a study of religiosity and weight was conducted by Bharmal and researchers (2013) among 3,228 mostly immigrant Asian Indians living in California. Religious affiliations of the sample were 60 % Hindu, 20 % Sikh, 6 % Muslim ($n=120$), and 15 % other or agnostics. Religiosity was assessed using a scale composed of self-rated religiosity, religious beliefs, and religious participation. While religiosity was positively related to BMI in Hindus and Sikhs, it was unrelated to BMI in Muslims (OR=0.69, 95 % CI 0.28–1.70, controlling for acculturation, time in the USA, age, gender, marital status, education, health status, and smoking status). Researchers explained this by the fact that Muslims do not drink alcohol (which is associated with weight gain) and pray five times a day, which is associated with changes in body position (a form of exercise).

Summary: Four studies have examined the associations between religiosity and weight or BMI in Muslims (Table 10.1). One found a significant decrease in weight during Ramadan fasting, and one found that religiosity in Arab American college students was positively related to being overweight. Two studies found no association between religiosity and weight, one among college students in Jordan and one in Asian Indian Muslims in California. Seven studies compared the body weight of Muslims with that of non-Muslims. Two found that Muslim Arab American college students and Muslims in Israel were significantly more likely to be overweight than non-Muslims, and one found that Muslim women in Bangladesh had significantly higher body mass index (BMI) than non-Muslims. Two studies found that Muslims had lower BMI than non-Muslims, i.e., one study from Israel finding lower BMI among Muslim women compared to Jewish women and one study finding that Muslim female college students in Jordan had lower weight than Christian female students in America. Likewise, one study found that BMI was lowest among Muslim American women who wear traditional Muslim dress and veil compared to non-Muslim American women, and another study found that Muslim and Christian adolescent girls in Israel had roughly equal BMI and both had lower BMI than Druze girls. Again, the research demonstrates no consistent pattern of findings.

Sexual Behavior

Sexual behavior is a private activity among Muslims and carries with it serious moral overtones, given that any sexual activity outside of marriage is forbidden. Thus, Muslims may not readily admit to such behavior, and willingness to do so may be affected by the gender and dress of the person conducting the interview (Blaydes and Gillum 2013). Extramarital sexual activity is of particular importance to health given its relationship to the spread of sexually transmitted diseases, especially HIV. Our systematic review identified only one study prior to 2010 that had examined relationships between religiosity and extramarital sexual behavior in Muslims. A second study compared extramarital sexual activity between Hindu and Muslim male college students in Nepal. We now review both studies below.

Shirazi and Morowatisharifabad (2009) surveyed 200 male college students in Iran, assessing religiosity and self-reported sexual activity. Students were all unmarried or never married, had completed at least 2 years of college, and were Shiite Muslims (age range 20–27). Religious involvement was assessed with a 4-item scale: frequency of prayer, frequency of fasting during Ramadan, talking with others about religious concerns, and frequency of following religious rules. Students were also asked about past sexual relationships, norms about sexual relationships, attitudes toward sexual relationships, and self-efficacy in avoiding sex until married. Of the group, 20 % indicated sexual contact in the past. Religiosity was related to more conservative attitudes toward sex ($p < 0.001$), greater self-efficacy in avoiding sex ($p = 0.001$), and lower likelihood of past sexual contact ($p < 0.001$) (uncontrolled).

Adhikari and Tamang (2009) compared extramarital sexual activity in 573 Hindu and Muslim male students attending 12 colleges in Kathmandu, Nepal. Participants were ages 15–24 years, 88 % unmarried, and most (91 %) had taken a course in school on reproductive health. About half (41 %) lived with family, 19 % alone, and 40 % with friends. Overall, 39 % said they had experienced premarital sexual intercourse. Multivariate analysis indicated that Hindu students were three times more likely than Muslim students to report having had premarital sex ($OR = 2.99$, $p < 0.05$).

Missed Studies. We missed numerous studies in our 2010 review, especially those comparing Muslims and non-Muslims on extramarital sexual activity. Many of these studies were conducted in non-Muslim-majority African countries, so they did not show up in the studies we selected from our 2010 systematic review (which was largely limited to those from Muslim-majority countries). Religion has now become a focus in many studies since it may influence the spread of HIV infection and AIDS in sub-Saharan Africa.

Religiosity. In a study of 858 adults ages 15–59 in rural Senegal, Lagarde and colleagues (2000) examined factors related to protection against AIDS among Muslims (76 %) and Christians. In the overall sample, importance of religion was not related to being faithful to one's spouse or intending to be faithful to protect against AIDs (adjusting for age, education, marital status, religion, and migration status).

However, a number of important AIDS prevention-related variables were less frequent among those who were more religious, such as considering AIDS a major health problem, intending to change behavior to protect against AIDS, and believing that condom use was not forbidden by their religion.

Investigators studying Jewish and Muslim mothers in Israel found a similar negative effect of religion on practices to prevent the consequences of extramarital sexual activity, including the intention to vaccinate their daughters for human papillomavirus (a sexually transmitted virus that leads to cervical cancer) (Ben Natan et al. 2011). Muslims in that study had lower intention to vaccinate their daughters than did Jews. This might be explained by the belief that advocating the use of condoms for protection and vaccination against HPV, while helping to prevent AIDS and cervical cancer, means giving implicit permission to have sexual relations outside of marriage, which is strictly forbidden (haram) in Islam.

In a study previously described, Herzog (2003) examined the relationship of religiosity to perceived seriousness of a wide range of crimes in a random sample of 987 Israeli adults (633 Jews, 198 Arab Muslims). Religiosity was measured by a single item that categorized respondents as secular, religious, or very religious. Among Arab Muslims, who were more likely than Jews to believe that illegal sexual relations was a serious crime, greater religiosity was surprisingly not associated with this belief, as it was among Jews.

Trinitapoli and Regnerus (2006) analyzed data from the second wave of the Malawi Diffusion and Ideational Change Project in rural Malawi ($n=978$, all men). The largest percentage of any religion in the sample was Muslim (23 %), compared to Pentecostal (20 %), Mission Protestant (19 %), African Independent Church (14 %), Catholic (19 %), and other (5 %). At that time, this was the largest dataset available that had measured religiosity and characteristics related to HIV transmission. Religious affiliation and frequency of religious attendance were assessed, along with several extramarital sexual activity variables: extramarital partner in the past 12 months reporting sexually transmitted infection (STI), likelihood of already being infected with HIV, and likelihood of being infected in the future. Religiosity (attendance at religious services) was significantly and inversely related to having an extramarital partner in the past 12 months and to having an STI.

Mohammadi and colleagues (2006) surveyed a random sample of 1,385 males aged 15–18 in Tehran, Iran, examining correlates of sexual behavior. Most participants (98 %) were Muslim and 79.7 % indicated that they were religious (vs. somewhat religious or not religious). An index of premarital sexual relations was developed based on six questions. Those who were more religious were significantly less likely to have permissive attitudes toward premarital sexual behavior. Similarly, religiosity was significantly and inversely related to having had sexual contact/experience (23.2 % of religious, 43.4 % of somewhat religious, 51.5 % of not religious). A logistic regression model that controlled for other predictors revealed that those who said they were only somewhat or not religious were 64 % more likely to have had sexual contact than those who were religious (OR = 1.64, 95 % CI 0.98–2.73, $p<0.10$, trend).

Jaafar and associates (2006) surveyed 389 Malaysian and Indonesian adolescents who reported that they had premarital sex at least one time or more (179 boys and 210 girls, ages 13–20). Adolescents were also asked how important religion was in their life and whether they believed in God. Interestingly, 93 % believed in God and 87 % said they believed that God would punish those who did wrong or sinned (as expected in this largely Muslim population). However, 65 % described themselves as *not religious*. Although the relationship between sexual activity and religion or religiosity was not examined, this is a very low rate of religiosity for youth in this part of the world. The finding suggests that religiosity was lower in this group of sexually active adolescents compared to their peers.

Gilbert (2008) examined the influence of Islam on preventing AIDS among 234 Muslim college students in the West African country of Senegal (ages 18–33, 73 % male). Religiosity was assessed using two 6-item scales that focused on Islamic religious beliefs and practices. Results indicated that religiosity was positively related to abstinence from sex ($B = +0.12$, $p < 0.01$). Furthermore, in contrast to previous reports, religiosity was not associated with a lower likelihood of using condoms.

Yasan and associates (2009) examined predictors of premarital sexual behaviors in 638 college students in Turkey (60 % male). Religiosity was measured, but in an atypical fashion. Participants were categorized as "non-religion" (no religious belief), "another religious belief" (practices a religion other than Islam), "non-religiosity" (does not practice acts of Islamic worship but has religious belief), "liberal religiosity" (sometimes performs daily Islamic acts and has religious belief), and "conservative religiosity" (engages in daily Islamic worship). For masturbation, compared to conservative religious Muslims, those who were "non-religion" were 11 times more likely (OR = 10.9, 95 % CI 2.5–47.6); those who were not Muslim were six times more likely (OR = 6.0, 95 % CI 2.4–14.2); and those who were of liberal religiosity were 2.6 times more likely (OR = 2.6, 95 % CI 1.3–5.4). For foreplay/sexual intercourse, compared to those who were conservative religious Muslims, those in the non-religion group were 13 times more likely (OR = 13.4, 95 % CI 3.2–56.0); those who were not Muslim were 16 times more likely (OR = 16.2, 95 % CI 4.7–56.2); and liberally religious were nine times more likely (OR = 8.9, 95 % CI 2.6–29.9). Analyses were controlled for socioeconomic status, living area, sexual orientation, and gender.

Muslims vs. *Non-Muslims*. In the Lagarde et al. (2000) study cited above from Senegal, Muslim men were significantly more likely than Christian men to intend to be (or become) faithful in order to be protected from AIDS (55 % vs. 39 %, $p = 0.01$), although among women, there was no difference between Muslims and Christians. There was also no significant difference between Muslims and Christians among either men or women in percentage that reported casual sex in the past 12 months (in men, 22 % vs. 24 %, and in women, 5 % vs. 5 %).

Addai (2000) examined data from the 1993 Ghana Demographic and Health Survey to explore relationships between religion and premarital sex in 4,562 women ages 15–49. Results indicated that Muslim women in Ghana were least likely to have had premarital sex (57.8 %) compared to Protestants (82.6 %), Catholics (78.9 %), and other Christian participants (76.8 %). Among women who were never married, there was no difference in premarital sex between Muslims and Christians or those affiliated with other religious groups. However, among currently married or previously married women, Muslims were significantly less likely to report having had premarital sex compared to all other religious groups. Likewise, in the Herzog (2003) study cited above, recall that Muslims were more likely than Jews to feel that illegal sexual relations were a serious crime ($B=+0.18$, $p<0.05$).

Gray (2004) examined the prevalence of HIV infection in 38 sub-Saharan African countries, correlating it with the percentage of Muslims that made up each country. All countries had a minimum of 1 million inhabitants. Predictors were percentage of Muslims, population density, percentage of urban population, annual per capita purchasing power, and year of first recorded AIDS case. Percentage of the population ages 15–49 with HIV infection was the dependent variable. The statistical model with the five variables above accounted for 69 % of the variance in HIV prevalence. Of the five predictors, however, only two were significantly related to HIV infection rates: percentage of a country's population that was Muslim predicted lower HIV infection rates ($B=-0.52$, $p=0.0005$) and annual per capita purchasing power predicted higher infection rates ($B=+0.64$, $p=0.0002$).

In the Trinitapoli and Regnerus (2006) study cited above of 978 men from rural Malawi, Muslims were *more likely* to have an extramarital partner (15.0 % vs. 4.2 % for Pentecostal Christians) and were more likely to report a sexually transmitted infection (21.8 % vs. 7.4 % Pentecostals). When other variables were controlled (religious attendance, previous marriage, age, and region of residence), however, Muslim affiliation was no longer a significant predictor of sexual behavior.

Soldan and colleagues (2007) examined predictors of sexual behavior among a random sample of 715 sexually active men in rural Malawi (surveyed in 2000–2001 for determining HIV risk). The majority of men were Muslim (86.4 %) and the others were mostly Christian (13.6 %). Regression models controlling for age, income, and occupation and migration status revealed that there was no difference between Muslims and Christians in the likelihood of ever having paid for sex or in the use of condoms during sex. However, Muslim men were significantly more likely to have more sexual partners than Christian men ($B=+0.44$, $p<0.05$), even after controlling for men with more than one wife.

Coleman and Testa (2008) surveyed 3,007 students aged 15–18 attending secondary schools in London, UK, examining sexual knowledge, attitudes, and behaviors. None of the schools were religious schools. Included in the sample were 679 Muslims (26 %), 967 Christians (36 %), 582 Hindus (22 %), and 418 with no religious affiliation (16 %). Prevalence of having had sexual intercourse differed between religious groups. Among males, prevalence was 49.7 % in Christians, 40.9 % in those with no religious affiliation, 30.9 % in Muslims, and 23.9 % in Hindus ($p<0.001$). Among females, prevalence was 41.3 % among those with no religious affiliation, 34.6 % of Christians, 12.5 % of Hindus, and 9.0 % of Muslims ($p<0.001$). Christians and Muslim girls were least likely to use contraception (55.0 % and 53.6 %, respectively). Among women, 13.3 % ($n=39$) reported having gotten pregnant or contracted a sexually transmitted disease, with the majority occurring in Christian girls ($n=26$).

Koffi and Kawahara (2008) analyzed data on religion and sexual behavior in 3,041 never-married people ages 15–24 living in the Cote d'Ivoire, the country in West Africa with the highest HIV infection rates. The sample was 54 % male, and most participants were either Christian (50.4 %) or Muslim (30.7 %). Sexual abstinence was the main outcome variable. "Primary" abstinence was defined as never having had sexual intercourse, and "secondary" abstinence was defined as having had sex but not within the past 12 months. Results stratified by gender indicated that among abstinent males (primary or secondary), religious affiliation was as follows: 48.2 % Christian, 36.5 % Muslims, and 15.2 % "other" ($p<0.01$). Among women who were abstinent, 53.9 % were Christian, 30.4 % were Muslim, and 15.5 % were "other." Logistic regression was used to control analyses for age, education, place and region of residence, attitude, and AIDS-related knowledge. Among males, those in the "other" religious category (including those with no religion, other religion, and Animists) were significantly less likely than Catholics (the reference group) to engage in sexually abstinent behavior. There were no significant differences in sexual abstinence between Muslims and any Christian group in either males or females, after these other variables were controlled.

Recent Research. We identified four studies that have examined this subject since our 2010 review, two conducted in sub-Saharan African countries.

Religiosity. In a study previously described, Kagimu and colleagues (2011) examined factors related to new HIV infections among 1,224 Muslim youth ages 15–24 (50 % male) attending 30 mosques surrounding a hospital in Uganda. Religiosity was assessed using the Brief Multidimensional Measurement of Religiousness/Spirituality scale (Fetzer Institute). As an objective indicator of religiosity, researchers also determined whether the respondent had a "Sujda" (a spot on forehead due to frequent praying and bowing head to touch ground). High-risk sexual behaviors that increase risk of HIV were assessed. Results indicated that Muslims who had a Sujda were less likely to have ever had sex (66 % vs. 76 % without a Sujda, $p<0.001$, no controls). Likewise, wearing a Muslim cap was associated with a lower risk of having had sex (65 % vs. 77 %, $p=0.01$). Sex outside of marriage was also lower among those with a Sujda (40 % vs. 53 %, $p=0.01$). Having a single lifetime sexual partner (vs. more than one lifetime partner) was also more common among those who watched religious TV regularly (29 % vs. 17 %, $p<0.005$), frequently attended mosque prayers (23 % vs. 16 %, $p=0.02$), frequently participated in other mosque activities (31 % vs. 18 %, $p=0.01$), wore a Muslim cap (24 % vs. 11 %, $p=0.005$), and strongly tried to implement religious teachings (55 % vs. 40 %, $p<0.05$). Using a condom was *positively* associated with several religious activities (watching religious programs, trying hard to love God, participating in mosque activities).

Rahman and associates (2012) examined factors related to premarital sexual activities in 1,032 secondary school students in Kelantan, Malaysia (57 % female, ages 13–17, all Muslim). Religious practice was assessed by a single question that asked about "neglecting religious practice (daily prayers)." Attitude toward premarital sexual activities was the outcome. Results indicated that compared to those who never neglected their daily prayers, those who neglected their daily prayers were over twice as likely to have permissive attitudes toward premarital sexual activities, after controlling for age, gender, and knowledge (OR = 2.02, 95 % CI 1.49–2.73, $p < 0.001$).

Muslims vs. *Non-Muslims.* Clark (2010) analyzed data from a prospective study of religion and sexual behaviors in Malawi. The sample consisted of 722 married men surveyed in 1998 and again in 2001. Extramarital sexual partnerships (EMSP) were the focus of the study. In both 1998 and 2001, 9 % of men reported having extramarital affairs within the past year. Religious affiliation (in 1998 and 2001) and attendance at religious services (in 2001 only) were both measured. Religious affiliation was categorized as Protestant (52–55 %), Catholic (18 %), Muslim (21–22 %), or "other" (7–8 %). Analyses using logistic regression that controlled for age, education, religious attendance, and socioeconomic status indicated that in 1998, Muslims were *more likely* to have an EMSP compared to Catholics ($B = +1.51$, $p < 0.05$), whereas in 2001, Muslims were *less likely* than Catholics to have an EMSP ($B = -1.27$, $p < 0.05$). Although the percentage of Muslims who made up those having EMSP increased from 24 % in 1998 to 34 % in 2001, the percentage of Catholics increased even more from 10 to 28 % (while Protestants dropped from 59 to 33 %). No explanation for these changes was given.

Finally, Adamczyk and Hayes (2012) analyzed cross-national data from more than 30 mostly developed countries to determine whether the Muslim percentage of a country's population was associated with having sex outside of marriage. Data were available from each country on persons ages 15–64. The analysis for premarital sex focused on the 418,140 who had been married or were currently married, and for extramarital sex, focused on the 327,752 married respondents who were currently married and indicated they had sexual relations within the past year. Religious affiliation was 39 % Christian, 23 % Muslim, 27 % Hindu, 4 % Buddhist, and 2 % no religion. Overall, 53 % of married or ever-married participants indicated that they had experienced premarital sex, whereas only 1 % of currently married respondents admitted to having extramarital sex. At the individual person level, hierarchical logistic regression was used to control for demographic, work, and family variables. Results indicated that Muslims were 53 % less likely than Christians to have had premarital sex (OR = 0.47, $p < 0.001$). At the country level, percentage of the population Muslim was related to a slightly lower likelihood of having premarital sex (OR = 0.98, $p < 0.001$). The same pattern was present for extramarital affairs. Muslims were 45 % less likely than Christians to have had such affairs when married (OR = 0.55, $p < 0.001$), although percentage of Muslims at the country level (after controlling for individual-level relationships) was unrelated to having extramarital affairs.

Summary. At least nine studies have examined the relationship between religiosity and extramarital sexual activity in Muslim-majority populations. Of those, seven (78 %) reported significant inverse relationships (Table 10.1). At least 12 studies have compared Muslims with members of other religious groups, with eight (67 %) finding less extramarital sexual activity in Muslims, one finding greater extramarital sexual activity among Muslims in Malawi, and three reporting no difference or mixed findings between Muslims and those from other religious affiliations. In general, then, premarital and extramarital sex is less common in Muslims compared to other religious groups. As in Christians, greater religiosity is related to lower rates of premarital and extramarital sex in Muslims. However, under-reporting among Muslims may be an issue given the strong prohibition against such activity. Also, strong beliefs against extramarital sex may lead to resistance against taking measures to prevent the spread of sexually transmitted diseases.

Summary and Conclusions

In general, healthy behaviors are more common and unhealthy behaviors are less common in Muslims who are more deeply religious. First, the research indicates lower rates of cigarette smoking among those who are more religious (seven of ten studies). There is not much difference in smoking behavior between Muslims and other religious groups, although Muslims in general are less likely to smoke (three of eight studies) given the fatwa against smoking. Very little research has examined relationships between religiosity and exercise, diet, or weight among Muslims, although what research exists is not particularly positive, suggesting that this area of health behavior needs improvement. Religious Muslims may view exercise as less of a priority since it takes time away from work, academic pursuits, or religious activity. Socioeconomic factors may also play a role since poorer Muslims may not have time for exercise. The eating habits of Muslims are not always balanced, with strong cultural factors influencing the kind of foods eaten and views toward an ideal body weight, especially for women. Finally, risky sexual activity outside of marriage is inversely related to religiosity among Muslims in the vast majority of studies (seven out of nine) and is also less common in Muslims (compared to other religious groups). However, strong prohibitions against extramarital sexual activity may prevent Muslims from taking precautions to prevent the spread of sexually transmitted diseases.

References

Adamczyk, A., & Hayes, B. E. (2012). Religion and sexual behaviors: Understanding the influence of Islamic cultures and religious affiliation for explaining sex outside of marriage. *American Sociological Review, 77*(5), 723–746.

Addai, I. (2000). Religious affiliation and sexual initiation among Ghanaian women (2000). *Review of Religious Research, 41*(3), 328–343.

Adelekan, M. L., Abiodun, O. A., Imouoklhome-Obayan, A. O., Oni, G. A., & Ogunremi, O. O. (1993). Psychosocial correlates of alcohol, tobacco and cannabis use: Findings from a Nigerian university. *Drug and Alcohol Dependence, 33*, 247–256.

Adhikari, R., & Tamang, J. (2009). Premarital sexual behavior among male college students of Kathmandu, Nepal. *BMC Public Health, 9*, 241.

Afifi Soweid, R. A., Khawaja, M., & Salem, M. T. (2004). Religious identity and smoking behavior among adolescents: Evidence from entering students at the American University of Beirut. *Health Communication, 16*(1), 47–62.

Al-Kandari, Y. Y. (2003). Religiosity and its relation to blood pressure among selected Kuwaitis. *Journal of Biosocial Science, 35*(3), 463–472.

Al-Sahab, B., Tamim, H., Mumtaz, G., Khawaja, M., Khogali, M., Afifi, R., Nassif, Y., & Yunis, K. A. (2008). Predictors of breast-feeding in a developing country: Results of a prospective cohort study. *Public Health Nutrition, 11*(12), 1350–1356.

Bachir, R., & Chaaya, M. (2008). Maternal smoking: Determinants and associated morbidity in two areas of Lebanon. *Maternal and Child Health Journal, 12*(3), 298–307.

Batnizky, A. K. (2011). Cultural constructions of "obesity": Understanding body size, social class and gender in Morocco. *Health & Place, 17*, 345–352.

Ben Natan, M., Aharon, O., Palickshvili, S., & Gurman, V. (2011). Attitude of Israeli mothers with vaccination of their daughters against papilloma virus. *Journal of Pediatric Nursing, 25*, 70–71.

Bharmal, N., Kaplan, R. M., Shapiro, M. F., Kagawa-Singer, M., Wong, M. D., Mangione, C. M., Divan, H., & McCarthy, W. J. (2013). The association of religiosity with overweight/obese body mass index among Asian Indian immigrants in California. *Preventive Medicine, 57*(4), 315–321.

Biddle, S. J. H., & Asare, M. (2011). Physical activity and mental health in children and adolescents: A review of reviews. *British Journal of Sports Medicine, 45*, 886–895.

Blaydes, L., & Gillum, R. M. (2013). Religiosity-of-interview effects: Assessing the impact of veiled enumerators on survey response in Egypt. *Politics and Religion, 6*(3), 459–482.

Bond A (2013). Fattest countries in the world revealed: Extraordinary graphic charts the average body mass index of men and women in every country (with some surprising results). *Mail Online*: *Health*, March 29. Retrieved October 7, 2013, from http://www.dailymail.co.uk/health/article-2301172/Fattest-countries-world-revealed-Extraordinary-graphic-charts-average-body-mass-index-men-women-country-surprising-results.html

Bonne, K., Vermeir, I., Bergeaud-Blackler, F., & Verbeke, W. (2007). Determinants of halal meat consumption in France. *British Food Journal, 109*, 367–386.

Bradby, H., Williams, R., Bradby, H., & Williams, R. (2006). Is religion or culture the key feature in changes in substance use after leaving school? Young Punjabis and a comparison group in Glasgow. *Ethnicity & Health, 11*(3), 307–324.

Chaturvedi, H., Phukan, R., & Mahanta, J. (2003). The association of selected sociodemographic factors and differences in patterns of substance use: A pilot study in selected areas of Northeast India. *Substance Use & Misuse, 38*(9), 1305–1322.

Clark, S. (2010). Extra-marital partnerships and male friendships in rural Malawi. *Demographic Research* 22,1–28.

Cohen, M., & Azaiza, F. (2007). Health-promoting behaviors and health locus of control from a multicultural perspective. *Ethnicity & Disease, 17*(4), 636–642.

Coleman, L. M., & Testa, A. (2008). Sexual health knowledge, attitudes and behaviors: Variations among a religiously diverse sample of young people in London, UK (2008). *Ethnicity & Health, 13*(1), 55–72.

Dima-Cozma, C., & Cozma, S. (2012). Religion and medicine or the spiritual dimension of healing. *Journal for the Study of Religions and Ideologies, 11*(Spring), 31–48.

Divsalar, K., Nejadnaderi, S., Nakhaee, N., & Rouhani, S. (2010). Religious attitude associated with general health and smoking in Iranian students. *Journal of Addiction and Health, 2*(1–2), 1–7.

Dunkel, T. M., Davidson, D., & Qurashi, S. (2010). Body satisfaction and pressure to be thin in younger and older Muslim and non-Muslim women: The role of Western and non-Western dress preferences. *Body Image, 7*, 56–65.

Fatoye, F. O. (2003). Psychosocial correlates of substance use amongst secondary school students in south western Nigeria. *East African Medical Journal, 80*(3), 154–158.

Ford, E. S., Bergmann, M. M., Kroger, J., Schienkiewitz, A., Weikert, C., & Boeing, H. (2009). Healthy living is the best revenge: Findings from the European prospective investigation into cancer and nutrition-Potsdam study. *Archives of Internal Medicine, 169*, 1355–1362.

Ghouri, N., Atcha, M., & Sheikh, A. (2006). Influence of Islam on smoking among Muslims. *British Medical Journal, 332*, 291–294.

Gilbert, S. S. (2008). The influence of Islam on AIDS prevention among Senegalese university students. *AIDS Education and Prevention, 20*(5), 399–407.

Gray, P. B. (2004). HIV and Islam: Is HIV prevalence lower among Muslims? *Social Science & Medicine, 58*, 1751–1756.

Herzog, S. (2003). Religiosity and perceptions of crime seriousness by Jewish and Muslim respondents in Israel. *Deviant Behavior, 24*, 153–174.

Hossain, M. G., Bharati, P., Aik, S., Lestrel, P. E., Abeer, A., & Kamarul, T. (2012). Body mass index of married Bangladeshi women: Trends and association with socio-demographic factors. *Journal of Biosocial Science, 44*(4), 385–399.

Islam, S. M. S., & Johnson, C. A. (2003). Correlates of smoking behavior among Muslim Arab-American adolescents. *Ethnicity & Health, 8*(4), 319–337.

Jaafar, J., Istiqomah, W., & Afiatin, T. (2006). The relationship between religiosity, youth culture, and premarital sex among Malaysian and Indonesian adolescents. *Asia Pacific Journal of Social Work and Development, 16*(2), 5–18.

Kagimu M, Guwatudde D, Rwabukwali C, Kaye S, Walakira Y, Ainomugisha D (2011). Religiosity for promotion of behaviors likely to reduce new HIV infections in Uganda: A study among Muslim youth in Wakiso district. Journal of Religion and Health, December 28 [E-pub ahead of print] DOI 10.1007/s10943-011-9563-8

Kahan, D. (2003). Islam and physical activity: Implications for American sport and physical education. *Journal of Physical Education, Recreation & Dance, 74*(3), 48–54.

Kahan, D. (2007). Overweight and its relationship to Middle Eastern American college students' sociodemographics and physical activity. *Research Quarterly for Exercise and Sport, 78*(3), 248–256.

Kahan, D. (2009). Quantity, type, and correlates of physical activity among American Middle Eastern university students. *Research Quarterly for Exercise and Sport, 80*, 412–423.

Kalter-Leibovici, O., Chetrit, A., Lubin, F., Atamna, A., Alpert, G., Ziv, A., Abu-Saad, K., Mura, H., Eilat-Adar, S., & Goldbourt, U. (2011). Adult-onset diabetes among Arabs and Jews in Israel: A population-based study. *Diabetic Medicine, 29*(6), 748–754.

Kamal, S. M. M., Islam, M. A., & Rahman, M. A. (2011). Sociopsychological correlates of smoking among male university students in Bangladesh. *Asia-Pacific Journal of Public Health, 23*, 555–567.

Khader, Y. S., & Alsadi, A. A. (2008). Smoking habits among university students in Jordan: Prevalence and associated factors. *Eastern Mediterranean Health Journal, 14*(4), 897–904.

Khan, M. M., Aklimunnessa, K., Kabir, M. A., Kabir, M., & Mori, M. (2006). Tobacco consumption and its association with illicit drug use among men in Bangladesh. *Addiction, 101*(8), 1178–1186.

Khan, M. M., Khan, A., Kraemer, A., & Mori, M. (2009). Prevalence and correlates of smoking among urban adult men in Bangladesh: Slum versus non-slum comparison. *BMC Public Health, 9*, 149.

Knoops, K. T., de Groot, L. C., Kromhout, D., Perrin, A. E., & Moreiras-Varela, O. (2004). Mediterranean diet, lifestyle factors, and 10-year mortality in elderly European men and women: The HALE project. *Journal of the American Medical Association, 292*, 1433–1439.

Koffi, A. K., & Kawahara, K. (2008). Sexual abstinence behavior among never-married youths in a generalized HIV epidemic country: Evidence from the 2005 Cote d'Ivoire AIDS indicator survey. *BMC Public Health, 8*, 408.

Kvaavik, E., Batty, G. D., Ursin, G., Huxley, R., & Gale, C. R. (2010). Influence of individual and combined health behaviors on total and cause-specific mortality in men and women: The United Kingdom Health and Lifestyle Survey. *Archives of Internal Medicine, 170*, 711–718.

Lagarde, E., Enel, C., Seck, K., Gueye-Ndiaye, A., Piau, J. P., Pison, G., Delaunay, V., Ndoye, I., & Mboup, S. (2000). Religion and protective behaviors towards AIDS in rural Senegal. *AIDS, 14*, 2027–2033.

Latzer, Y., Azaiza, F., & Tzischinsky, O. (2009). Eating attitudes and dieting behavior among religious subgroups of Israeli-Arab adolescent females. *Journal of Religion and Health, 48*, 189–199.

Lee, C. D., Sui, X., & Blair, S. N. (2009). Combined effects of cardiorespiratory fitness, not smoking, and normal waist girth on morbidity and mortality in men. *Archives of Internal Medicine, 169*, 2096–2101.

Lerner-Geva, L., Boyko, V., Blumstein, T., & Benyamini, Y. (2010). The impact of education, cultural background, and lifestyle on symptoms of the menopausal transition: The Women's Health at Midlife Study. *Journal of Women's Health, 19*, 975–985.

Merom, D., Sinnreich, R., Aboudi, V., Kark, J. D., & Nassar, H. (2012). Lifestyle physical activity among urban Palestinians and Israelis: A cross-sectional comparison in the Palestinian-Israeli Jerusalem Risk Factor Study. *BMC Public Health, 12*, 90.

Mohammadi, M. R., Mohammad, K., Farahani, F. K., Alikhani, S., Zare, M., Tehrani, F. R., Ramezankhani, A., & Alaeddini, F. (2006). Reproductive knowledge, attitudes and behavior among adolescent males in Tehran, Iran. *International Family Planning Perspectives, 32*(1), 35–44.

Muhamad, N., & Mizerski, D. (2013). The effects of following Islam in decisions about taboo products. *Psychology & Marketing, 30*, 357–371.

Naing, N. N., & Ahmad, Z. (2001). Factors related to smoking habits of male secondary school teachers. *Southeast Asian Journal of Tropical Medicine & Public Health, 32*(2), 434–439.

Nakhaee, N., Divsalar, K., & Jadidi, N. (2009). Religious involvement and cigarette smoking among Iranian university students. *International Journal of Psychiatry in Medicine, 39*(2), 189–198.

Ozcan, Y. Z., & Ozcan, K. M. (2002). Determinants of youth smoking—Evidence from Turkey. *Substance Use & Misuse, 37*(3), 313–336.

Pampel, F. C. (2005). Patterns of tobacco use in the early epidemic stages: Malawi and Zambia, 2000–2002. *American Journal of Public Health, 95*(6), 1009–1015.

Penedo, F. J., & Dahn, J. R. (2005). Exercise and well-being: A review of mental and physical health benefits associated with physical activity. *Current Opinion in Psychiatry, 18*(2), 189–193.

Perk, G., Ghanem, J., Aamar, S., Ben-Ishay, D., & Bursztyn, M. (2001). The effect of the fast of Ramadan on ambulatory blood pressure in treated hypertensives. *Journal of Human Hypertension, 15*(10), 723–725.

Rahman AA, Rahman RA, Ibrahim MI, Ali SH, Salleh H, Muda WAMW (2012). Factors associated with attitude toward premarital sexual activities among school-going adolescents in Kelantan, Malaysia. Asia-Pacific Journal of Public Health

Regenstein, J. M., Chaudry, M. M., & Regenstein, C. E. (2003). The kosher and halal food laws. *Comprehensive Reviews in Food Science and Food Safety, 2*(3), 111–127.

Rguibi, M., & Belahsen, R. (2006). Fattening practices among Moroccan Sharawi women. *Eastern Mediterranean Health Journal, 12*, 619–624.

Shirazi, K. K., & Morowatisharifabad, M. A. (2009). Religiosity and determinants of safe sex in Iranian non-medical male students. *Journal of Religion and Health, 48*(1), 29–36.

Soldan, V. A. P., deGraft-Johnson, J. E., Bisika, T., & Tsui, A. O. (2007). Social, economic and demographic determinants of sexual risk behaviors among men in rural Malawi: A district-level study. *African Journal of Reproductive Health, 11*(2), 33–46.

Tahlil, T., Woodman, R. J., Coveney, J., & Ward, P. R. (2013). The impact of education programs on smoking prevention: A randomized controlled trial among 11 to 14 year olds in Aceh, Indonesia. *BMC Public Health, 13*, 367.

Trinitapoli, J., & Regnerus, M. D. (2006). Religion and HIV risk behaviors among married men: Initial results from a study in rural Sub-Saharan Africa. *Journal for the Scientific Study of Religion, 45*(4), 505–528.

Vucina, T., & Becirevic, I. Z. (2007). Risk factors and protective factors for adolescent substance use. *Review of Psychology, 14*, 59–72.

Walseth, K., & Fasting, K. (2003). Islam's view on physical activity and sport Egyptian women interpreting Islam. *International Review for the Sociology of Sport, 38*(1), 45–60.

Williams, E. D., Nazroo, J. Y., Kooner, J. S., & Steptoe, A. (2010). Subgroup differences in psychosocial factors relating to coronary heart disease in the UK South Asian population. *Journal of Psychosomatic Research, 69*, 379–387.

Woofenden, H. (2012). A call to prayer: A cross-cultural examination of religious faith, modesty, and body image. *Undergraduate Review, 8*(article 15), 81–87.

Yasan, A., Essizoglu, A., & Yildirim, E. A. (2009). Predictor factors associated with premarital sexual behaviors among university students in an Islamic culture. *International Journal of Sexual Health, 21*, 145–152.

Yong, H. H., Hamann, S. L., Borland, R., Fong, G. T., & Omar, M. (2009). Adult smokers' perception of the role of religion and religious leadership on smoking and association with quitting: A comparison between Thai Buddhists and Malaysian Muslims. *Social Sciences in Medicine, 69*(7), 1025–2031.

Yong HH, Savvas S, Borland R, Thrasher J, Sirirassamee B, Omar M (2013). Secular versus religious norms against smoking: Which is more important as a driver of quitting behaviour among Muslim Malaysian and Buddhist Thai smokers? *International Journal of Behavioral Medicine, 20*(2), 252–258.

Zohrabian, A., & Philipson, T. J. (2010). External costs of risky health behaviors associated with leading actual causes of death in the U.S.: A review of the evidence and implications for future research. *International Journal of Research in Public Health, 7*, 2460–2472.

Chapter 11
Religion and Physical Health in Muslims

Since studies suggest that Muslims who are more deeply religious experience better mental health, social health, and healthier lifestyles, we might expect that physical health would also be better for Muslims who are more religious. Psychological and social factors are known to have a strong influence on physical health as a result of psychosomatic or mind–body influences. Likewise, as noted in the last chapter, poor health behaviors account for a large proportion of population-based disease and chronic illness. We now examine whether religiosity is related to more or less physical illness in Muslims, including heart disease, hypertension, cerebrovascular disease, dementia, diabetes, cholesterol/triglycerides, immune and endocrine functions, perceptions of their own health, and overall mortality.

Heart Disease

No physiological system is more affected by psychosocial and behavioral factors than the cardiovascular system, with the heart at its center. An intricate system of parasympathetic and sympathetic nerves—with primary inputs from the brain—surrounds and penetrates deep into cardiac muscle tissue, carefully regulating the timing and force of contractions. Religious involvement, because it may affect emotions, social functioning, and behaviors that impact the heart (e.g., cigarette smoking, diet, weight, alcohol use), then, ought to be related in one way or another to diseases of this organ. However, despite the fact that ischemic heart is the most common cause of disability (Murray et al. 2012) and death in the world (Lozano et al. 2012), almost no research has examined the relationship between religiosity and heart disease in Muslims. Our 2010 systematic review uncovered only two such studies on coronary artery disease (CAD): one examining the effects of religiosity (Burazeri et al. 2008a) and one assessing the effects of the Ramadan fast (Chamsi-Pasha and Ahmed 2004).

H.G. Koenig and S. Al Shohaib, *Health and Well-Being in Islamic Societies: Background, Research, and Applications*, DOI 10.1007/978-3-319-05873-3_11,

To our knowledge, only one study has examined the relationship between religiosity per se and heart disease in Muslims. Burazeri and colleagues (2008a) conducted a case–control study involving 457 consecutively admitted patients with nonfatal acute coronary syndrome (ACS, i.e., myocardial infarction) to the University Hospital in Tirana, Albania, between 2003 and 2006. These cases were compared to a population-based sample of 632 controls. Muslims made up 77 % of cases and 66 % of controls. Religious activity was assessed with three items that measured frequency of religious attendance, frequency of prayers, and frequency of fasting during Ramadan or Easter. Age- and sex-adjusted odds ratios in Muslims ($n=782$) revealed that those who attended religious services were 47 % less likely to have ACS compared to those who never attended (OR = 0.53, 95 % CI 0.36–0.79, $p<0.01$). Those who prayed at least 2–3 times per week were 48 % less likely to have ACS than those who never prayed (OR = 0.52, 95 % CI 0.32–0.82, $p=0.01$). Finally, those who always fasted during Ramadan were 72 % less likely to have ACS compared to those who never fasted (OR = 0.28, 95 % CI 0.13–0.58, $p<0.01$). Similar relationships were found in Christians (except for fasting). A significant linear trend was present in these relationships for both Muslims and Christians.

Ramadan. Chamsi-Pasha and Ahmed (2004) examined the effects of the Ramadan fast on heart disease in 86 Muslims (63 % male) in Jeddah, Saudi Arabia, given concerns that fasting might precipitate cardiac dysfunction. Muslims eat prior to sunup and then after sundown during Ramadan, fasting from food and water from sunup to sunset (about 12 h). Depending on how strictly the fast is adhered to, this may influence the intake of medications and affect metabolic stability. Patients in this study had a wide range of serious heart conditions: 53 % with CAD, 27 % with valvular heart disease, 15 % with congestive heart failure, and 5 % with arrhythmias. Physiological measures were collected on the third day prior to the start of Ramadan and then again on the last day of Ramadan. Most patients (86 %) were able to fast throughout the entire month of Ramadan without ill effects. Outcome measures were NYHA class, along with biochemical and hematological indices. No significant changes were found on any of these outcomes during the Ramadan fast.

Muslims vs. Non-Muslims. The next four studies compared rates of heart disease in Muslims with other religious groups (Hindus, Christians, Jews). Gupta and colleagues (2002) examined risk factors and CAD in 1,415 males (19.2 % Muslim) and 797 females (11.4 % Muslim) living in India. Researchers found that CAD was significantly higher in Hindu compared to Muslim males when diagnosed by either EKG changes only (4.3 % vs. 0.7 %, respectively, $p<0.01$, uncontrolled) or by a combination of EKG changes and clinical history (7.1 % vs. 1.8 %, $p<0.005$). Nonsignificant trends in a similar direction were also present in females.

Roshi and associates (2005) examined the characteristics of 331 men (average age 59) and 146 women (average age 63) admitted to a university hospital with acute myocardial infarction (ACS) in Tirana, Albania. Participants were matched with 389 men and 227 women visiting the hospital (mean age 60). The majority of male cases (74 %) and female cases (67 %) were Muslims, while the remainder of participants was Christian. Analyses were controlled for age, education, occupation, marital status, smoking, alcohol, physical activity, BMI, diet, medical history, and family history. No significant differences were found on religious affiliation between cases with ACS and controls in either men or women (although there was a weak nonsignificant trend in men for Muslims to be more common among cases than controls, OR = 1.32, $p = 0.10$).

Kark and colleagues (2006) analyzed data on coronary events (CAD) among 76,200 Palestinian Arabs and 226,500 Jews ages 25–74 in Jerusalem between 1995 and 1997. Outcome was CAD events (fatal and nonfatal). Men and women were analyzed separately. Among male Palestinian Arabs, CHD events were 796 per 100,000 (95 % CI 680–912) compared to 503 per 100,000 (95 % CI 460–546) in Jews. Among female Palestinian Arabs, CHD events were 295 per 100,000 (95 % CI 230–360) compared to 125 per 100,000 (95 % CI 105–144) in Jews. Researchers concluded that rates of CAD events in Palestinian Arabs were higher than in Jews and, in fact, were higher than CAD rates found in 21 other developed countries.

A second report by Burazeri's research group (2008b) examined religious affiliation and ACS among Albanians in the same sample that was described earlier. Cases were 370 consecutive male patients (mean age 59) and 97 female patients (mean age 63) admitted with nonfatal ACS to the University Hospital in Tirana, Albania. As in the earlier report, ACS was diagnosed based on EKG and clinical criteria. Cases were matched with 452 men (mean age 53) and 237 women (mean age 54) without CAD from the community. The age- and sex-adjusted odds ratio (OR) indicated that ACS was 80 % more common in Muslims than in Christians (OR = 1.8, 95 % CI 1.4–2.3, $p < 0.01$). Even after controlling for marital status, family size, education, income, employment, social position, emigration of relatives, financial loss, and other CAD risk factors, the relationship persisted (OR = 1.6, 95 % CI 1.1–2.3, $p = 0.02$). Researchers concluded that ACS was more common in Muslims than in Christians.

Missed Studies. Several studies were missed by our 2010 review, all either examining the effects of fasting during Ramadan on cardiac outcomes or comparing rates of heart disease between Muslims and non-Muslims.

Ramadan. Al Suwaidi and colleagues (2004) analyzed clinical data from a retrospective chart review involving 2,160 congestive heart failure patients in Qatar admitted during a 10-year period (1991–2001). Findings indicated no difference in number of hospitalizations or significant change in any physiological measure while fasting during Ramadan. Al Suwaidi and colleagues (2005) next examined the effects of Ramadan fasting in 465 stable cardiac patients identified from medical centers in Qatar, Kuwait, UAE, and Bahrain (mean age 56, 78 % male). Only the abstract of this study was available for review, so details are lacking. Participants were assessed 1 month before Ramadan, during Ramadan, and 1 month after Ramadan. Results indicated that 91 % felt fine during the Ramadan fast and 7 % felt worse. Most were compliant with their cardiac medications (83 %) and dietary instructions (69 %). Researchers concluded, as did Chamsi-Pasha and Ahmed (2004) above, that the effect of Ramadan fasting on patients with stable cardiac disease was minimal. These findings confirmed earlier research by Temizhan and associates

(1999) from Turkey who found that acute coronary events were not more common during Ramadan compared to before and after Ramadan between 1991 and 1997.

However, different results were reported from a later prospective study by Al Suwaidi and colleagues (2006) that involved 1,019 patients admitted to the coronary care unit (CCU) of a general hospital in Qatar (78 % Muslim) during the month of Ramadan. Among those admitted to the CCU, 162 were fasting on the day of admission. Fasting and non-fasting patients were compared. While there was no difference in terms of age, the percentage of patients presenting with acute myocardial infarction was significantly higher among those who were fasting compared to those who were not fasting (79.6 % vs. 47.0 %, $p<0.001$). Fasting patients were more likely to have cardiac symptoms during mealtimes (i.e., 5:00–6:00 AM and 5:00–6:00 PM).

Muslims vs. Non-Muslims. Muir (1960) compared rates of CAD (per 1,000/year) diagnosed at autopsy during the 1947 and 1957 Malaysian census ($n=1{,}206{,}000$) across ethnic groups. CAD rates were as follows: Chinese (0.026); Malay Muslims (0.024); Eurasians (0.100); European Christians (0.186); Indian/Pakistani Hindus, Christians, Buddhists, and Others (0.222); Indian/Pakistani Sikh (0.333); and Indian/Pakistani Muslims (0.435). Thus, CAD rates were highest in Muslims from India/Pakistan, which was ten times the rate of CAD in Muslims from Malaysia. Socioeconomic, education, and dietary factors almost certainly accounted for these differences.

Gopinath and associates (1995) surveyed 13,560 community-dwelling adults living in Delhi, India, diagnosing CAD based on clinical history during hospital admission or on EKG evidence using standard criteria. CAD (based on clinical evidence alone) was most prevalent among Sikhs (47.3 per 1,000), least prevalent in Muslims (22.8), and intermediate among Hindus (31.8) and Christians (31.2). However, silent CAD (based on EKG evidence alone) was highest in Muslims (89.5) and Sikhs (87.3) and lowest in Hindus (60.0) and Christians (25.0). Researchers concluded that the difference in CAD between religious groups could not be explained by conventional risk factors.

Studying 10,657 deaths that occurred in the Republic of Mauritius between 1989 and 1994, Vos and colleagues (1998) compared deaths from CAD between Hindus, Muslims, Chinese, and Christian Creoles (ages 30–64). Muslims make up 16 % of the population of this small country in the Indian Ocean off the coast of Madagascar, whereas the remaining population is Hindu (51 %) or Christian (32 %). Among men, Muslims had a similar standard mortality ratio (SMR) from CAD (SMR=93, 95 % CI 84–102) compared to Hindus (SMR=100), although SMR in Muslims was higher than in Christian Creoles (SMR=66, 95 % CI 60–72). Among women, SMR from CAD was also higher in Muslims (SMR=114, 95 % CI 96–132) compared to Christians (SMR=81, 95 % CI 70–92). To get a sense of how common this pattern might be in countries throughout the world, we examined rates of CAD in over 190 countries (World Health Rankings, 2011). Of the ten countries worldwide with the highest rates of CAD, five are Muslim-majority countries (Turkmenistan, Kyrgyzstan, Kazakhstan, Afghanistan, Uzbekistan); among the 25 countries with the lowest rate of CAD, only two are Muslim-majority countries (Maldives and

Brunei). Studies of South Asian immigrants (25–33 % Muslim) in the UK (Williams et al. 2009), in Canada (Anand et al. 2000), and in Israeli Arabs (Na'amnih et al. 2010) have likewise reported high rates of CAD in Muslim populations.

The findings above are consistent with those reported by Jabara and colleagues (2007) who compared cardiac risk factors in 444 Jewish women and 102 Palestinian Arab women (Muslim) who were admitted for cardiac catheterization at a Jewish medical center in Israel between 2000 and 2003. Arab compared to Jewish women were younger (63 vs. 68, respectively, $p<0.001$), had more children (6.5 vs. 3.7, $p<0.001$), were of lower socioeconomic status (SES; 83 % vs. 39 %, $p=0.001$), had more exposure to passive smoking (62 % vs. 28 %, $p<0.001$), had more use of olive oil (98 % vs. 65 %), and were more likely to have diabetes (61 % vs. 46 %, $p=0.01$). However, they were less likely than Jewish women to have hyperlipidemia (69 % vs. 79 %, $p<0.01$), a family history of CAD (40 % vs. 56 %, $p<0.05$), take hormone replacement therapy (5 % vs. 12 %, $p<0.05$), or drink alcohol (4 % vs. 26 %, $p<0.001$). Although Arab women were also less likely to engage in physical activity (12 % vs. 44 %, $p<0.001$), there was no difference in average BMI or prevalence of obesity between Arab and Jewish women. Researchers concluded that certain characteristics place Arab women at greater risk for CAD compared to Jewish women. In a related study published soon afterward that examined 40 Arab and 179 Jewish women being seen for CAD in Jerusalem, Salame and colleagues (2008) found that Arab women had more extensive CAD ($p=0.002$) despite their younger age and lower cigarette smoking. However, Arab women were more likely to have diabetes, to be obese, and to be physically inactive. Neither study above examined religiosity.

Recent Research. Several studies on religion and heart disease have been published since our 2010 systematic review. These include a study of the effects of Ramadan on atrial fibrillation, a study of cardiac risk factors in South Asians in the UK, a comparison of rates of heart disease among religions in the West Indies, and a qualitative report describing the spiritual experiences of Muslim heart attack survivors.

Ramadan. Salam and colleagues (2013) examined the effects of Ramadan fasting on the occurrence of atrial fibrillation (AF) among 1,718 patients hospitalized for AF from 1991 to 2010 in Qatar. Results of this retrospective chart review revealed that there was no difference in number of cases of AF hospitalized during the month before Ramadan ($n=136$), during Ramadan ($n=143$), or during the month after Ramadan ($n=151$) ($p=0.95$). The only difference found was that patients with a history of prior myocardial infarction were *less likely* to be hospitalized during Ramadan (7 %) compared to the month prior to Ramadan (15.4 %) or the month after Ramadan (19.9 %) ($p=0.01$).

Muslims vs. Non-Muslims. Williams and colleagues (2010) compared CAD risk factors between 1,065 South Asian (Sikh, Hindu, Muslim) emigrants and 818 white Europeans (Christian) in London, UK. Muslims (15.8 % of South Asians) were more likely to experience individual deprivation, overcrowding, financial strain, racism, and had high rates of depression and hostility (although were also the most religious group). Muslims also smoked more, ate less fruits and vegetables (but more low-fat products), were more sedentary, and engaged in less physical activity. Researchers pointed to these factors to help explain the higher CAD rates found in Muslim emigrants.

Chadee and associates (2013) retrospectively analyzed data from the medical records of 14,793 persons receiving government assistance in Trinidad and Tobago (West Indies), examining the prevalence of diabetes, hypertension, and heart disease. Religious affiliation was also recorded: 28 % Hindu, 16 % Catholic, 5 % Seventh Day Adventist (SDA), 45 % Other Christian, and 5 % Muslim ($n=646$). Comparison of self-reported rates of cardiac disease revealed a significant difference based on religious affiliation: Hindu 13.3 %, Muslims 10.5 %, Other Christians 6.5 %, Catholics 5.3 %, and SDA 3.7 % ($p<0.001$). A similar pattern was seen for both hypertension and diabetes.

In a qualitative study,[1] Momennasab and other researchers (2012) examined the spiritual experiences of Muslim survivors of myocardial infarction. They interviewed nine patients hospitalized in coronary care units in three hospitals located in Shiraz, Iran (four females and five males, ages 33–71). Five main themes emerged from the data: perceived threat to life, seeking spiritual support (connecting with God), religious values (reflection and introspection in preparing for life after death), increasing faith (new insights, thankfulness to God), and deepening spiritual realization (realization of risk, presence, and returning to life). Researchers developed a theoretical model that explained how perceived threat leads to seeking spiritual support and putting religious values into practice, which in turn leads to increasing faith and ultimately to recovery.

D-Dimer, C-Reactive Protein (CRP), Fibrinogen. We broaden our review here to include these CAD risk factors. CRP, D-dimer, and fibrinogen are inflammatory and coagulation markers in blood that predict a greater risk of CAD and cardiovascular disease (Danesh et al. 1998, 2001, 2004). Our 2010 systematic review identified three studies from Turkey that examined relationships between religious activity and these inflammatory or coagulation markers. Two of those studies examined the effects of the Ramadan fast on D-dimer, CRP, and fibrinogen (Aksungar et al. 2005, 2007). The last study from Turkey compared CRP levels in those who prayed five times daily to CRP levels in those who did not (Yilmaz et al. 2008). We briefly review these studies below.

Yilmaz and colleagues (2008) examined 46 persons over age 50 who had performed regular prayer five times daily for at least 10 years, comparing them to 40 controls over age 50 who did not pray. All participants were from Ankara, Turkey, and were Muslim. Blood samples taken from participants revealed that there was no difference in CRP level between those who prayed and those who did not.

Aksungar and colleagues (2005) drew blood samples from 24 healthy fasting volunteers (ages 21–35) in Turkey one week before Ramadan, on the 21st day of

[1] Although we rarely mention qualitative research studies in this volume, there are so few studies examining religiosity and heart disease in Muslims that we decided to include this study in our review.

Ramadan, and 20 days after Ramadan, examining levels of inflammatory and coagulation markers, including D-dimer and fibrinogen. D-dimer levels were significantly lower during Ramadan than either before or after Ramadan in both male and female subjects (both $p<0.001$), although no effect was seen on fibrinogen levels. In a second report from Aksungar's research group (2007), researchers followed the sample protocol as above, drawing blood prior to, during, and after Ramadan in 40 healthy volunteers who were fasting (ages 20–39, half men). They were compared to 28 healthy volunteers of similar age and gender. CRP levels decreased significantly during the Ramadan fast ($p<0.01$) and remained at lower levels when checked 20 days after the fast ended ($p<0.01$) in both men and women (CRP levels in non-fasting controls did not change).

Missed Studies and Recent Research: We could find no other research that examined relationships between inflammatory or coagulation makers and religiosity in Muslims, although we identified two studies that compared levels of these markers between Muslims and non-Muslims. Cook and colleagues (2001), studying 459 South Asians in London, UK, ages 40–59, found no differences in average fibrinogen levels between Muslims and Christians. The only other relevant study we could find examined CRP levels in 893 adult participants of the Malawi Longitudinal Study of Families and Health (average age 42, 70 % Muslim, 30 % Christian). In that study, researchers found significantly lower levels of CRP in Muslims compared to Christians (OR=0.68, 95 % CI 0.48–0.95, $p<0.05$) (Kohler et al. 2013). No explanation was given for this incidental finding.

Summary. Only one study has examined the relationship between religiosity and heart disease in Muslims, finding lower rates of ACS in those who were more religious. Six studies have examined the effects of the Ramadan fast on cardiac functions or cardiac events. Four reported no significant changes as a result of fasting, one reported significantly higher admission rates for acute myocardial infarction during Ramadan, and one found a lower rate of hospitalization for atrial fibrillation during Ramadan among those with a history of prior myocardial infarction (Table 11.1). Eight studies compared heart disease in Muslims with other religious groups. Four found higher rates in Muslims: one found higher rates in Hindus compared to Muslims; one found equal rates between Muslims and Christians; one found lower or higher rates of CAD in Muslims depending on how CAD was diagnosed; and one found the highest rates in Indian/Pakistani Muslim emigrants to Malaysia (but low rates in Malaysian Muslims). Two studies reported a worse cardiac risk-factor profile in Muslims compared to non-Muslims: one in Palestinian Arabs compared to Jews and one in South Asian Muslims compared to Hindus and other religious groups. Finally, one qualitative study found spiritual factors of crucial importance to Muslims surviving acute myocardial infarction.

With regard to inflammatory and coagulation markers that increase risk of heart disease, one study found a drop in CRP and a second study reported a drop in D-dimer during Ramadan (mechanism unclear), which should be good for cardiovascular health. No effect, however, was found on fibrinogen levels in two studies. One small study in Turkey found that frequency of prayer did not influence CRP

Table 11.1 Religiosity, cardiovascular, and neurological disease in Muslims

Authors (year)	Method	Sample size	Participants	Location	Controls	Findings
Heart disease						
Religiosity						
Burazeri et al. (2008a)	CC	424	Muslim adults	Albania	SC	P
Effects of Ramadan						
Temizhan et al. (1999)	RS	1,655	Adults, myocardial infarction	Turkey	None	NA
Chamsi-Pasha and Ahmed (2004)	Exp	86	Adults, serious heart disease	Saudi Arabia	None (?)	NA
Al Suwaidi et al. (2004)	RS	2,160	Adults, congestive heart fail	Qatar	None	NA
Al Suwaidi et al. (2005)	RS	465	Adults, stable heart disease	Middle East	None	NA
Al Suwaidi et al. (2006)	PC	1,019	Adults, CCU admissions	Qatar	None	NG
Salam et al. (2013)	RS	1,718	Adults, atrial fibrillation	Qatar	None	P
Heart disease risk *(inflammation/coagulation)*						
Religiosity						
Yilmaz et al. (2008)	CC	46	Praying adults, age >50	Turkey	Ctrl group	NA
Effects of Ramadan						
Aksungar et al. (2005)	Exp	24	Healthy adults, 21–35 years	Turkey	None	P
Aksungar et al. (2007)	Exp	40	Healthy adults, 20–39 years	Turkey	None	P
Hypertension *(HTN)/blood pressure*						
Religiosity						
Al-Kandari (2003)	CS	223	Adults, average age 30	Kuwait	MC	P
Al-Kandari (2011)	CS	1,472	Adults over 60	Kuwait	SC	P
Solman and Mohamed (2013)	RCT	40	Surgical patients, 18–60	Egypt	–	NA
Effects of Ramadan						
Bernieh et al. (1994)	Exp	11	Renal transplant recipients	Saudi Arabia	None	P
Perk et al. (2001)	Exp	17	Adults, stable HTN	Israel	None	NA
Saleh et al. (2004)	Exp	103	Obese adults	Egypt	None	P
Topacoglu et al. (2005)	RS	2,159	ER admissions for HTN	Turkey	None	NG
Ural et al. (2008)	Exp	45	Adults with HTN	Turkey	None	NG

Cerebrovascular disease						
Religiosity						
None						
Effects of Ramadan						
Akhan et al. (2000)	RS	1,579	Admissions with stroke	Turkey	None	NA
Bener et al. (2006)	RS	335	Admissions with stroke	Qatar	None	NA
Dementia/Alzheimer's						
Religiosity						
Inzelberg et al. (2013)	CS/RS	935	Arabic population > age 65	Israel	SC	P

CC case control, *Exp* experimental study examining effect of Ramadan fasting, *RS* retrospective chart review examining effect of Ramadan fasting, *CS* cross-sectional, *PC* prospective, *RCT* randomized clinical trial, *NA* no association, *P* significant positive association, (P) trend positive association ($0.05 < p < 0.10$), *NG* significant negative association, *M* mixed (both significant positive and negative findings), *C* complex association, *MC* multiple controls, *SC* some controls, *Q* qualitative report. CCU coronary care unit; HTN hypertension; ER emergency room levels. Concerning differences between Muslims and non-Muslims, one study from Malawi reported lower CRP levels in Muslims compared to Christians, and one study found no difference between Muslims and Christians with regard to fibrinogen levels. Given the limited research in this area, conclusions are difficult to make. However, higher rates of heart disease (four of eight studies) and a worse risk-factor profile in Muslims are of concern. Socioeconomic factors, no doubt, play at least some role in these differences.

Hypertension/Blood Pressure

Hypertension is a serious problem in Muslim-majority countries. Rates of hypertension in countries with more than 95 % Muslim range from 19 % (Jordan) to 36 % (Libya) (World Health Organization 2008). Our 2010 systematic review identified six studies that examined relationships between religion and blood pressure (BP) in Muslim-majority countries. The only study, however, to examine the relationships between level of religious involvement and BP in a Muslim population was that of Al-Kandari (2003) in Kuwait. Four of the remaining five studies examined the effects of Ramadan fasting on BP (each reporting a different finding), and the final study compared BP in Muslims and Hindus.

Al-Kandari (2003) interviewed 223 Kuwaitis in their homes, work, school, and wherever they were available, assessing religiosity and BP (53 % female, age range 18–75). BP was measured three times and the average of the measurements was used. Religiosity was assessed using self-reports of daily prayer and a 15-item scale assessing level of religious commitment (e.g., reading and memorizing parts of the Qur'an, giving alms to the poor, attending religious lectures, extra-religious activities, fasting, making Hajj to Mecca, and so forth). Frequency of prayer and the 15-item religiosity index were combined to form a single religious commitment scale. After researchers controlled for BMI, smoking, SES, gender, and age, religious commitment was inversely related to systolic BP ($B=-0.49, p<0.05$) and to diastolic BP ($B=-0.66, p<0.05$).

Ramadan. Four studies examined the effects of Ramadan fasting on BP. In the first study, as reviewed in chapter 10, Perk and associates (2001) examined the effects of the Ramadan fasting on 17 persons with treated hypertension (15 men, mean age 57) living in Israel. Ambulatory 24-h systolic and diastolic BP were measured before Ramadan and during the last week of Ramadan. No difference in average BP (mean, diastolic, or systolic) was found. Saleh and colleagues (2004) examined the effects of Ramadan fasting on BP in 103 obese volunteers (88 women, ages 15–52) living in Egypt. BP was measured before Ramadan, at the end of Ramadan, 4 weeks after the end of Ramadan, and then again 4 weeks later. Results (uncontrolled) revealed that both systolic and diastolic BP declined significantly ($p<0.05$) during Ramadan, an effect that persisted for up to 4 weeks after fasting ended.

The last two studies examined effects of the Ramadan fast on BP in Turkish Muslims. Topacoglu and associates (2005) retrospectively reviewed the medical records of adults admitted to a university-based emergency department (ED) from 2000 to 2004, identifying patients with hypertension and other medical disorders. A total of 130,506 patients were admitted to the ED during this period and 2,159 were admitted for hypertension. Results indicated that admission rates to the ED for hypertension during Ramadan were significantly higher than during the rest of the year ($p = 0.015$, uncontrolled). Finally, Ural and colleagues (2008) examined the effects of Ramadan fasting on average ambulatory 24-h BP in 45 patients with grade II–III treated hypertension in Kocaeli, Turkey (mean age 58, 67 % female). Ambulatory BP was measured during the month of Ramadan and again 1 month later. There was no significant difference in average 24-h BP during Ramadan and 1 month later. The only change was a rise in BP while having the morning meal during Ramadan (increased from 118/68 to 126/74, $p = 0.004$).

Muslims vs. Non-Muslims. Gupta and colleagues (2002), in a study described previously, surveyed a random sample of 1,415 males and 797 females in Jaipur, India, among whom were 272 Muslim males (19 %) and 91 Muslim females (11 %). Among males, Hindus had significantly higher diastolic BP than Muslims (81.2 vs. 79.0, $p < 0.001$) and a higher prevalence of hypertension (30.5 % vs. 25.8 %, $p < 0.05$). Among females, systolic BP was significantly higher in Hindus and the prevalence of hypertension was also higher compared to Muslims (35.2 % vs. 25.3 %).

Missed Studies. Several studies were missed by our 2010 review, including one on the effects of Ramadan fasting on BP and several studies comparing BP in Muslims and non-Muslims.

Ramadan. Bernieh and colleagues (1994) studied the effects of the Ramadan fast on cardiovascular indices in 11 renal transplant recipients (Saudi Arabia), who were assessed three times during the month prior to Ramadan, three times during the month of Ramadan, and three times during the month following Ramadan. All participants fasted from food and water the entire month from dawn to sunset. Few changes were noted, except there was a significant drop in mean lying BP from the month before Ramadan (112) to the time of Ramadan fasting (100) to the month after Ramadan (96) ($p = 0.01$), although researchers gave no explanation for this change.

Muslims vs. Non-Muslims. Several studies compared BP in Muslims and non-Muslims in different countries, including two that examined rates of preeclampsia in pregnant women. Seedat and colleagues (1978) measured BP in a random sample of 1,000 adults in Durban, India. Hypertension was defined as a systolic BP ≥ 160 or diastolic BP ≥ 95. Muslims had a hypertension rate of 16.7 % compared to 20.2 % in Dravidian Hindus and 23.5 % in Aryan Hindus. Other than noting that the prevalence of hypertension was lower in Muslims than Hindus, nothing else was said about the finding.

McKeigue and associates (1991) compared the median systolic BP across religious groups in a sample of 1,712 South Asians living in London, UK, and 1,268 native British Europeans (ages 40–69). Median systolic BP for Muslims ($n = 211$) was 120, compared to 121 in Christians (native Brits), 122 in Gujarati Hindus,

126 in Punjabi Hindus, and 128 in Sikhs ($p<0.001$, primarily between Sikhs/Punjabi Hindus and Muslims). Again, not much was said about the lower BP in Muslims. However, Muslims had low BP despite fairly high rates of smoking (30 %), low HDL/total cholesterol ratio (18.4 %), and high fasting triglycerides (1.85), all conducive to poorer vascular health. Could their religion have something to do with it?

Preeclampsia is a life-threatening condition in pregnant women that affects both the mother's and the fetus' health and is manifested by the onset of hypertension and protein in the urine often during the last trimester of pregnancy. Razzaque and associates (2005) studied 11,122 women (86 % Muslim) visiting a health center in Bangladesh during their third trimester of pregnancy between 1996 and 2002. Rates of high blood pressure and preeclampsia were compared across religious groups. Non-Muslims had higher rates of preeclampsia and high blood pressure per 100 pregnancies compared to Muslims (3.50 vs. 2.55, $p<0.05$, for preeclampsia and 4.19 vs. 3.15, $p<0.05$, for high blood pressure). In multivariate analyses controlling for inter-pregnancy interval, age, gravidity, pregnancy losses, education, and household space (SES), non-Muslims were still 48 % more likely than Muslims to have preeclampsia (OR = 1.48, $p<0.05$) and 54 % more likely to have high blood pressure (OR = 1.54, $p<0.01$). Again, the authors did not discuss or explain these findings.

Funai and colleagues (2005), however, reported different results. These investigators examined risk factors for preeclampsia in women having their first pregnancy (nulliparous) and in those having their second or more pregnancies (multiparous). The Jerusalem Perinatal Study followed a random population-based cohort of 82,436 women in Israel who delivered a baby between 1964 and 1976, among whom were 1,319 cases of preeclampsia. Religious affiliation (Muslim vs. Jewish) was one factor examined as a predictor of preeclampsia. Statistical analyses controlled for maternal and paternal age, admitting hospital, obstetric risk factors, maternal education, social class, rabbinical student status, employment outside the home, year of delivery, and season of the year. Results indicated no difference between Muslims and Jews on likelihood of developing preeclampsia during the first pregnancy. However, Muslims were 68 % more likely to develop preeclampsia during pregnancies beyond the first pregnancy (OR = 1.68, 95 % CI 1.13–2.52). Researchers hypothesized that high-risk Muslim women may be less likely than high-risk Jewish women to use birth control to avoid further births after their first preeclamptic pregnancy.

Maziak and associates (2007) analyzed data from the Aleppo Household Survey conducted in 2004 by the Syrian Center for Tobacco Studies. This survey involved a population-based random sample of 2,048 persons aged 18–65 in Aleppo, the second largest city in Syria. BP was also measured and hypertension defined as systolic BP greater than 140 or diastolic BP greater than 90. Smoking, BMI, and demographics were also assessed, as well as religion (Muslim vs. non-Muslim). Results indicated that Muslims were significantly more likely to have hypertension (41.2 % vs. 28.8 %, $p<0.05$), despite the fact that Muslims were less likely to smoke (38.2 % vs. 48.7 %, $p<0.05$) and had the same weight (BMI) as non-Muslims.

Tesfaye and researchers (2008) examined associations between cigarette smoking, khat chewing, and BP in a random population-based sample of 4,001 men and women ages 25–64 in Addis Ababa, Ethiopia. Also assessed was religious affiliation, with 93.4 % being Ethiopian Orthodox Christian and 6.6 % being Muslim. BP was measured using a standard digital device and the average of three readings was used. After controlling for BMI, waist–hip ratio, level of physical activity, employment status, and salt intake using regression analysis, results indicated that Christians had significantly higher mean systolic BP than Muslims ($B = +3.1$, $p = 0.02$), but no difference on mean diastolic BP. In contrast to the previous study, systolic BP was lower in Muslims despite the fact that Muslims were significantly *more likely* to smoke cigarettes and regularly chew khat than Christians (OR = 2.7, 95 % CI 1.9–3.9).

Recent Research. Since our 2010 review, several relevant studies have been published.

Religiosity. Al-Kandari (2011) surveyed 1,472 adults over age 60 living in six home care units supported by the Kuwaiti Ministry of Social Affairs, examining relationships between religiosity and health (average age of participants was 77). Religiosity was assessed using a single item that asked respondents to rate their religiosity on a scale from 0 (low) to 10 (high); for analysis, participants were divided into low and high religiosity groups. Research nurses measured systolic and diastolic BP in the usual manner (taking three measurements and using the average). Also assessed were social support, somatic symptoms, self-rated general health, and health within the past year. Uncontrolled analyses revealed that both systolic and diastolic BP were significantly lower in the high religious group compared to the low religious group (systolic 152.8 vs. 155.8 and diastolic 95.2 vs. 97.6, respectively, both $p < 0.05$). Somatic symptoms were also significantly lower and both social support and self-rated health (SRH) were significantly higher in the high religious vs. the low religious group. The significant differences in both systolic and diastolic BP between high and low religious groups persisted after controlling for social support and SRH.

In one of the few randomized clinical trials that have examined the effects of a religious intervention on physical health outcomes in Muslims, Solman and Mohamed (2013) studied the effects of Zikr meditation and jaw relaxation on postoperative pain, anxiety, and cardiovascular functions (including BP). Researchers randomized 40 Egyptian patients aged 18–60 before major abdominal surgery to either the intervention or a control group that received usual pre- and postoperative care (wound dressing, medications). The intervention was explicitly religious and involved Islamic prayer followed by 5 min of deep breathing and 10 min of jaw relaxation. This was immediately followed by 15 min of remembrance of Allah by saying the following phrases each 33 times—"sub Hanna Allah" (God is the holiest), "Al-ḥamdu lillāh" (all praise to God), "Allahu-akbar" (God is the greatest of all), and "lailaha-ila Allah" (there is no God but Allah)—while keeping count on a tasbih (kind of rosary).

Those in the intervention group were trained during a single session prior to surgery, including how to complete a pain rating scale and the Hamilton anxiety scale. On Day 1 (6–8 h after surgery), all participants were asked to complete the pain and anxiety scales as a baseline assessment and then those in the intervention group were asked to practice the Zikr meditation and jaw relaxation for 30 min. Immediately after the intervention, participants were asked to again rate their pain and anxiety, and BP and other physiological measurements were taken. On Day 2 (24–30 h after surgery) participants were asked to again rate their pain/anxiety and physiological measurements were taken. Those in the intervention group were again asked to practice the Zikr meditation/jaw relaxation for 30 min and then immediately afterwards rate their pain/anxiety and have their BP and other physiological parameters measured. Results indicated that while pre–post assessment of pain and anxiety levels in the intervention group decreased significantly, no effect was seen on BP, heart rate, or respiration.

Muslims vs. Non-Muslims. In a study of arsenic exposure in drinking water and hypertension, Islam and colleagues (2012) examined a random population-based sample of 1,004 persons ages 30 or over living in rural Bangladesh. Participants were interviewed in their homes, and BP was measured using the standard procedure recommended by the World Health Organization (the lowest of three measurements). Hypertension was defined as a systolic BP of 140 or higher or a diastolic BP of 90 or higher. Demographic characteristics were also assessed, including religious affiliation (76 % Muslim vs. 24 % Hindu). Results indicated that Muslims had lower systolic and diastolic BP than Hindus (110.1 vs. 115.7 for systolic and 73.0 vs. 76.6 for diastolic, respectively). Percent of Muslims with systolic or diastolic hypertension was also lower than in Hindus (6.1 % vs. 12.6 % for systolic and 9.9 % vs. 16.0 % for diastolic, respectively). Regression analysis revealed that Hindus were over twice as likely to have hypertension compared to Muslims (OR=2.5, 95 % CI 1.5–4.2). Researchers explained that this was because Hindus weighed more than Muslims (50.0 % of Hindus vs. 29.5 % of Muslims were obese, i.e., BMI>21 according to their definition).

Summary. We found only two studies that examined the relationship between religiosity and BP in a Muslim population, both by the same investigator (Al-Kandari) and both finding significant inverse relationships (lower BP in the more religious) (Table 11.1). In addition, one study found that Muslim meditation (Zikr) had no effect on BP following major abdominal surgery, although the intervention was not a very strong one (two 30-min sessions). At least five studies have now examined the effects of Ramadan fasting on BP, with a variety of findings. Two reported a reduction of BP during Ramadan fasting, one found no effect, one reported an increase in admissions to the emergency room for hypertension during the month of Ramadan, and one found a small increase in BP at the time of the morning meal during Ramadan. More studies examining the relationship between religiosity and BP in Muslims are clearly needed, given the widespread ramifications of this link.

Finally, at least eight studies have compared BP in Muslims and non-Muslims. Six of eight found lower BP in Muslims. Four studies found higher BP in Hindus or Sikhs vs. Muslims, and one found higher BP in Ethiopian Orthodox Christians vs. Muslims in Ethiopia. Two studies examined rates of preeclampsia in pregnant women: one from Bangladesh finding a lower BP and lower rates of preeclampsia in Muslims compared to non-Muslims and one study in Israel finding a higher rate of preeclampsia in Muslim women beyond their first pregnancy compared to Jewish women. One study from Syria also found that Muslims were more likely to have hypertension than non-Muslims. We note that there are many factors, cultural and genetic, that influence levels of BP among Muslims besides their religious beliefs. This applies especially to comparisons between Muslims and non-Muslims in developing countries around the world.

Cerebrovascular Disease

Stroke is a devastating disease that can instantly impact a person's physical and cognitive functioning. Stroke is related to high blood pressure, and there are also correlations between stroke and psychosocial stress, anxiety, and depression. Among the ten countries of the world (out of 192) with the highest death rate from stroke, Muslim-majority countries make up four of the ten (if Ivory Coast is included, along with Azerbaijan, Kyrgyzstan, and Albania) (World Health Organization 2011a). Among the 30 countries with the lowest stroke rate, Muslim-majority countries make up only two (Qatar and Bahrain). Our 2010 systematic review identified three studies that examined religion and cerebrovascular disease in Muslims, two examining the effects of the Ramadan fast on incidence of stroke. The final study compared stroke rates in Muslims and Christians in Greece. No studies have yet examined the effects of religiosity (level of religious involvement) on stroke rate in Muslims.

Ramadan. Akhan and associates (2000) examined the effects of Ramadan fasting on admission to hospitals in the Isparta Province (Turkey) from 1991 to 1995. Participants (1,579 persons with stroke) were divided into admissions that occurred during the month of Ramadan and admissions during other months of the year. Results indicated that there were 21 cases/month of cerebral infarct during Ramadan and 20.6 cases per month during the rest of the year. For cerebral hemorrhage, the rate was 6.8 cases during Ramadan compared to 5.6 cases in other months of the year ($p = 0.80$, not significant). There was also no difference in age of onset of stroke during the month of Ramadan compared to other months of the year.

In the second study, Bener and associates (2006) retrospectively reviewed a 13-year stroke database for patients hospitalized with stroke between 1991 and 2003 in Qatar. Patients were divided into four groups depending on the month when they were admitted with stroke: the month before Ramadan, the month of Ramadan, month after Ramadan, and average admissions per month throughout the year. During this 13-year period, 335 Muslims were admitted to the hospital (mean age 57). Average number of admissions for stroke for each of the four groups was 30 cases for month before Ramadan, 29 during Ramadan, 29 in the month after Ramadan, and 27 per month average throughout the year (no significant difference).

Muslims vs. Non-Muslims. Papadopoulos and colleagues (2006) examined 530 consecutive patients admitted with stroke between 1998 and 2002 from a rural area in northern Greece (Prefecture of Xanthi). The religious makeup of this region is 53 % Christian and 47 % Muslim. Based on the population of the district and the religious affiliation of patients admitted during the study period, researchers estimated that the incidence rate of stroke per 100,000 person-years was 173.9 for Christians and 87.2 for Muslims (RR = 1.99, 95 % CI 1.66–2.40, $p < 0.001$, uncontrolled). In other words, Christians were twice as likely to suffer from stroke compared to Muslims. This difference was for ischemic stroke only, not hemorrhagic stroke, and it was true in both men and women. Diabetes and atrial fibrillation were also less common in Muslims compared to Christians ($p = 0.02$ and $p < 0.001$, respectively). No differences in outcome of stroke were found between Muslims and Christians.

Studies Missed. Our recent review uncovered only one study missed by our 2010 review, and that study compared mortality from stroke in Muslims and non-Muslims. In a study cited previously, Vos and colleagues (1998) examined stroke mortality by religious group in the Republic of Mauritius from 1989 to 1994 in those aged 30–64. There were a total of 10,657 deaths among men and 5,008 deaths among women among those in the age range specified. The distribution of religions in the Republic according to the 1983 and 1990 census was 51 % Hindu, 32 % Christian, 16 % Islam, and 1 % miscellaneous. Results indicated that Muslims had the lowest proportional mortality ratio (PMR) from stroke (PMR = 77, 95 % CI 66–89) compared to Christian Creoles (PMR = 93, 95 % CI 85–101) and Hindus (PMR = 100, reference group). Sensitivity analysis of standard mortality ratios (SMR) from stroke revealed that Muslims (SMR = 49) had about two-thirds the mortality from stroke compared to Creole Christians (SMR = 78) and less than one-half that of Hindus (SMR = 100).

Recent Research. No additional studies after 2010 were identified.

Summary. Two studies found that fasting during the month of Ramadan does not increase the rate of stroke (Table 11.1), and two studies reported that Muslims experience a lower stroke rate than Christians or Hindus. No studies have yet examined the relationship between religiosity and stroke rate in Muslims, and this represents a serious research gap. While it is not known whether religiosity helps to prevent stroke in Muslims, it is well known that Muslims rely heavily on their religious beliefs when they experience a stroke (Omu et al. 2014).

Dementia/Alzheimer's Disease

We could find no studies that examined the relationship between religiosity and dementia or cognitive functioning in Muslims, either in our 2010 systematic review or in our recent review of studies prior to 2010. Given relatively young populations, most Muslim-majority countries have yet to deal with the problem of dementia that has increasingly plagued developed countries in the West. In fact, among the 192 countries of the world with the highest death rates from dementia, there are no Muslim-majority countries in the first 20 except Pakistan (which is #20). Likewise, of the 20 countries of the world with the lowest death rates from dementia, 10 are Muslim-majority countries (World Health Organization 2011b). Nevertheless, the proportion of people in developing countries with dementia (many with Muslim-majority populations) is expected to increase by 300 % over the next 40 years (United Nations 2004). Thus, dementia and Alzheimer's disease will soon become an issue for Muslim countries as their populations age. If greater religious involvement in Muslims can forestall the development of dementia or slow the progression of memory loss in those with dementia or normal aging, then documenting this could have substantial public health implications—especially in terms of predicting future healthcare needs of these populations.

Muslims vs. Non-Muslims. Among Muslims who are over age 65, cognitive impairment and dementia are not rare. Studies have reported higher, lower, or similar rates of dementia in Muslims compared to non-Muslims, depending on the method used to diagnose dementia or cognitive impairment and on the location where the study took place. In particular, high rates of dementia have been found among Muslim Arabs living in northern Israel, higher than in the surrounding Jewish population (Wadi-Ara region, in particular) (Afgin et al., 2012; Bowirrat et al., 2001).

For example, in a study of 767 community-dwelling Arabs over age 65 in Northern Israel, 444 had no cognitive problems (58 %), 234 (31 %) had mild cognitive impairment (MCI), and 89 (12 %) had Alzheimer's disease (Israeli-Korn et al. 2010). Rates of cognitive impairment also appear high among Muslims in Malaysia (Rushid et al. 2012) and especially among consanguineous Muslims in parts of India (Kaur and Balgir 2005). In contrast, low rates of Alzheimer's disease and dementia are found among the Yoruba in Ibadan, Nigeria, where about one-third the population is Muslim, compared to African-Americans in the Indiana (mostly Christian) (Hendrie et al. 2001). No research, to our knowledge, has yet compared rates of dementia or cognitive impairment between Muslims and non-Muslims in Muslim-majority countries.

Among Muslim Arabs in northern Israel, cognitive impairment appears particularly prevalent in those with high blood pressure. In one study, participants with MCI were 68 % more likely to have hypertension; those with Alzheimer's disease were over twice as likely to have hypertension (Israeli-Korn et al. 2010). If BP is lower in Muslims who are more religious (which at least two studies above suggest), this could be one mechanism by which religiosity helps to slow the decline in memory seen with age (or slow the progression of Alzheimer's disease).

Recent Research: We identified one study that recently reported an association between prayer and cognitive functioning among Arabs in Israel (to our knowledge, this is the only study to date that has examined the relationship between religiosity and cognitive function in Muslims). Inzelberg and colleagues (2013) at the Sagol Neuroscience Center conducted a door-to-door survey of 935 Israeli Arabic men and women over age 65 examining the relationship between number of hours praying per month during midlife (assessed retrospectively) and cognitive function. Logistic regression analysis was used to analyze the association between hours praying/month at midlife with likelihood of having MCI or Alzheimer's disease (AD). MCI ($n = 238$) and AD ($n = 92$) were identified using standard cognitive tests, indicating a combined prevalence of 35 %. Results indicated that 87 % of cognitively normal persons engaged in prayer at midlife compared to 71 % of those with MCI and 69 % of those with AD ($p < 0.0001$). Since most men (94 %) reported praying at midlife, relationships between prayer and MCI or AD could not be examined due to ceiling effects. Among women, however, after controlling for age and education, prayer at midlife was associated with a 45 % lower risk of MCI (OR = 0.55, 95 % CI 0.33–0.94, $p = 0.03$). There was no association with AD, and the actual amount of prayer was not associated with either MCI or AD.

In addition, at least one study has examined the effects of religiosity on Muslim lay persons' attitudes toward people with dementia. Cohen and colleagues (2009) found that Muslims who were more religious were more likely to feel compassion or sympathy for, or desire to help those with dementia. We should also mention that Sooki and associates (2011) found that the strongest predictor of good mental health in older Muslims (ages 52–110) was regular reciting of the Qur'an.

Summary. Only one study has examined the relationship between religiosity and cognitive functioning in Muslims (Table 11.1). That study found that prayer during midlife significantly reduced the likelihood of mild cognitive impairment after age 65 in Arabic women in Israel. No studies have compared Muslims and non-Muslims on level of cognitive functioning or rates of dementia in Muslim-majority countries, although some studies suggest higher rates of cognitive impairment and dementia among Muslims in northern Israel compared to the surrounding Jewish population and rates in Western countries.

Diabetes

Nielsen (1999) examined the prevalence rates of diabetes in Arab countries using the 1980 WHO diagnostic criteria. Results indicated a rising prevalence of diabetes in these countries. This was particularly noted for Saudi Arabia, where rates in those over age 55 rose from 11.0 % in 1982 to 22.0 % in 1997 for men ages 51–60, with a smaller increase for women (18.7 % in 1987 to 26.0 % in 1997). The researcher concluded that increasing diabetes was largely due to increasing affluence, urbanization, availability of food, and a sedentary lifestyle. In a qualitative study of 106 Muslim Kashmiri men with diabetes in Leeds, UK, participants believed that being overweight projected an image of prosperity and well-being to others within the community (which discouraged weight loss). The overall attitude toward their diabetes was "to enjoy life and 'leave the rest to Allah.'" Thus, there may be cultural and religious reasons for higher rates of diabetes in Muslims.

Our 2010 review identified no studies that examined the relationship between religiosity and diabetes in Muslims. However, four studies examined the effects of fasting during Ramadan on diabetic control and three studies compared rates of diabetes in Muslims and non-Muslims. We first review studies on Ramadan fasting and then those that compare Muslims and non-Muslims.

Ramadan. Salti and colleagues (2004) analyzed data collected by general practitioners, internists, and diabetologists involved in the care of patients with diabetes in 13 countries (Algeria, Bangladesh, Egypt, India, Indonesia, Jordan, Lebanon, Malaysia, Morocco, Pakistan, Saudi Arabia, Tunisia, and Turkey). One hundred practitioners were selected from each country and asked to interview and record clinical data on the next ten patients with diabetes that they saw immediately following the month of Ramadan. This method generated data on 12,243 patients with Type I diabetes (mean age 31) or Type II diabetes (mean age 54). Patients were asked if they fasted during Ramadan, with 42.8 % of Type I diabetics and 78.7 % of Type II diabetics indicating that they fasted at least 15 days during Ramadan. About one-fourth of those treated with oral hypoglycemics and one-third of patients on insulin changed their treatment dose during Ramadan. Outcome was self-reported episodes of hypo-/hyperglycemia that occurred during the year prior to Ramadan vs. during the month of Ramadan itself (where severe hypoglycemia was defined as hypoglycemia leading to hospitalization). Results indicated that severe hypoglycemic episodes were significantly more frequent during the month of Ramadan, for both Type I diabetics ($p=0.017$, uncontrolled) and Type II diabetics ($p=0.0001$). Researchers concluded that Muslims who fast during Ramadan should follow established treatment guidelines for diabetics, which are now available.

Khaled and associates (2006) examined the effects of Ramadan fasting on diabetic control in 60 obese females with Type II diabetes in Northwestern Algeria (average BMI = 35.4, mean age 51, mean duration of diabetes 5 years). Questionnaires were administered and blood drawn 1 month before Ramadan (pre-fasting), the third week of Ramadan, and after the end of Ramadan (post-fasting). Fasting blood sugar (mmol/L) decreased significantly from pre-fasting to the third week of Ramadan and post-Ramadan (8.85 to 7.37 to 7.12, $p<0.001$), as did HgbA1c level (7.35 to 6.52 to 6.36, $p<0.001$). Researchers concluded that the effect of Ramadan was an approximately 10–15 % improvement in glucose homeostasis.

M'guil and colleagues (M'Guil et al. 2008) examined the effects of Ramadan fasting on diabetic control in 120 Type II diabetics in Morocco (mean age 50–58, 52 % women, duration of diabetes 5 years). All had their diabetes under good control and planned to fast during the entire 30 days of Ramadan. Blood was obtained on the day prior to beginning the Ramadan fast, on day 15 and day 29 of the fast, and then 15 days after the fast ended. Blood glucose dropped slightly from before to during Ramadan (in women, $p<0.05$), but then increased 15 days after Ramadan ($p<0.01$, both men and women). Insulin levels increased from before to during Ramadan ($p<0.05$, both men and women) and then dropped after Ramadan ($p<0.01$, both men and women). HbgA1c did not change from before Ramadan to the 15th day of Ramadan. There were no serious adverse effects such as severe hypo- or hyperglycemia or hospitalization. Researchers concluded that Type II diabetics who follow their recommended diet and medication regimen do not experience significant hypoglycemia or neuroglycopenic symptoms during Ramadan.

The fourth study examining the effects of the Ramadan fast, conducted by Shariatpanahi and associates (2008), involved 55 men (mean age 34) with metabolic syndrome from a hospital in Tehran, Iran. Metabolic syndrome was defined as having three or more of the following: (1) abdominal obesity, (2) hypertriglyceridemia, (3) low HDL cholesterol, (4) high blood pressure, or (5) high fasting blood sugar. All men fasted the full 30 days during Ramadan. Blood was drawn before beginning the Ramadan fast and after the end of the 30-day fast. Results indicated a decrease in blood pressure from before to after Ramadan (both systolic and diastolic, $p<0.001$); a reduction in abdominal obesity, weight, and BMI (all $p<0.001$); an increase in insulin sensitivity ($p=0.001$); and a reduction in insulin resistance ($p=0.005$). All of these changes are known to have beneficial effects in those with metabolic syndrome.

Muslims vs. Non-Muslims. Three studies have compared Muslims and non-Muslims on rates of diabetes. In a study described earlier, Gupta and colleagues (2002) surveyed 1,415 males (19.2 % Muslim) and 797 females (11.4 % Muslim) in Jaipur, India, examining cardiovascular risk factors. Self-reported diabetes was reported by 1.4 % of Hindu males and 1.2 % of Hindu females, whereas no Muslims reported diabetes (0.0 % in males and females).

Papadopoulos and associates (2006), also cited earlier, retrospectively reviewed the medical records of 530 stroke cases between 1998 and 2002 admitted to a hospital in the Xanthi region of Thrace, Greece. Along with clinical information, religion was also abstracted from the medical record. Muslims and Christians were compared on a variety of clinical factors, including diabetes. Diabetes was defined as an abnormal fasting glucose, elevated glycosylated hemoglobin levels, or clinical history of diabetes. Results indicated that diabetes was less frequent in Muslims compared to Christians ($p=0.02$, uncontrolled).

Finally, Burazeri and colleagues (2008b) in a case–control study of 467 patients with acute coronary syndrome (ACS) and 737 controls in Albania (cited earlier) found no difference in diabetes between Muslims and Christians in the control group (5.6 % vs. 8.8 % among men and 8.8 % vs. 8.3 % among women). Such comparisons were not provided for ACS cases.

Studies Missed. No other studies examining religiosity and diabetes were identified in our recent review of this literature, although we did locate one study that compared Muslims and non-Muslims. Vijayakumar and associates (2009) compared the prevalence of Type II diabetes across religious groups in a random sample of 1,990 adults in Kerala, southern India (80 % middle class or poor). Diagnosis of diabetes was made if fasting blood sugar was ≥ 126 mg/dL or if the person was taking medication for diabetes. Religious group affiliation was Hindu ($n=883$, 44 %), Muslim ($n=272$, 14 %), and Christian ($n=406$, 20 %). Percentage of each group with diabetes was 11.0 % for Hindus, 20.2 % for Muslims, and 21.9 % for Christians. Although these differences appear significant (Hindus vs. Muslims/Christians), no statistics were provided in the report. The researchers did not discuss these findings, although they did report that diabetes was more frequent among those of higher SES and greater obesity, so if religion was related to the ability to afford food, then this may have influenced results.

Recent Research. Several studies have addressed religion and diabetes in Muslims since 2010: one examining the relationship between religiosity and diabetes, one analyzing the effects of Ramadan fasting on diabetic control, and two comparing rates of diabetes in Muslims and non-Muslims.

Religiosity. In a study already reviewed, Kalter-Leibovici and associates (2011) examined risk factors for adult-onset diabetes in a random national sample of 544 Arabs and 548 Jews in Israel. Among those risk factors was religiosity, which was measured by categorizing participants as secular, traditional, or religious. Although statistical comparison was not performed, only 1.7 % of diabetic Arabs ($n = 114$) were secular compared to 8.9 % of nondiabetic Arabs ($n = 430$). Similarly, 71.7 % of diabetic Arabs categorized themselves as religious compared to 46.3 % of non-diabetic Arabs. Thus, diabetes appeared to be positively related to being religious in Israeli Arabs.

Ramadan. Gaborit and colleagues (2011) interviewed 101 Muslim diabetic patients in Marseille, France, concerning their practices during Ramadan. HgA1c levels were also measured and patients' charts reviewed. Interviews and examinations were performed during the 3 months prior to Ramadan. In addition, 101 general practitioners (GPs) (not physicians of patients in the study) were interviewed regarding their recommendations to diabetic patients during Ramadan fasting. Most patients came from countries around the Mediterranean, primarily from Algeria, and had been living in France for an average of 36 years. Over half (52 %) had never attended primary school and could not read, and the majority (78 %) worked manual labor. Religious involvement was common: 71 % prayed five times daily, 95 % ate halal food exclusively, and 28 % had made a pilgrimage to Mecca. About two-thirds (64 %) had discussed fasting during Ramadan with their physician and over half ($n = 36$) were told that fasting was dangerous and was forbidden. More than half ($n = 19$) of those forbidden to fast said they fasted anyway against medical advice. Patients who fasted during Ramadan ($n = 52$) and those who did not fast during Ramadan but had fasted in the past ($n = 40$) were compared (those who had never fasted were excluded). Those who did not fast during Ramadan were also less likely to pray five times per day compared to those who fasted (60 % vs. 88 %, $p < 0.005$). Patients in the non-fasting group were older (64 vs. 56, $p = 0.02$), had diabetes for a longer time (16 vs. 10 years, $p = 0.002$), and were more likely to be taking insulin (73 % vs. 44 %, $p < 0.01$). Despite this, those in the non-fasting group had lower HgA1c levels compared to those in the fasting group (7.8 vs. 8.7, $p = 0.04$). Among GPs, only 2 % said they had received any medical training on Ramadan fasting, 77 % had never read any medical information on the subject, only 54 % typically advised their diabetic Muslim patients not to fast, and 15 % said they'd never talked with diabetics patients about Ramadan fasting.

Muslims vs. Non-Muslims. Albache and colleagues (2010) analyzed data from a population-based survey of 1,168 persons aged 25 and older in Aleppo, Syria, examining factors related to Type II diabetes in the population. Religious affiliation was recorded as Arab Muslim (93 %) vs. other. Although there was no difference in prevalence of impaired glucose testing or self-reported diabetes between Muslims and non-Muslims, newly diagnosed diabetics (fasting blood sugar >126 mg/dL) were more common in Muslims than non-Muslims (5.4 % vs. 0.2 %, $p<0.01$, uncontrolled). When gender, age, SES, BMI, weight–height ratio, and physical activity were controlled for in a regression model, religious affiliation was not among variables that significantly predicted new onset diabetes.

In the Kalter-Leibovici et al. (2011) study cited above, the prevalence of diabetes in Arabs was 21 % compared to 12 % in Jews. A multivariate regression model controlling for gender, BMI, family history of diabetes, and cumulative dietary energy density revealed that Arabs were 70 % more likely to have adult-onset diabetes (Type II) than Jews (OR = 1.70, 95 % CI 1.19–2.43, $p<0.005$).

Summary. To our knowledge, only one study has examined the relationship between religiosity and diabetes in Muslims, finding that Arab diabetics in Israel tended to be more religious than Arab nondiabetics. Four studies have examined the effects of fasting during Ramadan on diabetic control (Table 11.2). Three of those found that Ramadan fasting had positive effects (decreased blood sugar, decreased HgbA1c, increased insulin, increased insulin sensitivity), and one reported harmful effects (severe hypoglycemia). Note that all four studies found a lowering of blood sugar during Ramadan fasting, requiring that this be carefully monitored.

Given issues related to greater weight and lower levels of exercise, Muslims might be at greater risk for developing diabetes and poorer control of diabetes. One study reported a dramatic increase in diabetes in Saudi Arabia between 1982 and 1997 (doubling of the rate in men and over one-third increase in women). However, other research is not that clear. Of six studies reviewed here, two found higher rates of diabetes in Muslims compared to Hindus or Jews, two found lower rates of diabetes in Muslims compared to Hindus or Christians, and two found no difference in prevalence of diabetes between Muslims and non-Muslims. Only one of those six studies was in a Muslim-majority country (Syria) and it found no difference in diabetes between Muslims and non-Muslims when other factors were controlled.

Cholesterol and Triglycerides

Several studies have found elevated cholesterol levels in Arab countries, especially over the past four decades as diet has become more Westernized (Musaiger 2002). This is especially true for Arabs in the USA (Jaber et al. 1995; Hatahet et al. 2002). Our 2010 systematic review identified one study that examined the association between religiosity and blood lipid levels and six studies on the effects of Ramadan fasting on blood cholesterol or triglyceride levels.

Religiosity. In a study reviewed earlier, Yilmaz and associates (2008) surveyed 46 patients over age 50 in Turkey who had been praying regularly for at least

Table 11.2 Religiosity, diabetes, and cholesterol/triglycerides in Muslims

Authors (year)	Method	Sample size	Participants	Location	Controls	Findings
Diabetes						
Religiosity						
Kalter-Leibovici et al. (2011)	CS	544	Adult Arabs	Israel	None	NG
Effects of Ramadan						
Salti et al. (2004)	CS/RS	12,243	Diabetic patients in 13 Arabic countries		None	NG
Khaled et al. (2006)	Exp	60	Obese women, Type II	Algeria	None	P
M'guil et al. (2008)	Exp	120	Type II diabetics	Morocco	None	P
Shariatpanahi et al. (2008)	Exp	55	Men with metabolic syndrome	Iran	None	P
Cholesterol/triglycerides						
Religiosity						
Yilmaz et al. (2008)	CS	45	Patients over age 50	Turkey	Ctrl group	NA
Effects of Ramadan						
Adlouni et al. (1997)	Exp	32	Healthy men	Morocco	None (?)	P
Afrasiabi et al. (2003)	Exp	28	Men, high lipids	Iran	None	P
Rahman et al. (2004)	Exp	20	College students	Bangladesh	SC	P
Saleh et al. (2004)	Exp	103	Healthy obese	Egypt	None	P
Aksungar et al. (2005)	Exp	24	Healthy volunteers	Turkey	None	P
Aksungar et al. (2007)	Exp	40	Healthy volunteers	Turkey	Ctrl group	P
Khaled et al. (2006)	Exp	60	Obese female diabetics	Algeria	None	NG
Barkia et al. (2011)	Exp	25	Healthy volunteers	Tunisia	None	NG

See Table 11.1 for definitions of abbreviations in this table

10 years and matched them to 40 patients over age 50 who did not pray regularly. Blood samples were taken from these 86 patients and total serum cholesterol (TC) levels were measured and compared between the two groups. No difference was found between those who prayed regularly and those who did not.

Ramadan. Afrasiabi and associates (2003) examined the effects of Ramadan fasting on serum lipid levels in 28 healthy men with high blood lipid levels (hyperlipidemia) in Tabriz, Iran. These men were compared to ten healthy men with normal lipid levels who did not participate in the Ramadan fast. All were instructed to eat a low-calorie, low-fat diet during the testing period (from 20 days before Ramadan to 1 month afterward). Blood lipid levels were measured at baseline, 1 day before onset of the Ramadan fast, immediately after Ramadan, and 1 month afterward. In the fasting group, researchers found that there was a significant decrease in energy intake and nutrient materials during the month of Ramadan. Low-density lipoprotein (LDL), triglyceride, and total cholesterol (TC) decreased significantly during Ramadan in fasting men, but there was no change in non-fasting men. Investigators concluded that fasting during the month of Ramadan by hyperlipidemic men significantly improved their lipid profiles.

Rahman and colleagues (2004) examined fasting serum lipids before, after, and 1 month after Ramadan fasting in 20 healthy Bangladeshi male college students. Although fat intake and body weight increased significantly between the baseline evaluation and 1 month after Ramadan, high-density lipoprotein (HDL) cholesterol (the "good" cholesterol) also increased significantly during this period and remained significantly higher after controlling for other relevant variables.

Saleh and colleagues (2004) examined the effects of the Ramadan fast on blood lipid levels in 103 healthy obese volunteers ages 15–52 in Egypt. Blood lipid levels were measured at baseline prior to Ramadan, at the end of Ramadan, and 4 weeks and 8 weeks after Ramadan. Results indicated that total cholesterol, triglycerides, HDL, LDL, TC/HDL, and LDL/HDL ratio all significantly improved by the end of Ramadan, and these effects persisted for 4 weeks after the fast ended. These results are consistent with the positive effects of Ramadan fasting on blood lipid levels reported by the two other research teams above.

In a fourth study, reviewed previously, Aksungar and associates (2005) examined serum lipid levels (total cholesterol, triglycerides, HDL, LDL) in 24 healthy fasting volunteers aged 21–35 in Turkey. Blood was taken 1 week before Ramadan, on the 21st day of Ramadan, and 20 days following the end of Ramadan. Results indicated no significant change in total cholesterol, triglycerides, or LDL cholesterol, although HDL cholesterol increased during Ramadan and remained high at the 20-day follow-up in both males (49 to 56 to 47 mg/mL, $p<0.001$) and females (57.4 to 66.5 to 66.9, $p<0.001$). In a second report by this research group (Aksungar et al. 2007), investigators examined blood lipid levels in 40 healthy volunteers (50 % male, ages 20–39). In addition, 28 healthy age and BMI-matched non-fasting controls were also included. Blood was drawn 1 week before Ramadan, during the last week of Ramadan, and 3 weeks after Ramadan. Again, no significant changes were seen in total cholesterol (TC), triglycerides, or LDL levels. However, the TC/HDL ratio

(HDL risk factor) decreased significantly in both male and female fasting participants (males: 3.56 to 2.47 to 3.02, $p<0.05$; females: 3.45 to 2.12 to 2.95, $p<0.05$), whereas there was no change in the non-fasting group. As other researchers had found before them, Aksungar and his group concluded that the Ramadan fast exerted positive effects on lipid profile.

Finally, in a study also reviewed earlier, Khaled and colleagues (2006) examined 60 obese female volunteers with Type II diabetes seen in a diabetology center in Algeria. Average BMI was 35.4 (high), mean age was 51, and average length of diabetes was 5 years. Blood was drawn 1 month before Ramadan, on the third week of Ramadan, and 3 weeks after the fasting period ended. Investigators found that there was a significant improvement in patients' diabetic profile, lowering their blood sugar and reducing their HgA1c. However, total serum cholesterol increased during fasting (13.9 %, $p<0.001$), as did serum triglycerides (16.95, $p<0.003$) and LDL cholesterol (22.39 %, $p<0.0001$). Researchers concluded that while Ramadan fasting improved patients' diabetic control, it significantly worsened their lipid profile.

Missed Studies. Our current review identified four additional studies missed in our 2010 review, including one that focused on fasting during Ramadan and three that compared cholesterol levels in Muslims and non-Muslims.

Ramadan. Adlouni and colleagues (1997) studied 32 healthy adult Muslim men in Morocco, comparing lipid levels before and after Ramadan fasting. Although only the abstract of the research was available to us, researchers reported a significant decrease in total serum cholesterol (7.9 %, $p<0.001$) and LDL cholesterol (11.7 %) and an increase in HDL cholesterol (14.3 %, $p<0.001$) during the month of Ramadan. Serum triglycerides decreased even more (30.0 %, $p<0.001$). Some of these changes persisted throughout the month following Ramadan (increased HDL, decreased LDL). Researchers attributed lipid changes to alterations in diet with a reduction in fat intake during Ramadan fasting.

Muslims vs. Non-Muslims. McKeigue and associates (1991) examined 1,712 South Asians and 2,042 Europeans ages 40–69 living in London, UK, comparing cardiovascular risk factors between Muslims ($n=211$) and other religious groups. Age-adjusted total cholesterol (TC) levels (mmol/L) were significantly different between native Brits (largely Christian), Sikhs, Punjabi Hindus, Gujarati Hindus, and Muslims (6.12 vs. 6.01 vs. 5.94 vs. 5.45 vs. 5.95, respectively, $p<0.001$). HDL levels (the good cholesterol) were also significantly different between these groups (1.24 vs. 1.22 vs. 1.17 vs. 1.14 vs. 1.04, respectively, $p<0.001$). Fasting triglyceride levels were also significantly different (1.48 vs. 1.73 vs. 1.74 vs. 1.49 vs. 1.85, $p=0.02$). Thus, HDL cholesterol was lowest and triglyceride level highest in Muslims (i.e., a generally poor lipid profile).

Abou-Rbiah and Weitzman (2002) compared cardiovascular risk factors in 271 Bedouin diabetics with that of 201 Jewish diabetics being seen at primary care clinics in the Negev, Israel. Bedouins were significantly younger than Jews (52.8 vs. 65.6, $p<0.0005$), and duration of diabetes was shorter (7.3 vs. 9.3 years, $p<0.0005$).

Total cholesterol level was significantly lower in Muslim Bedouins compared to Jews (5.4 vs. 6.0, $p<0.0005$, uncontrolled), as was LDL cholesterol (bad cholesterol) (3.3 vs. 5.4, $p<0.0005$). There were no differences in HDL cholesterol or triglyceride levels.

Finally, Schulpis and associates (2006) compared lipid levels of mothers from three ethnic groups delivering infants in Greece: Greeks ($n=3,118$), Albanians ($n=3,050$), and Muslim Asians ($n=2,966$). Although religious affiliations were not given for Greeks and Albanians, the majority of Greeks are Greek Orthodox Christian (98 %) and the majority of Albanians (57 %) are Muslim. After 4–6 h of fasting and just before entering the delivery room, blood was obtained from the mothers for analysis. Total cholesterol, triglyceride, HDL, LDL, and VLDL (mmol/L) differed significantly between the three groups. For TC, Asian Muslims had lower levels than either Greeks or Albanians (5.09 vs. 5.20 and 7.10, respectively, $p<0.001$, uncontrolled). Both LDL and VLDL cholesterol (bad) were lowest in Asian Muslims compared to Greeks or Albanians ($p<0.001$). HDL cholesterol was also highest among Asian Muslims compared to Greeks and Albanians (1.60 vs. 1.40 and 1.31, $p<0.001$). Researchers explained these differences as being due to genetic, religious, or dietary factors (Muslims being forbidden to eat pork).

Recent Research. We could locate only one study since 2010 that examined religion and cholesterol in Muslims and that study focused on changes in lipid levels during Ramadan (the eighth such study). Barkia and colleagues (2011) examined lipid levels before, during, and after Ramadan in 25 healthy volunteers (19 males) aged 22–55 in Tunisia. Blood was taken 0–2 days prior to the onset of Ramadan fasting (BR), 2 weeks (R-2) and 4 weeks (R-4) after the fast began, and then 1 month after Ramadan (AR). Total cholesterol increased from 4.4 (BR) to 4.5 (R-2) to 5.0 (R-4) and 4.9 (AR) ($p<0.01$, uncontrolled). LDL cholesterol increased likewise from 2.9 (BR) to 2.9 (R-2) to 3.5 (R-4) and 3.4 (AR) ($p<0.01$). Triglyceride and HDL levels did not change. Researchers explained that changes in diet during Ramadan, including a significant increase in polyunsaturated fatty acids and cholesterol intake, helped to explain the worsening lipid profile observed.

Summary. Only one study has examined the relationship between religiosity and cholesterol level in Muslims. That study found no difference in lipid levels between those over age 50 in Turkey who prayed five times daily and those who did not. Eight studies have examined the effects of the Ramadan fast on cholesterol levels, with six of eight studies reporting either a lowering of total cholesterol and LDL cholesterol (bad) or an increase in HDL cholesterol (good) (Table 11.2). The remaining two studies found a worsening of cholesterol levels during Ramadan among obese female Type II diabetics in Algeria and among healthy volunteers in Tunisia. In addition, three studies compared cholesterol levels in Muslims and non-Muslims: two reporting a better lipid profile (lower bad cholesterol or higher good cholesterol) in Muslims and one finding a worse lipid profile in South Asian Muslims living in the UK compared to other religious groups.

Immune Function

One of the primary physiological mechanisms that connects mental health with physical health is the immune system, given the effects that stress or negative emotions can have on immunity. If religious involvement reduces psychological distress, then we would also expect it to positively influence immune functions. Our 2010 systematic review identified three studies that examined religiosity and immune function, all investigating the effects of the Ramadan fast.

Latifynia and colleagues (2007) obtained blood samples before and after Ramadan in 24 healthy adult males in Tehran, Iran, examining effects on neutrophil (white blood cell) functioning. No changes were found causing researchers to conclude that fasting during Ramadan did not have a negative effect on immunity. A later study by this group involving 21 healthy male students ages 18–35 confirmed the finding and extended it to circulating immune complex activity (no change during Ramadan).

As described previously, Aksunger and colleagues (2007) examined the effects of fasting during Ramadan on immune function in 40 healthy Muslim volunteers aged 20–38 (50 % women). The immune indicator assessed was the pro-inflammatory cytokine, interleukin-6 (IL-6). Blood samples were taken 1 week before Ramadan, the last week of Ramadan, and three weeks after Ramadan. IL-6 levels decreased significantly during Ramadan and remained low up to 3 weeks after Ramadan. In males, IL-6 levels dropped from about 4.5 pg/mL down to 2.0 during Ramadan ($p < 0.001$) and increased to 3.5 at 3 weeks after Ramadan (still lower than baseline at $p < 0.05$). In women, IL-6 levels dropped from about 5.0 pg/mL at baseline before Ramadan to 2.2 during Ramadan ($p < 0.001$) and increased to about 3.0 at 3 weeks after Ramadan (still lower than baseline at $p < 0.05$). Researchers concluded that fasting during Ramadan has positive effects on immune function (i.e., reduces levels of inflammation).

Missed Studies. Missed in our 2010 review was a study that examined risk factors associated with low CD4 lymphocyte counts in HIV-positive women and a study that compared antibody response to typhoid vaccination, both comparing Muslims and non-Muslims.

Abimiku and associates (2009) measured CD4 counts in the blood of 187 pregnant HIV-positive women in Nigeria (average age was 27, 92 % married, 81 % Christian, 17 % Muslim). CD4 lymphocyte counts of less than 200 cells/mm^3 indicate the transition from being HIV-positive to having an official diagnosis of AIDS (autoimmune deficiency syndrome). Results indicated that Muslims were 70 % more likely than Christians (OR = 1.70, $p = 0.03$) to have CD4 counts of 200 or lower, controlling for age, occupation, number of pregnancies, condom use, vaginal discharge, and vaginal ulcers. Researchers hypothesized that Muslim women may be less likely to come to a prenatal clinic at a specialist hospital until they are very sick, which may be partly due to men being the dominant decision-makers in Muslim families and controlling access to health care.

Table 11.3 Religiosity and immune function, endocrine function, cancer, self-rated health, and mortality in Muslims

Authors (year)	Method	Sample size	Participants	Location	Controls	Findings
Immune function						
Religiosity						
None						
Effects of Ramadan						
Latifynia et al. (2007)	Exp	24	Healthy males	Iran	None	NA
Latifynia et al. (2008)	Exp	21	Healthy males	Iran	None	NA
Aksunger et al. (2007)	Exp	40	Healthy volunteers	Turkey	Ctrl group	P
Endocrine function						
Religiosity						
None						
Effects of Ramadan						
Al-Hadramy et al. (1988)	Exp	10	Healthy volunteers	Saudi Arabia	None	C
Malhotra et al. (1989)	Exp	11	Pregnant Muslims	UK	Ctrl group	C
Haouari et al. (1998)	Exp	36	Healthy males	Tunisia	None	NA
Dikensoy et al. (2009)	Exp	36	Pregnant Muslims	Turkey	Ctrl group	NG
Lahdimawan et al. (2013)	Exp	27	Healthy volunteers	Indonesia	None	P
Cancer						
None						
Self-rated health						
Sujoldzic et al. (2006)	CS	1,282	Adolescents	Bosnia	MC	P
Kodzi et al. (2011)	CS	2,606	Adults over age 50	Kenya	MC	NG
Mortality						
Lerch et al. (2010)	RS	43.5 million	Adults ages 25+	Switzerland	MC	P

See Table 11.1 for definitions of abbreviations in this table

Majumder and other researchers (2009) examined the immune response to typhoid vaccination in 984 persons aged 12 or older in Calcutta, India (63 % Muslim and 37 % Hindu). Average age of participants was 34 years and 54 % were female. Antibody levels to typhoid were assessed pre- and post-vaccination. In Muslims, antibody level increased from 1.78 EU/ml pre-vaccination to 77.48 post-vaccination, whereas in Hindus, antibody level increased from 1.21 to 57.34. The difference, however, was not statistically significant ($p=0.30$).

Recent Research. We could locate no studies on religion and immune function published since 2010.

Summary. Very little research has examined the effects of religiosity on immune function in Muslims. Three studies examined the effects of the Ramadan fast on immune function: two finding no change in neutrophil functioning or circulating immune complex activity and the third study reporting a decrease in IL-6 levels (improved immune function) during Ramadan fasting (Table 11.3). Two studies compared immune functions in Muslims with those in non-Muslims: one finding lower CD4 lymphocyte counts (worse immune function) in pregnant HIV-positive Muslim women compared to Christian women and the other study finding no difference between Muslims and Hindus in antibody response to typhoid vaccine. Much further research in Muslim populations is needed to determine how religiosity affects immune function.

Endocrine Function

Stress hormones are known to modulate immune function and so may be part of the mechanism by which religious involvement affects physical health. Our 2010 review identified no studies in Muslim populations that examined relationships between religiosity and stress hormones (cortisol, epinephrine, norepinephrine).

Missed Studies. Missed, however, were at least four studies investigating the effects of fasting during Ramadan on endocrine functions, three of them examining change in cortisol levels. Of particular interest is the effect of Ramadan fasting on cortisol rhythm (the normal increase and decrease of cortisol secretion from adrenal glands during the day and nighttime), since many Muslims alter their sleep habits during Ramadan, sometimes staying up much of the night.

Al-Hadramy and colleagues (1988) at King Abdulaziz University, Jeddah, Saudi Arabia, examined the alterations in morning and midnight cortisol levels in ten healthy fasting adults during Ramadan. Four of these adults showed an alteration of cortisol rhythm during the last two weeks of Ramadan fasting showing a reversal of morning/midnight cortisol ratio. Researchers concluded that fasting and sleep pattern changes during the Ramadan fast could alter cortisol rhythms throughout the day and night with unclear consequences for health.

Haouari and colleagues (1998) examined the effects of the Ramadan fast on endocrine function in 36 healthy male volunteers from Tunisia (mean age 24).

Blood was drawn at 9:00, 13:00, 17:00, 21:00, 00:00, and 5:00 on the 7th day before the onset of Ramadan and then again on the 7th and 21st day of fasting. Insulin and cortisol levels were determined in the usual manner (radioimmunoassay). Average 24-h insulin levels decreased from before Ramadan to the 7th day of fasting and then increased slightly at the 21st day (50.3 μU/L to 38.4 and then to 43.2, respectively, $p<0.001$). Peak time of insulin secretion also shifted by 8 h from 21:00 peak to 05:00 peak. Average 24-h cortisol levels dropped slightly from 335.5 mg/L before Ramadan to 296.2 on the 7th day of fasting and increased back up to 320.8 by the 21st day (no significant change). Peak times of cortisol secretion also did not change. Researchers concluded that the changes in insulin and cortisol were not pathological and demonstrated adaptation during the course of Ramadan fasting.

The last two studies examined the effects of Ramadan fasting on endocrine changes in healthy pregnant women. Malhotra and colleagues (1989) examined endocrine changes during Ramadan in 11 pregnant Asian Muslims seen at a hospital clinic in Birmingham, England. All women were from Pakistan or Bangladesh, all women fasted during the entire month of Ramadan, and all had a normal pregnancy in the 28th–37th week. These were compared to 11 non-fasting women from Pakistan or Bangladesh in their 29th week with healthy pregnancies. Two blood samples were drawn in cases and controls. For cases fasting during Ramadan, a blood sample was taken in the morning after 8–14 h of fasting since the last meal at sunset the day before and a second sample was taken in the evening following 15–22 h of fasting before the first meal after sunset. A single blood sample was drawn in the morning from control women who did not eat for 9–14 h overnight only. Results indicated that while all biochemical values were the same in the morning between Ramadan fasting and control women, plasma glucose, insulin, carnitine, and lactate all fell during the day, while 3-hydroxybutyrate, triglycerides, and nonesterified fatty acids rose. By the end of the Ramadan-fasting day, none of the 11 fasting women had all biochemical tests within the normal range. Researchers concluded that while they did not observe any clinical harm, they were concerned about the metabolic changes from normal that were observed in fasting women.

Finally, Dikensoy and associates (2009) investigated the effects of Ramadan fasting on maternal cortisol levels in 36 women with healthy pregnancies of 20 weeks or more duration (average age 23) and compared them to levels in 29 healthy pregnant women of 20 weeks or more who were not fasting during Ramadan (average age 24). The study took place in Turkey at Gaziantep University. Maternal blood was taken one week prior to Ramadan and on the 20th day of fasting. Fetal growth and amniotic fluid were also measured by ultrasonography. Similar measures were made in non-fasting control women. Results indicated no difference in any fetal measures. However, serum cortisol levels increased significantly from before Ramadan to day 20 of fasting ($p<0.05$), and this increase was not present in the control group.

Recent Research. We could find only one study published since 2010, and this again focused on Ramadan fasting. Lahdimawan and colleagues (2013) explored effects on endorphin and endocannabinoid levels of Ramadan fasting in 27 healthy male volunteers ages 18–22 living in Indonesia. Blood was drawn 7 days before Ramadan and on day 7 and day 21 of Ramadan fasting. Results indicated a significant increase from before Ramadan to early and later in Ramadan for serum endorphin (3,676 to 7,884, $p<0.001$), serum endocannabinoid (27.6–28.1, $p=0.003$), PBMC (peripheral blood mononuclear cell) endorphin (1,951–3,220, $p<0.001$), PBMC endocannabinoid (8.6–13.6, $p<0.001$), and macrophage endorphin (1,872–3,458, $p<0.001$). There was a decrease, however, in macrophage endocannabinoid (2.8–2.6, $p<0.001$). Endorphins and endocannabinoids are hormones known to affect and modulate the stress response. Researchers did not discuss the meaning of these changes, but none seemed to be particularly harmful.

Summary. Even less is known about the relationship between religiosity and endocrine function in Muslims as is known about religiosity and immune function. The only studies examining religion and endocrine functions examine the effects of Ramadan fasting (five of them) (Table 11.3). No studies have examined relationships between level of religious involvement (religiosity) and stress hormones of any kind. Ramadan fasting does not appear to have major effects on cortisol in either healthy adults or healthy pregnant women. One study found a slight increase in serum cortisol in pregnant women, two studies found a decrease in insulin levels (one in pregnant women), and one study found an increase in serum endorphin and endocannabinoid levels in healthy volunteers. Overall, while caution has been advised especially in pregnant women (Almond and Mazumder 2011), no major endocrine changes appear to occur during Ramadan fasting.

Cancer

On the one hand, Muslims might be expected to have lower rates of cancer because of less cigarette smoking, decreased alcohol use, and less risky sexual behaviors. On the other hand, Muslims might also have higher rates of cancer due to high consanguinity or might present later with more advanced disease due to decreased access to care and/or lower rates of screening (which may worsen prognosis). Some of these possibilities are likely due to socioeconomic or cultural factors and have little to do with religiosity (except religious beliefs that foster fatalistic attitudes toward cancer).

Unfortunately, we were unable to find a single study during our 2010 systematic review that examined relationships between religiosity and the development or the prognosis of cancer in Muslims. Five studies, however, compared cancer risk or mortality in Muslims with non-Muslims. One study compared the prevalence of cervical intraepithelial neoplasia (CIN, a precancerous lesion of the cervix) in women from Saudi Arabia to that found in women from Western countries. A second study from India examined human papillomavirus (HPV) infection rates between Hindus and Muslims (HPV infection increases the risk of cervical cancer).

The three remaining studies compared death rates from specific cancers between Muslims and non-Muslims in India and Pakistan. We now review these studies.

Altaf (2001) conducted a retrospective study of 3,088 pap smears performed at King Khalid National Guard Hospital in Jeddah, Saudi Arabia, from 1990 to 1997, identifying 97 (3.14 %) abnormal cervical smears. Of women with abnormal smears, 85 % were Muslim. The prevalence of cervical intraepithelial neoplasia (CIN 1 and CIN 2) was 1.2 %, which is lower than in other developed countries (2.6 %). The prevalence of CIN 3 was also lower than in other developed countries (0.2 % vs. 0.5 %). Low rates of extramarital sex and fewer sexual partners likely account for these lower rates of CIN.

Yeole and colleagues (2000) compared death rates from head/neck cancer between Christians ($n=355$), Hindus ($n=4{,}514$), and Muslims ($n=1{,}193$) in Bombay, India. Cases of head/neck cancer were identified between 1987 and 1991 and followed up for 5 years through 1996. Survival was associated with religious affiliation. Christians had poorer 5-year survival compared to Hindus and Muslims (24.6 % vs. 31.7 % and 36.1 %, respectively, $p<0.001$). Analyses controlled for age, marital status, site, extent of disease, and treatment. Results indicated that Christians were 30 % more likely than Hindus to die during follow-up (OR=1.30, 95 % CI 1.10–1.50, $p<0.05$), and Muslims were 20 % less likely than Hindus to do so (OR=0.80, 95 % CI 0.70–0.90, $p<0.05$).

In a second study from Yeole's research group (Yeole and Kumar 2004), they compared survival rates for those with esophageal, stomach, pancreas, and lung cancer between Christians, Hindus, and Muslims in Bombay, using similar methodology as in the first study. There were no differences in survival rate between religious groups for pancreatic or lung cancer. However, uncontrolled analyses indicated that Muslims were more likely than Hindus or Christians to survive 5 years with esophageal cancer (13.4 % vs. 9.6 % and 4.0 %, respectively, $p<0.01$), and a similar trend was found for stomach cancer survival (11.3 % vs. 7.9 % and 3.3 %, respectively, $p<0.05$). Multivariate survival analysis revealed that Muslim were significantly less likely to die of both esophageal cancer and stomach cancer during the 5-year follow-up compared to Hindus (HR=0.81, 95 % CI 0.70–0.93, $p<0.05$, for both cancers). In neither study did researchers discuss these differences in survival.

Duttagupta and colleagues (2004) examined factors related to human papillomavirus (HPV-16 and HPV-18) infection and abnormal cytology (atypical cells of undetermined significance [ASCUS] and squamous intraepithelial lesions [SIL]) in 1,044 women in West Bengal, India. HPV infection and abnormal cervical cells are more common in those with multiple sexual partners. Religious affiliations of participants in the study were Hindu (51.3 %), Muslim (45.6 %), and Christian (3.1 %). Rates of HPV-16 infection were 8.8 % in Muslims, 6.6 % in Hindus, and 3.1 % in Christians. For HPV18 infection, rates were 0.9 % in Hindus, 0.8 % in Muslims, and 0 % in Christians. With regard to abnormal cytology, ASCUS was present in 6.2 % of Christians, 5.6 % of Muslims, and 4.3 % of Hindus, whereas SIL was present in 3.1 % of Muslims, 2.8 % of Hindus, and 0 % of Christians. The statistical significance of these differences was not given. However, researchers concluded that Muslims and Hindu women in India are equally susceptible to HPV-16 and HPV-18 infection and for development of abnormal cervical cytology.

Bhurgri and associates (2006) compared incident cases of lung cancer registered at the Karachi (Pakistan) Cancer Registry in Christians, Hindus, and Muslims for the years 1995–2004. Lung cancer was the most common cancer in Pakistani men during the entire period, although it was less common among women by a ratio of 8:1. No difference in lung cancer rate was found between Hindus, Muslims, and Christians.

Missed Studies. Numerous studies were missed by our 2010 systematic review. All involved comparisons of cancer rate or mortality between Muslims and non-Muslims.

In a study conducted in 1954, Wynder (1969) and colleagues found low rates of cervical cancer among Muslims compared to Hindus in India (although few study details were given, and the difference was attributed to circumcision in male Muslims).

Jussawalla and colleagues (1981) examined the distribution of breast cancer among women in Bombay, India, comparing Christians, Muslims, and Hindus. New cases of breast cancer were identified from the Bombay Cancer Registry between 1970 and 1975 ($n = 1{,}796$). Of these, 1,118 were Hindus (62.2 %), 252 were Muslim (14.0 %), 218 were Christian (12.1 %), and 146 were Parsis (8.1 %). Investigators compared this breakdown with religious affiliations in the general population of the region, which was 67.6 % Hindu, 13.7 % Muslims, 7.0 % Christians, and 1.3 % Parsis. Adjusting rates for age revealed that breast cancer was more common among Parsis women (46.0 per 100,000) and Christians (31.0) compared to Muslims (24.4) and Hindus (18.4). Of the 1,796 cases registered, however, only 1,230 were histologically proven cases of breast cancer. Among those cases, distribution by religious group was 64.9 % Hindu, 12.0 % Muslim, 12.8 % Christian, and 7.5 % Parsi, still proportionally higher in Parsis and Christians. Statistical analyses were not reported.

Rao and colleagues (1994) compared breast cancer patients ($n = 689$) seen at a single hospital in Bombay from 1980 to 1984 with 711 women controls who attended the same hospital with benign breast lesions or gynecological problems, matching cases and controls by age and location of residence. No difference was found between cases and controls on religion (77.9 % cases vs. 79.5 % controls were Hindu, 13.9 % vs. 13.6 % were Muslim, and 5.4 % vs. 4.8 % were Christian).

Bhurgri and associates (2003) compared age-standardized rates of oral and pharyngeal cancer across demographic and social characteristics in Karachi, Pakistan. Source of information was the Karachi Cancer Registry between 1995 and 2002. Oral/pharyngeal cancer rates by religion were 94.5 %/96.8 % in Muslims, 1.7 %/0.9 % in Christians, 1.8 %/1.8 % in Hindus, and 0.7 %/0.5 % in Parsis. Although researchers did not discuss these distributions, they were not substantially different from rates of religious affiliation in the general population (95 % Muslim, 1.6 % Christian, 1.6 % Hindu, and 0.5 % Parsi).

Another study by Yeole's research group (Yeole et al. 2004) examined 5-year survival rates in 4,865 women with cancers of the breast, cervix, or ovary registered between 1992 and 1994 in the Bombay Cancer Registry. No difference was found by religious group for breast or ovarian cancers, although Christians with cervical cancer tended to have a worse survival rate (20.4 %) compared to Hindus (44.8 %), Muslims (50.0 %), and other religious groups (39.3 %) ($p=0.08$, uncontrolled). Furthermore, survival rates were much lower than in Christian-majority countries in Europe, where 5-year cervical cancer survival ranges from 62 to 71 %. In a fourth report from Yeole (2005), they reported survival rates for cancers of the larynx and lung identified between 1992 and 1994, again using the Bombay Cancer Registry. A total of 675 patients with laryngeal and 1,230 with lung cancer registered during this period were followed up through 1999. Five-year survival rates for laryngeal cancer were compared between Hindus ($n=465$), Muslims ($n=131$), and Christians ($n=48$), finding a trend favoring Muslims (33.3 %) over Hindus (29.8 %) and Christians (17.1 %) ($p=0.08$). For lung cancer, however, the trend was more pronounced and statistically significant. Five-year survival for Muslims ($n=227$), Hindus ($n=842$), and Christians ($n=103$) were 17.5 %, 12.3 %, and 5.8 %, respectively ($p=0.0005$).

Swaminathan and colleagues (2009) examined the epidemiology of a wide range of cancers (cervix, breast, stomach, mouth, esophagus, lung, ovary) in South India using the Ambilikkai Cancer Registry for the period from 2003 to 2006. Incidence rates were compared across Hindus, Muslims, and Christians. Little difference in rates was observed for cancers of the stomach, mouth, esophagus, and lung. However, cancers of the cervix tended to be lowest in Muslims (13.4 %) compared to Christians (15.5 %) or Hindus (24.4 %). Cancers of the breast, however, were lowest in Hindus compared to Muslims or Christians (10.8 % vs. 12.3 % and 16.5 %, respectively). Finally, cancers of the ovary were lowest in Christians compared to Hindus and Muslims (2.0 % vs. 3.3 % and 7.0 %, respectively). Investigators explained that the lower cervical cancer rate in Muslims was due to male circumcision, and the higher breast cancer rate in Christians was due to later age of marriage and fewer children. No explanation was given for the higher rates of ovarian cancer in Muslims (although the numbers for this calculation were small).

Other studies have compared Muslims, Hindus, and Christians on rates of oral squamous cell carcinoma (South India) (Subapriya et al. 2007), head and neck cancer (East India) (Basu et al. 2008), and breast cancer (South India) (Meshram et al. 2009). None of these studies found significant differences between religious groups.

Recent Research. Several studies have been published since our 2010 systematic review. All, however, compared cancer rates in Muslims with non-Muslims.

Kohler and Preston (2011) analyzed causes of death in the entire population of Bulgaria from 1993 to 1998, comparing causes across the following religious-ethnic groups: Bulgarian Christians ($n=5,474,818$), Roma Christians ($n=91,239$), Turkish Muslims ($n=506,588$), Muslim Pomaks ($n=68,835$), and Roma Muslims ($n=60,844$). Gender- and age (30–60 and 60–90)-stratified analyses were conducted. Among men aged 30–60, cancer as a cause of death (per 1,000) was most common among Roma Christians (2.5) and Roma Muslims (2.4) and was least common among Turkish Muslims (1.7) and Bulgarian Christians (1.8). For men in the 60–90 age group, death from cancer was again highest in Roma Christians (9.2) and Roma Muslims (7.9) and lowest in Turkish Muslims (6.6) and Muslim Pomaks (7.6). In women aged 30–60, cancer mortality was highest in Roma Christians (1.2) and Bulgarian Christians (1.1) and lowest in Muslim Turks (0.8) and Muslim Pomaks (0.9). For women aged 60–90, cancer deaths were most common in Bulgarian Christians (4.3) and Roma Christians (4.2) and least common in Muslim Turks (2.8) and Muslim Pomaks (3.0). Smoking and alcohol-related cancer deaths partly explain these differences.

Saha and Pathak (2012) examined social factors influencing the prevalence of esophageal cancer in 23,851 patients (17,889 Hindus and 5,962 Muslims) in the state of West Bengal, India. Participants were those referred for upper gastrointestinal endoscopy. The prevalence of esophageal cancer in Hindus was 0.97 % (174 of 17,889) compared to 1.24 % (74 of 5,962) in Muslims, although the difference was not compared statistically. Researchers attributed this small difference to Muslims being less likely to eat a vegetarian diet and more likely to chew tobacco.

Haroon and colleagues (2012) examined breast cancer survival rates among 285 women in Western India, of whom 60 died during follow-up. Using logistic regression to examine predictors of survival, researchers found early cancer stage and Hindu religion (vs. Muslim) as predictors of greater survival. Details are lacking given that only the study abstract was available.

Dikshit and associates (2012) examined death rates from cancer in India from 2001 to 2003. Death from cervical cancer (the leading cause of cancer death among women in both rural and urban areas of India) was lower in Muslim compared to Hindu women. The age-standardized mortality ratio (SMR) in Muslim women was 0.68 (99 % CI 0.64–0.71) compared to 1.06 (99 % CI 1.05–1.08) in Hindus. Lower cancer deaths in Muslim women were also found for cancers of the lip, oral cavity, and pharynx (SMR = 0.80). However, death rate was higher in Muslim women for cancers of the breast (SMR = 1.43) compared to Hindu women (SMR = 0.92). Muslim men had higher SMRs for most cancers compared to Hindus or other religious groups, especially for cancers of the stomach, larynx, trachea, and lung (overall SMR = 1.26 in Muslim men vs. 0.97 in Hindu men).

Although cervical cancer rates are much lower in Muslims, there is concern that Muslim women may be less receptive to receiving or allowing their daughters to receive the HPV vaccine, because of their greater religiosity compared to non-Muslims (Ben Natan et al. 2011). However, a recent study of 1,166 secondary school teachers in Malaysia (69 % Muslim) found that while 96 % said that religion was very important to them, nearly 80 % agreed to have the vaccine (and more than 70 % said they were willing to vaccinate their daughters) (Ling et al. 2012).

Summary. No studies in Muslims have examined the relationship between religiosity and the risk of developing cancer or its prognosis (Table 11.3). This represents another major research gap, given that cancer is the second most common cause of death in many countries (after heart disease). The only research we found compares survival rates or rates of cancer or precancerous lesions between Muslims and non-Muslims. Nineteen such studies were identified, of which 15 were conducted in India, two in Pakistan, and one each in Saudi Arabia and

Bulgaria. Of those, seven (37 %) found that Muslims had lower rates of cancer or longer survival with cancer, two (11 %) found higher rates of esophageal cancer and poorer survival for breast cancer, and two found more or less cancer in Muslims depending on gender and type of cancer. Eight studies found no difference (42 %). Muslim women consistently have lower rates of cervical cancer than non-Muslim women, although breast cancer rates appear equal and survival worse in Muslims. In general, Muslims with esophageal, lung, or head/neck cancer tend to have better 5-year survival rates, although some studies report higher esophageal cancer rates and higher mortality from lung cancer. These differences are thought to be largely due to hygiene (circumcision), sexual behavior, smoking and alcohol use, and socioeconomic factors influencing access to health services. Nothing, however, is known about how religiosity affects cancer development or survival in Muslims.

Self-Rated Health

As noted in Chap. 6, self-rated health (SRH) is an easily measured construct that closely reflects a person's actual physical health and is a strong predictor of mortality. The subjective nature of SRH, however, makes it dependent in part on a person's perception of their health. Perception, in turn, can be strongly influenced by negative emotional states (such as depression, which can cause a person to perceive their health as worse than it actually is) or by positive emotional states (which can do the opposite). After conducting 46 in-depth interviews with adult Muslim Arab emigrants to the USA, Abdulrahim and Ajrouch (2010) concluded that ratings of SRH were based on both actual physical health and psychological well-being. Our systematic review in 2010 uncovered no studies that examined the relationship between SRH and religiosity in Muslim-majority populations. We did, however, identify one study that compared SRH between Muslim Arabs and Jews living in Israel.

In a study reviewed earlier, Baron-Epel and colleagues (2008) examined indicators of social capital and SRH in a random population-based sample of 985 Muslim Arabs and 3,365 Jews over age 18 in Israel. SRH was assessed by a single question asking about general health status, with responses ranging from "not good at all" (1) to "very good" (5). Optimal SRH was categorized as good or very good (4 or 5). With regard to religiosity, participants categorize themselves as religious (1) vs. traditional or secular (0). Muslim Arabs were much more likely to be religious than Jews (42.3 % vs. 16.1 %, $p<0.0001$). Uncontrolled analyses revealed that Jews and Muslim Arabs were equally likely to indicate their health was optimal (good or very good) (52 % vs. 50 %, respectively), despite the fact that Muslim Arabs had less education, lower income, and higher unemployment than Jews (all $p<0.0001$). We can only speculate that the greater religiosity in Muslim Arabs might have compensated for these socioeconomic inequalities, although the relationship between religiosity and SRH was not examined.

Missed Studies. We missed several studies in our 2010 review, although only one examined religiosity and SRH in a Muslim-majority sample. The rest compared SRH in Muslims and non-Muslims.

Religiosity. Sujoldzic and associates (2006) compared SRH across three groups of emigrant adolescents ages 15–18 originally from Bosnia–Herzegovina but now living in Bosnia ($n=359$, 100 % Muslim), Croatia ($n=301$, 81 % Christian), and Austria ($n=198$, 57 % Christian). Immigrants were compared to "host" adolescents (non-emigrants) living in Bosnia–Herzegovina ($n=424$, 93 % Muslim). SRH was measured by a question asking how adolescents would rate their overall physical health: excellent (1) to poor (4). Religiosity was assessed by religious attendance and self-rated religious devotion. Uncontrolled analysis indicated that religiosity was significantly higher and SRH significantly better among emigrants living in Croatia (largely Christian) compared to emigrants living in Bosnia (all Muslim) and the non-emigrant host population (mostly Muslim). Regression models controlling for perceived discrimination, peer violence, adult violence, gender, age, SES, protective factors, psychosocial factors (depression, anxiety, self-esteem, somatic stress), and objective health problems revealed that religiosity in the overall sample was related to significantly better SRH ($B=-0.10$, $p<0.001$). Bosnian emigrants to Croatia (largely Christian) continued to have significantly better SRH than the Bosnian host population (largely Muslim) ($B=-0.10$, $p<0.01$). Although researchers did not discuss the differences between religious groups, they did stress the protective role that religiosity played.

Muslims vs. Non-Muslims. Cockerham and colleagues (2004) examined health behaviors and SRH in a population-based random sample of 2,000 adults ages 18 or over living in Kazakhstan (38–44 % Muslim) and 2,000 adults ages 18 or over in Kyrgyzstan (74–85 % Muslim). Muslims and non-Muslims were compared on SRH (measured as 0 = bad or rather bad and 1 = quite good or good). In Kazakhstan, there was no significant difference in SRH between Muslims and non-Muslims after adjusting for demographic factors. However, in Kyrgyzstan, Muslims were over three times more likely to rate their health as good compared to non-Muslims (OR = 3.07, 95 % CI 1.64–5.73, $p<0.001$). Researchers attributed the better SRH in Muslims to lower rates of alcohol use and cigarette smoking.

Khawaja and associates (2006) examined relationships between religious affiliation and health status in population-based random sample of 1,294 adolescents aged 13–19 in Beirut, Lebanon. The survey covered three communities: Nabaa (NA, $n=488$), Hay el-Sellom (HS, $n=324$), and Bourj el-Barajneh (BB, $n=482$). Residents of HS and BB were Muslim (100 %), whereas those in NA were largely Christian (77 %), allowing a comparison between Muslims and Christians. SRH was measured by a question asking if their physical health was better, the same, or worse compared to other people (0 = better, 1 = same or worse). After controlling for age, gender, social community, and income, researchers found that Muslim adolescents in the BB community were significantly more likely to rate their health as "same or worse" compared to Christians in the NA community (OR = 3.68, 95 % CI 2.05–6.63, $p<0.05$). Muslims in the HS community, however, were equally likely as Christians in the NA community to rate their health as same or worse. The investigators explained that the political and economic exclusionary policies concerning Palestinian refugees who made up the BB community may have translated into worse perceived health status.

Abdulrahim and Baker (2009) analyzed data on a random sample of 1,016 community-dwelling Arab Americans in the Detroit, Michigan area (Detroit Arab American Study). SRH was again assessed by a single question with five response options that were dichotomized into "excellent, very good, or good" vs. "fair or poor." Although neither religion nor religiosity was examined, Arabic-speaking immigrants were significantly more likely to rate their health as fair or poor compared to US-born Arabs, controlling for gender, age, education, and income (OR=3.52, 95 % CI 1.82–6.81). Researchers attributed this finding to less acculturation.

Mini (2009) examined relationships between SRH and sociodemographic factors, including religion, in a population-based random sample of 1,766 persons over age 60 living in Kerala, India (64 % Hindu, 19 % Christian, 18 % Muslim). SRH was measured using a single question with responses dichotomized into good (excellent, very good, good, or fair) and poor (poor). SRH, together with single questions asking about physical mobility and whether the person was suffering from an illness, were combined to create a 3-item indicator of overall health status. Uncontrolled analysis indicated that Christians were least likely to rate their physical health as poor (29.5 %) compared to Hindus (38.9 %) and Muslims (38.2 %) ($p<0.05$). Controlling for marital status, place of residence, education, employment status, and economic independence, analyses revealed that Hindus and Muslims were significantly more likely than Christians to indicate poor overall health (OR=2.13, 95 % CI 1.63–2.80, $p<0.001$, and OR=3.42, 95 % CI 2.36–4.95, $p<0.001$, respectively). Although researchers noted this difference, they did not discuss or try to explain it.

Recent Research. We identified three studies that examined SRH in Muslims since our 2010 review: one that measured religiosity and the other two comparing Muslims and non-Muslims.

Religiosity. Kodzi and colleagues (2011) reported findings on 2,606 persons aged 50 or older in Nairobi, Kenya, examining relationships between social factors and SRH. Religious affiliation and religious participation (attending religious services more than once/week vs. not) were determined. SRH was measured in the usual fashion with a single question that asked, "In general, how would you rate your health today?" (very good, good, moderate, bad, very bad). Of the sample, 84 % were Christian, 12 % were Muslim, and 4 % were not affiliated with a religious group. Overall, 17 % attended religious services more than once/week. In uncontrolled analyses, Muslims were 34 % less likely than other groups to report good SRH (OR=0.66, $p=0.001$). Likewise, those attending religious services more than once/week were also less likely than less frequent attendees to report good SRH (OR=0.72, $p=0.001$). In multivariate analyses controlling for gender, age, marital status, financial conditions, schooling, tribe, social engagement, and more objective measures of physical health status, religiosity (> weekly attendance) continued to predict worse SRH (OR = 0.79, $p < 0.05$), although Muslim affiliation did not.

Muslims vs. Non-Muslims. Khoo (2010) analyzed data from two cohorts of the Longitudinal Survey of Immigrants to Australia study, examining relationships between personal characteristics and health status. The first cohort (Cohort 1) consisted of 5,192 emigrants who arrived in 1993–1995, while the second cohort (Cohort 2) consisted of 3,124 emigrants who arrived in 1999–2000 (both cohorts were selected using a random sampling scheme). Cohort 1 and Cohort 2 consisted of 24 % and 31 % Muslims, respectively, most coming from the Middle East. SRH was measured by a single question with responses ranging from very good (1) to very poor (5). Although the relationship between SRH and religion or religiosity was not examined, researchers did examine the relationship with place from where participants migrated. If we consider immigration from the Middle East as a proxy for Muslim religion, then differences in SRH between Muslims and non-Muslims can be compared. Results indicated no significant difference in self-rated poor health status between those coming from the Middle East vs. elsewhere (5 % vs. 3–6 %, respectively, for Cohort 1; 8 % vs. 4–14 %, respectively, for Cohort 2).

Finally, Singh and associates (2013) surveyed a population-based national sample of 34,831 persons aged 60 or over living in India, examining relationships between social and demographic factors and SRH. SRH was measured in the usual fashion and was dichotomized into poor (poor) vs. good (excellent, very good, good, fair). Religious affiliation of participants was 84 % Hindu, 9 % Muslim, and 6 % other. Uncontrolled analysis revealed that Muslims were more likely than either Hindus or those with other religious affiliations to rate their health as poor (in males, 28.9 % vs. 20.8 % and 20.7 %, respectively, $p < 0.001$; in females, 36.0 % vs. 24.7 % and 26.2 %, respectively, $p < 0.001$). After controlling for age, marital status, education, employment, income, economic independence, social group, living situations, place of residence, and region of India, Muslim males continued to be at higher risk for rating their health as poor compared to other religious groups (OR = 1.38, 95 % CI 1.22–1.57, $p < 0.001$). An even stronger relationship was found in Muslim females (OR = 1.50, 95 % CI 1.33–1.69). Researchers noted that Muslims were more disadvantaged in terms of education and economic status (especially women) compared to other religious groups in India.

Summary. Two studies have now examined the relationship between religiosity and SRH in Muslims, although neither was in Muslim-majority populations (Table 11.3). In one study, religiosity (measured by frequency of religious attendance and importance of religious devotion) was positively related to better SRH among immigrant and host adolescents in Bosnia–Herzegovina. In the other study, religiosity (measured by religious attendance) was negatively related to SRH among older adults in Kenya (although only 12 % of the population was Muslim). Eight studies have compared SRH in Muslims and non-Muslims. Of those, four (50 %) reported worse SRH in Muslims, three found no differences between Muslims and non-Muslims, and one reported better SRH in Muslims compared to non-Muslims in Kyrgyzstan.

Although it is not clear why half of the studies found worse SRH in Muslims, this may have something to do with education and socioeconomic factors that influence access to healthcare and could affect perception of health as well.

Mortality

The best and most objective way to determine if religiosity affects physical health in Muslims is to examine its relationship to mortality. No studies, however, have yet examined relationships between religiosity and longevity in Muslim-majority countries. The absence of prospective cohort studies examining the impact of religious involvement on mortality in Muslims represents another serious gap in the research literature. Numerous studies, though, have compared mortality in Muslim vs. non-Muslim populations. Our 2010 systematic review uncovered five such studies, four of the five examining infant or child mortality and three of those in third-world poverty-stricken countries (India, Bangladesh, Ghana).

In the first study, Saksena and Srivastava (1980) examined perinatal mortality in a random sample of 5,506 births in Lucknow, India, comparing Muslims and Hindus (population of Lucknow is 21 % Muslim and 75 % Hindu). There were 282 stillbirths and 136 deaths during the 1st weeks after birth. Perinatal mortality in Muslims was significantly higher than in Hindus (no other details are available since only abstract was available to us).

Miah (1993) analyzed data from the Bangladesh Fertility Survey that compared death rates during infancy/childhood between Hindus and Muslims in women with low parity (0–3 births, $n=1,772$), medium parity (4–5 births, $n=934$), and high parity (six or more births, $n=1,984$). This was the first comprehensive survey in Bangladesh (90 % Muslim, 10 % Hindu) to examine factors related to infant/child death. Controlling for other predictors of mortality, religious affiliation was unrelated to infant/child death in low- and high-parity women. However, among medium-parity women, deaths were significantly less among Muslim women compared to Hindu women ($B=-0.23$, $p<0.05$), with Muslim affiliation being the second strongest predictor of survival in this group. Researchers explained this finding as due to social and economic factors and improved access to healthcare by Muslims; however, some of those factors were controlled for in the regression model.

In a second study from Bangladesh, Hurt and colleagues (2004) examined characteristics predicting adult mortality in 14,803 married women over age 45 and their husbands living in a rural area 35 miles southeast of Dhaka (capital of Bangladesh). Among men, uncontrolled analyses revealed that Hindus experienced significantly higher all-cause mortality than Muslims (RR = 1.22, 95 % CI 1.13–1.33). After adjusting for education, occupation, marital status, percentage of surviving children, and area of residence, Hindus continued to have a marginally higher death rate than Muslims (RR = 1.12, 95 % CI 1.00–1.25). The same pattern was seen in women, where Hindus had a 30 % higher mortality than Muslims (RR = 1.30, 95 % CI 1.12–1.51) in uncontrolled analyses, although this effect diminished to nonsignificance after adjustment for other predictors (RR = 1.10, 95 % CI 0.89–1.36). In addition, men and women who received Qur'anic education, compared to those with no education, had lower death rates (RR = 0.85, 95 % CI 0.77–0.93, and RR = 0.76, 95 % CI 0.66–0.86, respectively). Although the effect in men was reduced to nonsignificance after other factors were controlled for, the relationship in women with Qur'anic education remained marginally significant (RR = 0.82, 95 % CI 0.66–1.00). Researchers explained the higher death rates among Hindus as due to their minority group status in Bangladesh leading to social exclusion.

Amitai and colleagues (2005) examined risk factors (including religion) that predicted infant mortality rates (IMR) in Israel between 1950 and 2000. There were 746 deaths in the year 2000, with an IMR of 5.4 per 1,000 live births. Death rates were significantly higher in Muslims (IMR = 9.2) and Druze (6.3) compared to Jews (3.9) and Christians (3.6). In fact, IMR in Muslims and Druze were higher than in Jews and Christians during every decade from 1950 to 2000. In later years (1990–2000), the primary cause of infant mortality in Muslims was due to congenital anomalies. Researchers explained that the high infant death rate from congenital factors in Muslims was caused by the high rate of consanguinity (33–45 %) and the low rate of abortions for fetal anomalies due to religious reasons.

Finally, Gyimah (2007) analyzed data from the 1998 and 2003 Ghana Demographic and Health Surveys to examine religious differences predicting survival in 7,142 children ages 0–5 years. Religious affiliations examined were Christian (65 %), Muslim (18 %), and Traditional Indigenous African (18 %). Overall survival was significantly higher in Christians compared to Muslims and Traditionalists (log rank test=14.9, $p < 0.001$). However, there were major socioeconomic differences between the three religions. Christians were more likely to have a household toilet, to drink treated water, and to have higher maternal education. There were also differences on maternal age at birth, birth order of children, and interval between births. After controlling for these factors using stepwise multiple regression, differences between religious groups disappeared. The researcher concluded that differences in child mortality between religious groups were "due to differential access to social and human capital rather than religious theology per se."

Missed Studies. Several studies were missed by our 2010 systematic review. All compared mortality in Muslims vs. non-Muslims and most examined infant and child mortality. No studies examined the effects of religiosity on mortality. Caldwell (1986) reported mortality rates by country around the world in 1982, examining infant mortality per 1,000 live births and life expectancy at birth. Adjustments were made for per capita GNP (gross national product). The eleven countries with the worst mortality, adjusted for GNP, in order from worse to better were Oman, Saudi Arabia, Iran, Libya, Algeria, Iraq, Yemen, Morocco, Ivory Coast, Senegal, and Sierra Leone. Every country listed was a Muslim-majority country, except Ivory Coast (37 % Muslim).

Similarly, in a prospective study of 4,934 babies of different ethnic groups in the UK, Bundey and colleagues (1991) found that perinatal mortality was highest in

Pakistanis (96 % Muslim). The primary cause of early death, however, was lethal congenital malformations, which accounted for about 50 % of all perinatal mortality in Pakistanis. Malformations were mostly due to autosomal recessive genes that occur only in consanguineous parents.

Defo (1996) examined socioeconomic, ethnic, and cultural factors related to infant and child mortality in Cameroon, where religious affiliations are 21 % Muslim, 70 % Christians, and 6 % Traditionalists. Traditionalists in Cameroon believe in a god (the "god of the ancestors") and worship the dead and the ancestors. Results indicated that infant and child mortality from birth to age 5 years was lowest in Protestant Christians ($B = -0.33$, $p < 0.01$) and Catholic Christians ($B = -0.22$, $p < 0.05$) compared to Traditionalists. Although a comparison between Christians and Muslims was not made, since the mortality rate in Muslims and Traditionalists was similar, Muslims likely also had higher infant/child mortality compared to Christians. Researchers explained that socioeconomic and educational factors influencing access to healthcare likely accounted for these differences.

Jones (2006), however, found that mortality rates relative to income in Muslim-majority countries declined significantly between 1982 and 2002 (since Caldwell's study of mortality in 1982), due in large part to increases in social development and advances in education.

Antai and associates (2009) examined religious differences in infant and child mortality in Nigeria based on the 2003 Nigeria Demographic and Health Survey, which interviewed a sample of 7,620 women ages 15–49 who delivered 6,029 babies during the 5-year period prior to the survey. Religious affiliations of mothers were Muslim (60 %), Christian (39 %), and Traditional (2 %). Compared to Christians, infant and child mortality was 37 % higher in Muslims (OR = 1.37, 95 % CI 1.18–1.58) and 139 % higher in Traditionalists (OR = 1.64–3.48) in uncontrolled analyses. However, after controlling for socioeconomic variables, the differences disappeared between Christians and Muslims and even reversed to some extent (OR = 0.77, 95 % CI 0.52–1.13, for Muslims compared to Christians). Researchers concluded that the differences were primarily due to use of maternal and child health services, especially prenatal care.

Recent Research. Since our 2010 review, several additional studies have now been published. One study from Switzerland compared the mortality of those indicating a religious affiliation with those who did not. This is the only study to examining the effects of religiosity on mortality in Muslims to date, and it is not a particularly strong one. All other studies compared mortality in Muslims and non-Muslims (again most examining infant and child mortality).

Religion vs. No Religion. Lerch and associates (2010) examined religious affiliation and mortality in Switzerland between 1991 and 2004 in a sample of nearly 44 million. In the year 2000, religious affiliations in Switzerland were 33.0 % Reformed Protestant, 41.8 % Catholic, 4.4 % Other Christian, 4.3 % Muslim (Other Religion), and 11.1 % no religion. Controlling for age, gender, marital status, education and occupational status, and nationality, analyses revealed that the risk of dying during a 10-year follow-up was lowest among the Other Religion group.

This was true for all three age groups examined—ages 25–44 (OR = 0.63, $p < 0.0001$), ages 45–64 (OR = 0.66, $p < 0.0001$), and ages 65 or over (OR = 0.65, $p < 0.0001$)—where Catholic was the reference group. Muslims (who made up 86 % of the Other Religion group) experienced about a one-third lower risk of dying during follow-up compared to Catholics. Protestants had an even higher risk of dying than Catholics (6–9 % higher risk), whereas Other Christians had a lower risk (13–22 %) than Catholics, but not nearly as low as the Other Religion group. In young and middle-aged adults, those with no religion had a higher risk of dying (21 % and 8 %, respectively, compared to Catholics), whereas older nonreligious adults had a slightly lower risk of dying (2 % lower than Catholics). Although not directly compared, those with no religious affiliation almost certainly had a higher mortality than Muslims in all age groups. Researchers speculated that the lower risk among Muslims might be because of their greater religiosity compared to the more secularized Catholics and Protestants in Switzerland.

Muslims vs. Non-Muslims. Bhalotra and associates (2010) discuss an emerging phenomenon in India that relates to differences in child survival by religious affiliation. Despite the lower SES of Muslims compared to upper-caste Hindus, and Muslim status as an ethnic minority (13–15 % of the Indian population), child survival among Muslims has become substantially higher than among Hindus. These researchers examine mortality rates based on the National Family Health Survey of India conducted between 1992 and 2006, which included 653,496 live births to 197,952 women. After controlling for birth order and urban–rural residence, analyses confirmed lower neonatal, infant, and child (ages 1–5) mortality among Muslims for male and female infants. Researchers concluded that "Muslims have an unobservable trait that is health-improving" (p. 198), noting that the strong social networks, better personal hygiene (due to washing prior to prayer), and the higher stature of women in Islam (yes, *higher stature*) might help to explain some of the survival advantage.

Kohler and Preston (2011) examined ethnic and religious factors affecting mortality in Bulgaria. This was a longitudinal study of the entire population of Bulgaria between the 1992 census and 1998 census. Mortality rates across five ethnic-religious groups were examined: Bulgarian Christians (majority), Christian Roma (gypsies), Muslim Turks, Muslim Bulgarians, and Muslim Roma. Among men ages 30–60 years, after controlling for calendar year, education, place of residence, marital status, and SES (standard of accommodation), Muslim Turks and Muslim Bulgarians were at significantly lower risk of dying during follow-up (16 % and 7 % lower risk, respectively) compared to Bulgarian Christians (BC) (reference group). Among men ages 60–90 years, Muslim Bulgarians also experienced a lower risk of dying (6 %) compared to BC, although Muslim Roma were at 33 % greater risk of dying compared to BC. Among women ages 30–60, there was no difference in risk of dying between Muslim Turks or Muslim Bulgarians and BC, although Muslim Roma were again 41 % more likely to die than BC. For women ages 60–90, Muslim Roma and Muslim Turks were at significantly greater mortality risk compared to BC (49 % and 3 %, respectively), whereas Bulgarian Muslims tended to have lower mortality than BC (5 %, $0.05 < p < 0.10$). For all gender and age groups,

Christian Roma had higher risk of dying than BC (from 12 to 62 %) (due to high smoking, low SES). Researchers explained that the lower risk of mortality in Muslims was due to lifestyle factors (less alcohol) and social relations (stronger support, lower suicide). The higher risk of dying in older Muslim women was mentioned but not discussed.

Singh and Tripathi (2013) examined maternal factors related to mortality in infants and children under age 5 years in India, analyzing data from the 2007 India National Family Health Survey that included information on 51,555 live births. Mortality rates were stratified by birth order and adjusted for gender, wealth, education, occupation, prenatal care, size of child at birth, place of delivery, immunization, and other factors. Compared to Hindus, Muslim infants and children were significantly less likely to die if they were the fourth or fifth child (OR=0.53, 95 % CI 0.35–0.88); there was no difference for first, second, or third child. Compared to Hindus, Christians were less likely to die if they were the 1st, 2nd, or 3rd child. Researchers did not explain these findings. Using data from the 1992–1993, 1998–1999, and 2005–2006 India National Family Health Survey, Kumar and colleagues (2013) also found that Muslims had a lower probability of neonatal death than Hindus.

Summary. As of 2013, based on our past and recent reviews, we found only one report examining religiosity and longevity in Muslims, and that study only compared Muslims to those without a religious affiliation in Switzerland (where Muslims make up less than 5 % of the population). Considerable research, however, has compared Muslims and non-Muslims, many focusing on infant/child mortality. Of fourteen such studies, six found significantly lower mortality in Muslims (four of the six in infants/children), five reported significantly higher mortality in Muslims (all in infants/children), two found no association (both in infants/children), and one reported mixed results (in adults). Most studies conducted prior to 1985 found that Muslims had worse infant/child mortality, which researchers explained as due to lower SES, lower education, and higher rates of congenital malformations as a result of consanguinity. More recent studies from India have reported significantly better infant/child survival in Muslims than in Hindus, so much so that researchers have suggested "an unobservable trait" in Muslims that improves infant/child health. Of the three studies examining adult mortality, two found significantly better survival in Muslims (Bangladesh and Switzerland) and one reported mixed findings (better survival in younger Muslim men, worse survival in older Muslim women) (Bulgaria). As noted above, among the more than 120 studies worldwide that have now examined the effects of religiosity on mortality, not one has been done in a Muslim-majority population.

Summary and Conclusions

Because of the links found between religiosity and better mental, social, and behavioral health in Muslims, there is every reason to expect that these benefits would spill over into better physical health as well. However, because of a lack of research on the relationship between religiosity and most areas of physical health in Muslims (as reviewed above), conclusions are difficult to make. There is tremendous opportunity, however, to conduct research that could fill the many gaps in our knowledge about the relationship between religiosity and heart disease, hypertension, stroke, dementia, cancer, immune function, endocrine function, SRH, and mortality. In fact, as noted in earlier chapters, much research is also needed on religiosity and mental, social, and behavioral health, especially in Muslim-majority populations. What is needed are motivated individuals at academic institutions who have the research training, credentials, and funding support to do that research. There are now resources available to help guide investigators on how to proceed (Koenig 2011).

References

Abdulrahim, S., & Ajrouch, K. (2010). Social and cultural meanings of self-rated health: Arab immigrants in the United States. *Qualitative Health Research, 20*(9), 1229–1240.

Abdulrahim, S., & Baker, W. (2009). Differences in self-rated health by immigrant status and language preference among Arab Americans in the Detroit metropolitan area. *Social Science & Medicine, 68*, 2097–2103.

Abimiku, A., Villalba-Diebold, P., Dadik, J., Okolo, F., Mang, E., & Charurat, M. (2009). Risk factors associated with low CD4+ lymphocyte count among HIV-positive pregnant women in Nigeria. *International Journal of Gynaecology and Obstetrics, 106*(3), 227–231.

Abou-Rbiah, Y., & Weitzman, S. (2002). Diabetes among Bedouins in the Negev: The transition from rare to a highly prevalent condition. *Israel Medical Association Journal, 4*, 687–689.

Adlouni, A., Ghalim, N., Benslimane, A., Lecerf, J. M., & Saile, R. (1997). Fasting during Ramadan induces a marked increase in high-density lipoprotein cholesterol and decrease in low-density lipoprotein cholesterol. *Annals of Nutrition and Metabolism, 41*, 242–249.

Afgin, A. E., Massarwa, M., Schechtman, E., Israeli-Korn, S. D., Strugatsky, R., Abuful, A., Farrer, L. A., Friedland, R. P., & Inzelberg, R. (2012). High prevalence of mild cognitive impairment and Alzheimer's disease in Arabic villages in Northern Israel: Impact of gender and education. *Journal of Alzheimer's Disease, 29*, 431–439.

Afrasiabi, A., Hassanzadeh, S., Sattarivand, R., Nouri, M., & Mahboob, S. (2003). Effects of low fat and low calorie diet on plasma lipid levels in the fasting month of Ramadan. *Saudi Medical Journal, 24*, 184–188.

Akhan, G., Kutluhan, S., & Koyuncuoglu, H. (2000). Is there any change of stroke incidence during Ramadan? *Acta Neurologica Scandinavica, 101*(4), 259–261.

Aksungar, F. B., Eren, A., Ure, S., Teskin, O., & Ates, G. (2005). Effects of intermittent fasting on serum lipid levels, coagulant status, and plasma homocysteine levels. *Annals of Nutrition and Metabolism, 49*(2), 77–82.

Aksungar, F. B., Topkaya, A. E., & Akyildiz, M. (2007). Interleukin-6, C-reactive protein and biochemical parameters during prolonged intermittent fasting. *Annals of Nutrition & Metabolism, 51*(1), 88–95.

Al Suwaidi, J., Bener, A., Gehani, A. A., Behair, S., Al Mohanadi, D., Salam, A., & Al Binali, H. A. (2006). Does the circadian pattern for acute cardiac events presentation vary with fasting? *Journal of Postgraduate Medicine, 52*(1), 30–33.

Al Suwaidi, J., Bener, A., Hajar, H. A., & Numan, M. T. (2004). Does hospitalization for congestive heart failure occur more frequently in Ramadan: A population-based study (1991–2001). *International Journal of Cardiology, 96*, 217–221.

Al Suwaidi, J., Zubaid, M., Al-Mahmeed, W. A., Al-Rashdan, I., Amin, H., Bener, A., Hadi, H. R., Helmy, A., Hanifah, M., & Al-Binali, H. A. (2005). Impact of fasting in Ramadan in patients with cardiac disease. *Saudi Medical Journal, 26*(10), 1579–1583.

Albache, N., Radwan, A. A., Samer, R., Fouad, F. M., Mzayek, F., & Maziak, W. (2010). Epidemiology of type 2 diabetes mellitus in Aleppo, Syria. *Journal of Diabetes, 2*, 85–91.

Al-Hadramy, M. S., Zawai, T. H., & Abdelwahab, S. M. (1988). Altered cortisol levels in relation to Ramadan. *European Journal of Clinical Nutrition, 42*, 359–362.

Al-Kandari, Y. Y. (2003). Religiosity and its relation to blood pressure among selected Kuwaitis. *Journal of Biosocial Science, 35*(3), 463–472.

Al-Kandari, Y. Y. (2011). Religiosity, social support, and health among the elderly in Kuwait. *Journal of Muslim Mental Health, 6*(1), 81–98.

Almond, D., & Mazumder, B. (2011). Health capital and the prenatal environment: The effect of Ramadan observance during pregnancy. *American Economic Journal: Applied Economics, 3*(4), 56–85.

Altaf, F. J. (2001). Pattern of cervical smear cytology in the western region of Saudi Arabia. *Annals of Saudi Medicine, 21*(1–2), 94–96.

Amitai, Y., Haklai, Z., Tarabeia, J., Green, M. S., Rotem, N., Fleisher, E., et al. (2005). Infant mortality in Israel during 1950–2000: Rates, causes, demographic characteristics and trends. *Paediatric and Perinatal Epidemiology, 19*(2), 145–151.

Anand, S. S., Yusuf, S., Vuksan, V., Sudarshan, D., Teo, K. K., Montague, P. A., Kelemen, L., Yi, C., Lonn, E., Gerstein, H., Hegele, R. A., & McQueen, M. (2000). Differences in risk factors, atherosclerosis, and cardiovascular disease between ethnic groups in Canada: The Study of Health Assessment and Risk in Ethnic groups (SHARE). *The Lancet, 356*, 279–284.

Antai, D., Ghilagaber, G., Wedren, S., Macassa, G., & Moradi, T. (2009). Inequities in under-five mortality in Nigeria: Differentials by religious affiliation of the mother. *Journal of Religion and Health, 48*(3), 290–304.

Barkia, A., Mohamed, K., Smaoui, M., Zouari, N., Hammami, M., & Nasri, M. (2011). Change of diet, plasma lipids, lipoproteins, and fatty acids during Ramadan: A controversial association of the considered Ramadan model with atherosclerosis risk. *Journal of Health, Population, and Nutrition, 29*(5), 486–493.

Baron-Epel, O., Weinstein, R., Haviv-Mesika, A., Garty-Sandalon, N., & Green, M. S. (2008). Individual-level analysis of social capital and health: A comparison of Arab and Jewish Israelis. *Social Science & Medicine, 66*(4), 900–910.

Basu, R., Mandal, S., Ghosh, A., & Poddar, T. K. (2008). Role of tobacco in the development of head and neck squamous cell carcinoma in an Eastern Indian population. *Asian Pacific Journal of Cancer Prevention, 9*, 381–386.

Ben Natan, M., Aharon, O., Palickshvili, S., & Gurman, V. (2011). Attitude of Israeli mothers with vaccination of their daughters against papilloma virus. *Journal of Pediatric Nursing, 25*, 70–71.

Bener, A., Hamad, A., Fares, A., Al-Sayed, H. M., & Al-Suwaidi, J. (2006). Is there any effect of Ramadan fasting on stroke incidence? *Singapore Medical Journal, 47*(5), 404–408.

Bernieh, B. O., Mohamed, A. O., & Wafa, A. M. (1994). Ramadan fasting and renal transplant recipients: Clinical and biochemical effects. *Saudi Journal of Kidney Diseases and Transplantation, 5*(4), 470–473.

Bhalotra, S., Valente, C., & Soest, A. V. (2010). The puzzle of Muslim advantage in child survival in India. *Journal of Health Economics, 29*, 191–204.

Bhurgri, Y., Bhurgri, A., Hussainy, A. S., Usman, A., Faridi, N., Malik, J., Zaidi, Z. A., Muzaffar, S., Kayani, N., Pervez, S., & Hasan, S. H. (2003). Cancer of the oral cavity and pharynx in Karachi—Identification of potential risk factors. *Asian Pacific Journal of Cancer Prevention, 4*, 125–130.

Bhurgri, Y., Bhurgri, A., Usman, A., Sheikh, N., Faridi, N., Malik, J., et al. (2006). Patho-epidemiology of lung cancer in Karachi (1995–2002). *Asian Pacific Journal of Cancer Prevention, 7*(1), 60–64.

Bowirrat, A., Treves, T. A., Friedland, R. P., & Korczyn, A. D. (2001). Prevalence of Alzheimer's type dementia in an elderly Arab population. *European Journal of Neurology, 8*, 119–123.

Bundey, S., Alam, H., Kaur, A., Mir, S., & Lancashire, R. (1991). Why do UK-born Pakistani babies have high perinatal and neonatal mortality rates? *Paediatric and Perinatal Epidemiology, 5*, 101–114.

Burazeri, G., Goda, A., & Kark, J. D. (2008a). Religious observance and acute coronary syndrome in predominantly Muslim Albania: A population-based case-control study in Tirana. *Annals of Epidemiology, 18*(12), 937–945.

Burazeri, G., Goda, A., Roshi, E., & Kark, J. D. (2008b). Religious affiliation and acute coronary syndrome: A population-based case–control study in Tirana, Albania. *European Journal of Public Health, 18*(3), 329–334.

Caldwell, J. C. (1986). Routes to low mortality in poor countries. *Population and Development Review, 12*(2), 171–220.

Chadee, D., Seemungal, T., Pereira, L. M. P., Chadee, M., Maharaj, R., & Teelucksingh, S. (2013). Prevalence of self-reported diabetes, hypertension and heart disease in individuals seeking State funding in Trinidad and Tobago, West Indies. *Journal of Epidemiology and Global Health, 3*, 95–103.

Chamsi-Pasha, H., & Ahmed, W. H. (2004). The effect of fasting in Ramadan on patients with heart disease. *Saudi Medical Journal, 25*(1), 47–51.

Cockerham, W. C., Hinote, B. P., Abbott, P., & Haerpfer, C. (2004). Health lifestyles in central Asia: The case of Kazakhstan and Kyrgyzstan. *Social Science & Medicine, 59*, 1409–1421.

Cohen, M., Werner, P., & Azaiza, F. (2009). Emotional reactions of Arab lay persons to a person with Alzheimer's disease. *Aging and Mental Health, 13*(1), 33–37.

Cook, D. G., Cappuccio, F. P., Atkinson, R. W., Wicks, P. D., Chitolle, A., Nakandakare, E. R., Sagnella, G. A., & Humphries, S. E. (2001). Ethnic differences in fibrinogen levels: The role of environmental factors and the B-fibrinogen gene. *American Journal of Epidemiology, 153*, 799–806.

Danesh, J., Collins, R., Appleby, P., & Peto, R. (1998). Association of fibrinogen, C-reactive protein, albumin, or leukocyte count with coronary heart disease: meta-analyses of prospective studies. *Journal of the American Medical Association, 279*(18), 1477–1482.

Danesh, J., Wheeler, J. G., Hirschfield, G. M., Eda, S., Eiriksdottir, G., Rumley, A., et al. (2004). C-reactive protein and other circulating markers of inflammation in the prediction of coronary heart disease. *New England Journal of Medicine, 350*(14), 1387–1397.

Danesh, J., Whincup, P., Walker, M., Lennon, L., Thomson, A., Appleby, P., Rumely, A., & Lowe, G. D. (2001). Fibrin d-dimer and coronary heart disease: A prospective study. *Circulation, 103*(19), 2323–2327.

Defo, B. K. (1996). Areal and socioeconomic differentials in infant and child mortality in Cameroon. *Social Science & Medicine, 42*(3), 399–420.

Dikshit, R., Gupta, P. C., Ramasundarahettige, C., Gajalakshmi, V., Aleksandrowicz, L., Badwe, R., Kumar, R., Roy, S., Suraweera, W., Bray, F., Mallath, M., Singh, P. K., Sinha, D. N., Shet, A. S., Gelband, H., & Jha, P; Million Death Study Collaborators (2012). Cancer mortality in India: a nationally representative survey. *Lancet, 379*(9828), 1807–1816.

Dikensoy, E., Balat, O., Cebesoy, B., Ozkur, A., Cicek, H., & Can, G. (2009). The effect of Ramadan fasting on maternal serum lipids, cortisol levels and fetal development. *Archives of Gynecology and Obstetrics, 279*, 119–123.

Duttagupta, C., Sengupta, S., Roy, M., Sengupta, D., Bhattacharya, P., Laikangbam, P., Roy, S., Ghosh, S., & Das, R. (2004). Are Muslim women less susceptible to oncogenic human papillomavirus infection? A study from rural eastern India. *International Journal of Gynecological Cancer, 14*(2), 293–303.

Funai, E. F., Paltiel, O. B., Malaspina, D., Friedlander, Y., Leutsch, L., & Harlap, S. (2005). Risk factors for pre-eclampsia in nulliparous and parous women: The Jerusalem Perinatal Study. *Paediatric and Perinatal Epidemiology, 19*, 59–68.

Gaborit, B., Dutour, O., Ronsin, O., Atlan, C., Darmon, P., Gharsalli, R., Pradel, V., Dadoun, F., & Dutour, A. (2011). Ramadan fasting with diabetes: an interview study of inpatients' and general practitioners' attitudes in the South of France. *Diabetes & Metabolism, 37*, 395–402.

Gopinath, N., Chadha, S. L., Jain, P., Shekhawat, S., & Tandon, R. (1995). An epidemiological study of coronary heart disease in different ethnic groups in Delhi urban population. *Journal of the Association of Physicians of India, 43*(1), 30–33.

Gupta, R., Gupta, V. P., Prakash, H., Sarna, M., & Sharma, A. K. (2002). Hindu-Muslim differences in the prevalence of coronary heart disease and risk factors. *Journal of the Indian Medical Association, 100*(4), 227–230.

Gyimah, S. O. (2007). What has faith got to do with it? Religion and child survival in Ghana. *Journal of Biosocial Science, 39*(6), 923–937.

Haouari, M., Haouari, F., Mbazaa, A., & Nagati, K. (1998). Physiological evaluation of serum glucose, insulin, total protein and cortisol levels in healthy fasting volunteers. *Practical Diabetes International Supplement, 15*(1), 83–84.

Haroon, A. S., Gupta, S. M., Tyagi, B. B., & Farhat, J. (2012). Epidemiology of breast cancer in female in Meerut, India: Patients characteristics and survival analysis. *Indian Journal of Public Health, 3*(2), 49–52.

Hatahet, W., Khosla, P., & Fungwe, T. V. (2002). Prevalence of risk factors to coronary heart disease in an Arab-American population in southeast Michigan. *International Journal of Food Sciences and Nutrition, 53*(4), 325–335.

Hendrie, H. C., Ogunniyi, A., Hall, K. S., & Baiyewu, O. (2001). Incidence of dementia and Alzheimer disease in 2 communities: Yoruba residing in Ibadan, Nigeria, and African Americans residing in Indianapolis, Indiana. *Journal of the American Medical Association, 285*, 739–747.

Hurt, L. S., Ronsmans, C., & Saha, S. (2004). Effects of education and other socioeconomic factors on middle age mortality in rural Bangladesh. *Journal of Epidemiology & Community Health, 58*(4), 315–320.

Inzelberg, R., Afgin, A. E., Massarwa, M., Schechtman, E., Israeli-Korn, S. D., Strugatsky, R., Abuful, A., Kravitz, E., Lindsay, A. F., & Friedland, R. P. (2013). Prayer at midlife is associated with reduced risk of cognitive decline in Arabic women. *Current Alzheimer Research, 10*(3), 340–346.

Islam, M. R., Khan, I., Attia, J., Hasan, S. M. N., McEvoy, M., D'Este, C., Azim, S., Akhter, A., Akter, S., Shahidullah, S. M., & Milton, A. H. (2012). Association between hypertension and chronic arsenic exposure in drinking water: A cross-sectional study in Bangladesh. *International Journal of Environmental Research and Public Health, 9*, 4522–4536.

Israeli-Korn, S. D., Masarwa, M., Schechtman, E., Abuful, A., Strugatsky, R., Avni, S., Farrer, L. A., Friedland, R. P., & Inzelberg, R. (2010). Hypertension increases the probability of Alzheimer's disease and of mild cognitive impairment in an Arab community in northern Israel. *Neuroepidemiology, 34*(2), 99–105.

Jabara, R., Namouz, S., Kark, J. D., & Lotan, C. (2007). Risk characteristics of Arab and Jewish women with coronary heart disease in Jerusalem. *Israel Medical Association Journal, 9*, 316–320.

Jaber, L. A., Slaughter, R. L., & Grunberger, G. (1995). Diabetes and related metabolic risk factors among Arab Americans. *Annals of Pharmacotherapy, 29*(6), 573–576.

Jones, G. W. (2006). A demographic perspective on the Muslim world. *Journal of Population Research, 23*(2), 243–265.

Jussawalla, D. J., Yeole, B. B., & Natekar, M. V. (1981). Histological and epidemiological features of breast cancer in different religious groups in Greater Bombay. *Journal of Surgical Oncology, 18*, 269–279.

Kalter-Leibovici, O., Chetrit, A., Lubin, F., Atamna, A., Alpert, G., Ziv, A., Abu-Saad, K., Mura, H., Eilat-Adar, S., & Goldbourt, U. (2011). Adult-onset diabetes among Arabs and Jews in Israel: A population-based study. *Diabetic Medicine, 29*(6), 748–754.

Kark, J. D., Fink, R., Adler, B., Goldberger, N., & Goldman, S. (2006). The incidence of coronary heart disease among Palestinians and Israelis in Jerusalem. *International Journal of Epidemiology, 35*(2), 448–457.

Kaur, M., & Balgir, P. P. (2005). APOE2 and consanguinity: A risky combination for Alzheimer's disease. *Journal of Alzheimer's Disease, 8*, 293–297.

Khaled, B. M., Bendahmane, M., & Belbraouet, S. (2006). Ramadan fasting induces modifications of certain serum components in obese women with type 2 diabetes. *Saudi Medical Journal, 27*(1), 23–26.

Khawaja, M., Abdulrahim, S., Afifi Soweid, R., & Karam, D. (2006). Distrust, social fragmentation and adolescents' health in the outer city: Beirut and beyond. *Social Science & Medicine, 63*, 1304–1315.

Khoo, S. E. (2010). Health and humanitarian migrants' economic participation. *Journal of Immigrant and Minority Health, 12*, 327–339.

Kodzi, I. A., Gyimah, S. O., Emina, J., & Ezeh, A. C. (2011). Religious involvement, social engagement, and subjective health status of older residents of informal neighborhoods of Nairobi. *Journal of Urban Health, 88*(Suppl 2), 5370–5380.

Koenig, H. G. (2011). *Spirituality and health research: Methods, measurement, statistics, and resources*. Conshohocken, PA: Templeton Foundation Press.

Kohler, I. V., & Preston, S. H. (2011). Ethnic and religious differentials in Bulgarian mortality, 1993–1998. *Population Studies, 65*(1), 91–113.

Kohler, I. V., Soldo, B. J., Anglewicz, P., Chilima, B., & Kohler, H. P. (2013). Association of blood lipids, creatinine, albumin, and CRP with socioeconomic status in Malawi. *Population Health Metrics, 11*(1), 4.

Kumar, C., Singh, P. K., Rai, R. K., & Singh, L. (2013). Early neonatal mortality in India, 1990–2006. *Journal of Community Health, 38*, 120–130.

Lahdimawan, A., Handono, K., Indra, M. R., & Prawiro, S. R. (2013). Effect of Ramadan fasting on endorphin and endocannabinoid level in serum, PBMC and macrophage. *International Journal of Pharmaceutical Science Invention, 2*(3), 46–54.

Latifynia, A., Vojgani, M., Gharagozlou, M. J., & Sharifian, R. (2008). Effect of Ramadan on neutrophil's respiratory burst (innate immunity) and circulating immune complex. *Journal of Ayub Medical College, Abbottabad, 20*(3), 128–131.

Latifynia, A., Vojgani, M., Jafarieh, H., & Abofazeli, T. (2007). Neutrophil respiratory burst (innate immunity) during Ramadan. *Journal of Biological Sciences, 7*(6), 997–1000.

Lerch, M., Oris, M., Wanner, P., Forney, Y., & Dutreuilh, C. (2010). Religious affiliation and mortality in Switzerland, 1991–2004. *Population, 65*(2), 217–250.

Ling, W. Y., Razali, S. M., Ren, C. K., & Omar, S. Z. (2012). Does the success of a school-based HPV vaccine programme depend on teachers' knowledge and religion? A survey in a multicultural society. *Asian Pacific Journal of Cancer Prevention, 13*, 4651–4654.

Lozano, R., Naghavi, M., Foreman, K., Lim, S., & Shibuya, K. (2012). Global and regional mortality from 235 causes of death for 20 age groups in 1990 and 2010: A systematic analysis for the Global Burden of Disease Study 2010. *Lancet, 380*, 2095–2128.

M'Guil, M., Ragala, M. A., El Guessabi, L., Fellat, S., Chraibi, A., Chebraoui, L., et al. (2008). Is Ramadan fasting safe in type 2 diabetic patients in view of the lack of significant effect of fasting on clinical and biochemical parameters, blood pressure, and glycemic control? *Clinical and Experimental Hypertension, 30*(5), 339–357.

Majumder, P. P., Staats, H. F., Sarkar-roy, N., Varma, B., Ghosh, T., Maiti, S., Narayanasamy, K., Whisnant, C. C., Stephenson, J. L., & Wagener, D. K. (2009). Genetic determinants of immune-response to a polysaccharide vaccine for typhoid. *The HUGO Journal, 3*(1–4), 17–30.

Malhotra, A., Scott, P. H., Scott, J., Gee, H., & Wharton, B. A. (1989). Metabolic changes in Asian Muslim pregnant mothers observing the Ramadan fast in Britain. *British Journal of Nutrition, 61*, 663–672.

Maziak, W., Rastam, S., Mzayek, F., Ward, K. D., Eissenberg, T., & Keil, U. (2007). Cardiovascular health among adults in Syria: A model from developing countries. *Annals of Epidemiology, 17*, 713–720.

McKeigue, P. M., Shah, B., & Marmot, M. G. (1991). Relation of central obesity and insulin resistance with high diabetes prevalence and cardiovascular risk in South Asians. *The Lancet, 337*, 382–386.

Meshram, I. I., Hiwarkar, P. A., & Kulkarni, P. N. (2009). Reproductive risk factors for breast cancer: A case–control study. *Online Journal of Health and Allied Sciences, 8*(3), 5.

Miah, M. M. R. (1993). Factors influencing infant/child mortality in Bangladesh: Implication for family planning programs and policies. *International Journal of Sociology of the Family, 23*(Autumn), 21–34.

Mini, G. K. (2009). Socioeconomic and demographic diversity in the health status of elderly people in a transitional society, Kerala, India. *Journal of Biosocial Science, 41*, 457–467.

Momennasab, M., Moattari, M., Abbaszade, A., & Shamshiri, B. (2012). Spirituality in survivors of myocardial infarction. *Iranian Journal of Nursing and Midwifery Research, 17*(4), 343–351.

Muir, C. S. (1960). Coronary heart disease in seven racial groups in Singapore. *British Heart Journal, 22*(1), 45–53.

Murray, C. J. L., Vos, T., Lozano, R., Naghavi, M., & Flaxman, A. D. (2012). Disability-adjusted life years (DALYS) for 291 diseases and injuries in 21 regions, 1990–2010: A systematic analysis for the Global Burden of Disease Study 2010. *Lancet, 380*, 2197–2223.

Musaiger, A. O. (2002). Diet and prevention of coronary heart disease in the Arab Middle East countries. *Medical Principles and Practice, 11*(Suppl 2), 9–16.

Na'amnih, W., Muhsen, K., Tarabeia, J., Saabneh, A., & Green, M. S. (2010). Trends in the gap in life expectancy between Arabs and Jews in Israel between 1975 and 2004. *International Journal of Epidemiology, 39*, 1324–1332.

Nielsen, J. V. (1999). Diabetes in the Arab world: Prevalence and risk factors. *Practical Diabetes International, 16*(3), 82–86.

Omu, O., Al-Obaidi, S., & Reynolds, F. (2014). Religious faith and psychosocial adaptation among stroke patients in Kuwait: A mixed method study. *Journal of Religion and Health, 53*(2), 538–551.

Papadopoulos, V., Tsakiridis, K., Filippou, D. K., Aggelopoulos, P., Nikiforidis, D., & Baltatzidis, G. (2006). Comparison of stroke among Christians and Muslims in Thrace, Greece. *Rural and Remote Health, 6*(2), 505.

Perk, G., Ghanem, J., Aamar, S., Ben-Ishay, D., & Bursztyn, M. (2001). The effect of the fast of Ramadan on ambulatory blood pressure in treated hypertensives. *Journal of Human Hypertension, 15*(10), 723–725.

Rahman, M., Rashid, M., Basher, S., Sultana, S., & Nomani, M. Z. (2004). Improved serum HDL cholesterol profile among Bangladeshi male students during Ramadan fasting. *Eastern Mediterranean Health Journal, 10*(1–2), 131–137.

Rao, D. N., Ganesh, B., & Desai, P. B. (1994). Role of reproductive factors in breast cancer in a low-risk area: A case–control study. *British Journal of Cancer, 70*, 129–132.

Razzaque, A., Da Vanzo, J., Rahman, M., Gausia, K., Hale, L., Khan, M. A., & Mustafa, A. H. M. G. (2005). Pregnancy spacing and maternal morbidity in Matlab, Bangladesh. *International Journal of Gynecology & Obstetrics, 89*, 541–549.

Roshi, E., Kamberi, A., Goda, A., & Burazeri, G. (2005). Myocardial infarction and religion: Hospital-based case–control study in Tirana, Albania. *Croatian Medical Journal, 46*(6), 977–983.

Rushid, A. K., Azizah, A. M., & Rohana, S. (2012). Cognitive impairment among the elderly Malays living in rural Malaysia. *Medical Journal of Malaysia, 67*(2), 186–189.

Saha, A. K., & Pathak, H. S. (2012). Epidemiological profile of oesophageal cancer in the Gangetic areas of West Bengal. *Journal, Indian Academy of Clinical Medicine, 13*(2), 107–115.

Saksena, D. N., & Srivastava, J. N. (1980). Biosocial correlates of perinatal mortality: Experiences of an Indian hospital. *Journal of Biosocial Science, 12*, 69–81.

Salam, A. M., Al Binali, H. A., Salim, I., Singh, R., Asaad, N., Qahtani, A., & Al Suwaidi, J. (2013). Impact of religious fasting on the burden of atrial fibrillation: A population-based study. *International Journal of Cardiology, 168*(3), 3042–3043.

Salame, S., Hochner-Celnikier, D., Chajek-Shaul, T., Manor, O., & Bursztyn, M. (2008). Ethnic gap in coronary artery disease: Comparison of the extent, severity, and risk factors in Arab and Jewish middle-aged women. *Journal of the Cardiometabolic Syndrome, 3*(1), 26–29.

Saleh, S. A., El-Kemery, T. A., Farrag, K. A., Badawy, M. R., Sarkis, N. N., Soliman, F. S., et al. (2004). Ramadan fasting: Relation to atherogenic risk among obese Muslims. *Journal of the Egyptian Public Health Association, 79*(5–6), 461–483.

Salti, I., Benard, E., Detournay, B., Bianchi-Biscay, M., Le Brigand, C., Voinet, C., et al. (2004). A population-based study of diabetes and its characteristics during the fasting month of Ramadan in 13 countries: Results of the epidemiology of diabetes and Ramadan 1422/2001 (EPIDIAR) study. *Diabetes Care, 27*(10), 2306–2311.

Schulpis, K. H., Gavrili, S., Vlachos, G., Karikas, G. A., Michalakakou, K., Demetriou, E., & Papassotiriou, I. (2006). The effect of nutritional habits on maternal-neonatal lipid and lipoprotein serum levels in three different ethnic groups. *Annals of Nutrition & Metabolism, 50*, 290–296.

Seedat, Y. K., Seedat, M. A., & Reddy, K. (1978). The prevalence of hypertension in the Indian population of Durban. *South African Medical Journal, 54*(1), 10–15.

Shariatpanahi, Z. V., Shariatpanahi, M. V., Shahbazi, S., Hossaini, A., & Abadi, A. (2008). Effect of Ramadan fasting on some indices of insulin resistance and components of the metabolic syndrome in healthy male adults. *British Journal of Nutrition, 100*(1), 147–151.

Singh, L., Arokiasamy, A., Singh, P. K., & Rai, R. K. (2013). Determinants of gender differences in self-rated health among older population: Evidence from India. *SAGE Open, 3*, 1–2. doi:10.1177/2158244013487914.

Singh, R., & Tripathi, V. (2013). Maternal factors contributing to under-five mortality at birth order 1 to 5 in India: A comprehensive multivariate study. *SpringerPlus, 2*, 284.

Solman, H., & Mohamed, S. (2013). Effects of Zikr meditation and jaw relaxation on postoperative pain, anxiety and physiologic response of patients undergoing abdominal surgery. *Journal of Biology, Agriculture and Healthcare, 3*(2), 23–38.

Sooki, Z., Shariff, K. H., & Tagharobi, Z. (2011). Role of Qur'an recitation in mental health of the elderly. *Quarterly of Qur'an & Medicine, 1*(1), 17–23.

Subapriya, R., Thangavelu, A., Mathavan, B., Ramachandran, C. R., & Nagini, S. (2007). Assessment of risk factors for oral squamous cell carcinoma in Chidambaram, Southern India: A case–control study. *European Journal of Cancer Prevention, 16*, 251–256.

Sujoldzic, A., Peternel, L., Kulenovic, T., & Terzic, R. (2006). Social determinants of health—Comparative study of Bosnian adolescents in different cultural contexts. *Collegium Antropologicum, 30*(4), 703–711.

Swaminathan, R., Selvakumaran, R., Esmy, P. O., Sampath, P., Ferlay, J., Jissa, V., Shanta, V., Cherian, M., & Sankaranarayanan, R. (2009). Cancer pattern and survival in rural district of South India. *Cancer Epidemiology, 33*, 325–331.

Temizhan, A., Donderici, O., Ouz, D., & Demirbas, B. (1999). Is there any effect of Ramadan fasting on acute coronary heart disease events? *International Journal of Cardiology, 70*, 149–153.

Tesfaye, F., Byass, P., Berhane, Y., Bonita, R., & Wall, S. (2008). Association of smoking and khat (Catha edulis Forsk) use with high blood pressure among adults in Addis Ababa, Ethiopia, 2006. *Preventing Chronic Disease, 5*(3), 1–11.

Topacoglu, H., Karcioglu, O., Yuruktumen, A., Kiran, S., Cimrin, A. H., Ozucelik, D. N., et al. (2005). Impact of Ramadan on demographics and frequencies of disease-related visits in the emergency department. *International Journal of Clinical Practice, 59*(8), 900–905.

United Nations (2004). World urbanization prospects: The 2001 revision. Retrieved October 7, 2013, from http://www.un.org/esa/population/publications/wup2001/wup2001dh.pdf

Ural, E., Kozdag, G., Kilic, T., Ural, D., Sahin, T., Celebi, O., et al. (2008). The effect of Ramadan fasting on ambulatory blood pressure in hypertensive patients using combination drug therapy. *Journal of Human Hypertension, 22*(3), 208–210.

Vijayakumar, G., Arun, R., & Kutty, V. R. (2009). High prevalence of Type 2 diabetes mellitus and other metabolic disorders in rural central Kerala. *Journal of the Association of Physicians of India, 57*, 563–567.

Vos, T., Gareeboo, H., & Roussety, F. (1998). Ethnic differences in ischaemic heart disease and stroke mortality in Mauritius between 1989 and 1994. *Ethnicity & Health, 3*(1/2), 45–54.

Williams, E. D., Nazroo, J. Y., Kooner, J. S., & Steptoe, A. (2010). Subgroup differences in psychosocial factors relating to coronary heart disease in the UK South Asian population. *Journal of Psychosomatic Research, 69*, 379–387.

Williams, E. D., Steptoe, A., Chambers, J. C., & Kooner, J. S. (2009). Psychosocial risk factors for coronary heart disease in UK South Asian men and women. *Journal of Epidemiology and Community Health, 63*, 986–991.
World Health Rankings (2011). Coronary heart disease: Death rate per 100,000 (age-standardized). Source: World Health Organization. Retrieved October 7, 2013, from http://www.worldlifeexpectancy.com/cause-of-death/coronary-heart-disease/by-country/
World Health Organization (2008). Blood pressure: Raised blood pressure (SBP > 140 or DBP > 90) by country. Global Health Observatory Data Repository. Retrieved October 7, 2013, from http://apps.who.int/gho/data/node.main.A875?lang=en
World Health Organization (2011a). World health rankings: Stroke. Retrieved October 7, 2013, from http://www.worldlifeexpectancy.com/cause-of-death/stroke/by-country/
World Health Organization (2011b). World health rankings: Alzheimer's/Dementia. Retrieved October 7, 2013, from http://www.worldlifeexpectancy.com/cause-of-death/alzheimers-dementia/by-country/
Wynder, E. L. (1969). Epidemiology of carcinoma in situ of the cervix. *Obstetrical and Gynecological Survey, 24*, 697–711.
Yeole, B. B. (2005). Respiratory cancer population-based survival in Mumbai, India. *Asian Pacific Journal of Cancer Prevention, 6*, 449–454.
Yeole, B. B., & Kumar, A. V. (2004). Population-based survival from cancers having a poor prognosis in Mumbai (Bombay), India. *Asian Pacific Journal of Cancer Prevention, 5*(2), 175–182.
Yeole, B. B., Kumar, A. V. R., Kurkure, A., & Sunny, L. (2004). Population-based survival from cancers of breast, cervix and ovary in women in Mumbai, India. *Asian Pacific Journal of Cancer Prevention, 5*, 308–315.
Yeole, B. B., Sankaranarayanan, R., Sunny, M. S. L., Swaminathan, R., Parkin, D. M., & Sunny, L. (2000). Survival from head and neck cancer in Mumbai (Bombay), India. *Cancer, 89*(2), 437–444.
Yilmaz, S., Kart-Koseoglu, H., Guler, O., & Yucel, E. (2008). Effect of prayer on osteoarthritis and osteoporosis. *Rheumatology International, 28*(5), 429–436.

Chapter 12
Understanding How Islam Influences Health

The vast majority of research reviewed in previous chapters (and summarized in Tables 12.1 and 12.2) suggests that greater religious involvement is related to better health in Muslims. This begs the question, "How do Islamic beliefs and practices influence health and well-being?" In this chapter we try to make sense of relationships between Islam and health based on the limited research that has now been conducted. We also broaden the discussion to go beyond the existing research and speculate on what underlying mechanisms and pathways might explain how Islamic beliefs and practices influence health. Because of the many common features between Islam and Christianity, we also utilize what we now know about relationships between religiosity and health found in Christian populations to provide clues about mechanism. While the relationship with mental and social health may be easier to understand, the connection between religiosity and physical health is less obvious yet equally important, and all have far-reaching consequences for the survival and flourishing of Islamic populations worldwide (see Part III).

Mental and Social Health

There are many pathways by which Islamic beliefs and practices could promote mental and social health. Foremost among these is that Islam helps people to cope better with stress, loss, and trauma and surrounds them with a community that provides support when they are in need. Islamic beliefs influence coping through a number of psychological and social mechanisms that we now discuss.

Positive Worldview. Islamic beliefs provide a positive worldview in which events are explainable and predictable. This contrasts with the secular belief that events occur completely at random and have no ultimate significance or meaning. The Islamic view is that if one does good and behaves morally, then this will be rewarded either in this life or in the next. God is in complete control of everything that happens to a person, is immensely merciful and forgiving, and can be trusted to desire

H.G. Koenig and S. Al Shohaib, *Health and Well-Being in Islamic Societies: Background, Research, and Applications*, DOI 10.1007/978-3-319-05873-3_12,

Table 12.1 Summary of findings on religiosity and health in Muslim populations

	Studies in Muslims		Findings (systematic)[a]		Findings (overall)	
All studies	Total no.	No. (% of total)	Positive[b] no. (%)	Negative no. (%)	Positive no. (%)	Negative no. (%)
Negative mental health						
Depression	444	13 (3)	12 (92)	0 (0)	15 (75)	1 (5)
Suicide	141	5 (4)	4 (80)	0 (0)	7 (78)	0 (0)
Anxiety	299	23 (8)	15 (68)	1 (5)	19 (68)	2 (7)
Psychosis	43	1 (2)	0 (0)	1 (100)	2 (50)	2 (50)
Alcohol use/abuse	278	2 (1)	2 (100)	0 (0)	9 (100)	0 (0)
Drug use/abuse	185	1 (1)	1 (100)	0 (0)	6 (100)	0 (0)
Positive mental health						
Well-being	326	8 (2)	8 (100)	0 (0)	20 (100)	0 (0)
Hope	40	1 (3)	0 (0)	0 (0)	0 (0)	0 (0)
Optimism	32	1 (3)	0 (0)	0 (0)	5 (71)	0 (0)
Meaning/purpose	45	0 (0)	0 (0)	0 (0)	3 (100)	0 (0)
Self-esteem	69	3 (4)	2 (67)	0 (0)	11 (73)	2 (13)
Sense of control	21	2 (10)	1 (50)	0 (0)	1 (25)	1 (25)
Personality traits						
Extraversion	50	2 (4)	1 (50)	0 (0)	3 (43)	0 (0)
Neuroticism	54	1 (2)	1 (100)	0 (0)	4 (57)	0 (0)
Conscientiousness	30	1 (2)	0 (0)	0 (0)	5 (80)	0 (0)
Agreeableness	30	1 (2)	1 (100)	0 (0)	5 (100)	0 (0)
Openness	26	1 (4)	1 (100)	0 (0)	3 (60)	0 (0)
Social health						
Social support	74	2 (3)	1 (50)	0 (0)	5 (83)	0 (0)
Marital stability	79	2 (3)	2 (100)	0 (0)	6 (100)	0 (0)
Delinquency/crime	104	3 (3)	2 (67)	1 (33)	9 (82)	1 (9)
Social capital	14	1 (7)	0 (0)	0 (0)	5 (50)	2 (20)

Cigarette smoking	137	5 (4)	3 (60)	0 (0)	7 (70)	0 (0)
Exercise	37	1 (3)	0 (0)	0 (0)	0 (0)	1 (33)
Diet	22	0 (0)	0 (0)	0 (0)	0 (0)	1 (100)
Weight	36	1 (3)	1 (100)	0 (0)	1 (25)	1 (25)
Sexual behavior	95	1 (1)	1 (100)	0 (0)	7 (78)	0 (0)
Physical health[c]						
Heart disease[d]	36	5 (14)	3 (60)	0 (0)	4 (40)	1 (10)
Hypertension	63	5 (8)	2 (40)	1 (20)	4 (50)	2 (25)
Cerebrovascular disease	9	2 (22)	0 (0)	0 (0)	0 (0)	0 (0)
Dementia/Alzheimer's disease	21	0 (0)	0 (0)	0 (0)	1 (100)	0 (0)
Diabetes	17	4 (24)	3 (75)	1 (25)	3 (60)	1 (20)
Cholesterol/triglycerides	24	7 (29)	5 (71)	1 (14)	6 (67)	2 (22)
Immune function[e]	45	3 (7)	1 (33)	0 (0)	1 (33)	0 (0)
Endocrine function	31	0 (0)	0 (0)	0 (0)	1 (20)	1 (20)
Cancer	29	0 (0)	0 (0)	0 (0)	0 (0)	0 (0)
Self-rated health	50	0 (0)	0 (0)	0 (0)	1 (50)	1 (50)
Mortality	121	0 (0)	0 (0)	0 (0)	1 (100)	0 (0)

[a]Based on 2010 systematic review documented in *Handbook of Religion and Health* (Oxford University Press 2001, 2012)

[b]"Positive" means significantly *better* on health outcome and "negative" means significantly *worse*

[c]Includes effects of Ramadan fasting

[d]Includes studies on coronary artery disease, cardiac surgery, cardiovascular functions, inflammatory (CRP), and coagulation (fibrinogen) markers

[e]Includes studies examining susceptibility to infection and viral load in blood, indirect measures of immune function

Table 12.2 Comparison of mental, social, behavioral, and physical health in Muslims vs. non-Muslims

	No. of studies	Better (%)	Worse (%)	Mixed (%)	Same (%)
Mental health[a]	3	67	33	0	0
Depression					
Suicide	7	43	14	14	29
Anxiety	7	14	86	0	0
Psychosis	2	100	0	0	0
Alcohol use/abuse	12	75	0	0	25
Drug use/abuse	6	50	0	0	50
Well-being	1	0	0	0	100
Optimism	3	0	67	33	0
Sense of control	6	33	17	33	17
Social health[a]					
Social support	2	100	0	0	0
Marital stability	2	50	50	0	0
Delinquency/crime	3	67	0	33	0
Social capital	4	50	50	0	0
Behavioral health					
Cigarette smoking	8	38	13	0	50
Exercise	6	17	67	17	0
Diet	4	25	50	25	0
Weight	7	57	43	0	0
Extramarital sex	12	67	8	8	17
Physical health					
Heart disease	10	20	40	20	10
Hypertension	8	75	25	0	0
Cerebrovascular disease	2	100	0	0	0
Dementia	0	0	0	0	0
Diabetes	6	33	33	0	33
Cholesterol/triglycerides	3	67	33	0	0
Immune function	2	0	50	0	50
Endocrine function	0	0	0	0	0
Cancer	19	37	11	11	42
Self-rated health	8	13	50	0	37
Mortality	14	43	36	7	14

[a]For hope, purpose in life, self-esteem, the five personality dimensions, and social support, we found no studies that compared Muslims and non-Muslims. In general, for areas of mental and social health, we focused on religiosity, not on comparison of Muslims and non-Muslims, so the review of that comparison may not be complete. For behavioral and physical health states, however, we did a complete review comparing Muslims and non-Muslims

only good for people. God is also just, however, and evil actions or lack of mercy will likewise have consequences both in this life and the next. Life does not end at death, but continues on for those who do good. In fact, life continues in a place that is much better than here on earth, where there is a continual sense of peace and joy in the presence of God and where individuals will reunite with loved ones who have died before and will die after them. Again, this is a positive worldview where events are predictable.

Meaning and Purpose. Islamic beliefs give meaning and purpose to both good and bad events and situations. Nothing is senseless. Everything has meaning because God has a purpose for the world, and God's will is supreme. Every individual is believed to have a part in helping to accomplish the Divine purpose, if they are willing to submit their lives to the rulership and will of God. This is especially true when accidents or sickness strikes and causes pain and disability, which God also has a purpose for. Sickness is there to test the person to see if he or she will bear the burden courageously and without complaint. Sickness can help to purify the person if he or she has done evil deeds or failed to do good deeds in the past. Sickness positions a person to do good by empowering their prayers (more so than the prayers of the healthy) to change situations both in their own lives and in the lives of others. These beliefs give the sick and those experiencing loss or trauma a new sense of purpose and meaning, and give new strength to bear suffering, which thereby reduces it.

Psychological Integration. Islamic beliefs and practices help believers to psychologically integrate traumatic events. Severely traumatized people, such as those with post-traumatic stress disorder, have had their worldview shattered by these disturbing experiences. They may have come close to death, witnessed the death of a loved one, been directly involved in a traumatic event with mass casualties, or had to suffer for a prolonged period without relief. These persons are constantly on edge, fearful, anxious, depressed, and often angry over the seeming senselessness of what has happened. They often turn to alcohol or drugs to numb or distance themselves from the tremendous pain that they cannot escape from. Religious beliefs give these events meaning, and with meaning comes a renewed sense that the world is predictable, that events in it are controllable, and that good will triumph in the end. This gives hope and motivation to continue to improve life rather than give up and despair.

Tools to Cope. Islamic beliefs and practices give people tools to deal with sickness, loss, and trauma, which empower those who might otherwise feel helpless and without alternatives. For example, prayer enables people to enlist the help of God and all the power that God has at His disposal to get them through a difficult situation, or to change their attitudes toward situations that do not change. The five daily prayers help to structure life and remind people to think about God and submit to God's will for their lives. Likewise, reading the Qu'ran provides comfort by reminding the person of God's promises and rewards that are available to all who faithfully live out these words of God. There is also belief in the power of verses in the Qu'ran to causing healing and wholeness and to counteract evil forces. Muslims, then, have resources to deal with any and all situations that they confront. Note, however, that daily religious practices alone (outside of a close intimate relationship with a caring, merciful God) may not be sufficient to prevent emotional distress, as has been shown in Christian populations (Bradshaw et al. 2008).

Satisfying Answers. Islamic beliefs provide answers to ultimate questions in life. Where did we come from, why are we here, and where are we going after death? Humans crave answers to these questions, especially when experiencing sickness or trauma that stimulates such thoughts. Science and medicine have no answers to these questions, nor will they ever have answers, since the scientific worldview sees events as happening at random and without any underlying purpose or meaning. Religious beliefs alone provide answers that satisfy these deep yearnings.

Healthy Decision-Making. Islamic beliefs provide guidance for decision-making on a day-to-day basis. These decisions involve how to treat family members, friends, and colleagues at work and how to use financial resources for the good of themselves and others. Those decisions help people to live useful and productive lives that are meaningful and fulfilling and that positively influence those around them in their community. These positive decisions, if repeated over and over again, produce character traits such as dependability, forgiveness, courage, honesty, hard work, self-discipline, humility, and patience. They influence the kinds of behaviors that people engage in that affect their mental and social health, including whether to steal, cheat, or engage in other criminal behavior and whether to engage in sexual practices outside of marriage or other immoral acts.

Social Support. Islamic beliefs and practices promote social support, both human and Divine. Attending prayer services at the mosque or going on Hajj allows for interactions with others that often result in supportive relationships. These relationships provide an opportunity to share religious belief and faith in God and provide supportive human interactions that are satisfying and life enhancing. Such relationships provide social support when people undergo stressful life experiences and sometimes even practical resources that are needed for survival.

Fostering Generosity. Finally, Islam encourages believers to do charitable acts by every means possible, whether that involves giving money or time for charitable purposes. People who work in charities have more satisfaction and self-esteem. They may find even more satisfaction in their charitable work than in a successful career (see example below). Islam stresses that people should contribute to charitable work, even if it is only a small act. Those who do so often end up making more friendships that are based on real value rather than simply on business terms. How much a person owns, the extent of their material possessions, or how much they have produced does not matter in Islam. Contributing to charity accomplishes many things not only on the individual level but also on the community level. Charity helps to combat poverty, reduce crime, and make those who are poor feel worthy, enhancing self-esteem and likely improving both mental and physical health, particularly when the poor themselves begin to contribute to charity.

For example, one of us (Saad) saw a patient in private practice who suddenly was in a better mood, with improved blood pressure and better blood sugar control. When asked what changes he had made in his life, he said that he had started to devote almost all of his time to a charitable organization. Despite being a successful businessman, his life had been full of stress resulting in high blood pressure and diabetes.

So, he decided to take early retirement in order to devote more time to the charity. He chaired an organization that takes care of prisoners and their families. When he saw these people, he realized how privileged he was. When he gave these people help and attention, he felt more valuable. When he called some wealthy people to help him in his task, they showed him more respect and attention compared to when he was calling them for business purposes. The generosity and other-directed actions that Islam promotes have many benefits.

Negative Influences on Mental and Social Health

Just as Islamic beliefs may have powerful positive influences on mental and social health, they can also have negative effects, especially when taken out of context. These too must be taken into account and balanced against the positive influences.

Attitude Toward Women. Islamic teachings, rooted in the strongly patriarchal culture in which they emerged, may be utilized by some to deny women their human rights. This is demeaning to women and actually counter to the intentions of the Prophet Muhammad who wished to safeguard women during an era when many did not have male protectors because of heavy casualties experienced during war. When women are not treated with respect and honor, not only is the mental and social health of women reduced, but all of society suffers.

Promote Anxiety. Emphasis in Islam on the weighing of good deeds and bad deeds as a determinant of eternal happiness in Paradise or eternal suffering in hell may foster anxiety among those who are vulnerable, particularly when death approaches and nothing can be done to receive forgiveness for past sins. Family members may also worry about this. Similarly, the stress that Islam places on praying five times daily and the emphasis on reading, reciting, and memorizing the Qu'ran may strengthen obsessive–compulsive traits in those who already have such a predisposition. Others within the Islamic community may view persons with these traits (or even obsessive–compulsive disorder) as being particularly devout, rather than as being someone with mental illness in need of treatment. Finally, one source of anxiety in Muslims who live in non-Muslim countries is their minority group status and the discrimination they face on a day-to-day basis.

Worsen Guilt. Even more common among Muslims may be the guilt they experience from failing to live up to the high moral standards set by Islam. It is difficult to be generous, forgiving, dependable, patient, faithful to spouse, prudent in eating, and compliant with regular religious practices as required in Islam. This may be discouraging to some, creating cynicism and hopelessness, which may lead to giving up or depression, and/or to ostracism from the Muslim community, which may further adversely affect mental and social health.

Exacerbate Psychosis. Emphasis placed on the supernatural in Islamic teachings (jinn, angels, etc.) may foster psychotic symptoms or delusional thinking, which can be difficult to differentiate from normative religious or culture-based beliefs. Such persons may be viewed by other Muslims as strange or different, but not in need of psychiatric care, and so are not referred for treatment in a timely manner. However, rather than inducing psychotic symptoms, it is much more likely that Islamic beliefs are simply a manifestation of psychotic illness. Given the wide prevalence of Islamic beliefs in Muslim populations, those beliefs become intertwined in the psychotic process itself. In general, then, it is not at all clear whether it is the Islamic beliefs and practices that are causing the anxiety, obsessive–compulsive symptoms, guilt, depression, or psychosis or whether the direction of causation is actually the opposite. In other words, individuals with these mental problems may simply express their symptoms in religious ways or, even more likely, may turn to religion for comfort when trying to cope with these symptoms. Thus, it is not Islam that is the problem but the underlying mental illness.

Delay Treatment. Reliance entirely on Islamic beliefs and practices for healing may delay effective diagnosis and treatment of serious mental illness. This is especially worrisome in severe depressive disorder (with the potential for suicide) or acute psychotic disorders (with the potential for violence and homicide). These conditions may be treated by Islamic healers or Imams and not referred for psychiatric care or may be referred too late in the course of the disease, allowing it to progress and worsen. The poor relationship between religion and at least Western psychiatry has created deep divisions and hostilities between the two healing traditions, which may prevent timely communication when cooperation is needed.

Criticize the Sick. Members of the person's religious community who are not familiar with the causes of mental illness may criticize persons with emotional problems for not being religious enough or not praying or reading the Qu'ran enough, thus adding condemnation and guilt to the person's suffering. While Islamic beliefs and practices may be sufficient in warding off emotional problems for the vast majority of people with stable mental health, they may be less helpful in reversing severe mental disorders driven largely by biological or developmental factors.

Justice over Mercy. This topic is sensitive, but one that must be addressed here. There are radical elements within Islam that emphasize the justice of God over His love, mercy, and forgiveness. In these circles, fighting and martyrdom for the cause of Islam is highly valued, as it was and still is in Christianity for those who stand up for their faith. However, when hatred and revenge is the motivation that drives these activities, we believe this is contrary to the will of God who is wholly and completely good. Likewise, the killing of innocents is nowhere condoned in either Christianity or Islam. While the original motivation in many of these radicalized elements has been the purification of Islam (a highly honorable goal), this has deteriorated in some cases to a drive that is largely political or based on a desire for power and control, not justice. While hatred and domination have been common driving forces in many religions at one time or another, this does not produce either individual or community health but only an endless cycle of revenge, war, and destruction.

We realize many of the negative effects described above are common to all major world religions, including Christianity (perhaps especially Christianity), so they are not at all unique to Islam. They involve the dark side of religion, which while a truly powerful force for health and well-being can also have the opposite effects.

In summary, Islamic beliefs and practices have the potential to influence many aspects of mental and social health, especially if those beliefs are taken seriously and integrated into daily life. In general, the limited research reviewed in earlier chapters suggests that Islamic beliefs neutralize negative emotions and increase positive emotions. They enhance personal and family relationships and expand social networks. They promote decisions that lead to both psychological and social health. Again, these are all likely to have powerful effects on physical health and well-being.

Behavioral Health

The core teachings of Islam emphasize respect for the body and discourage any behaviors that lead to poor physical health or adversely affect the health of the community. This is the reason why the Qur'an forbids the use of intoxicating substances that may interfere with prayer or incite arguments between people and disrupt social harmony. Likewise, the Qur'an discourages excesses of all kinds, whether this relates to eating and food consumption or to extravagant living practices. This also applies to having sexual relationships outside of marriage, which are strictly condemned in Islam. The Prophet Muhammad himself engaged in regular sport (archery, running) and encouraged his followers to maintain their physical health in order to enhance their ability to fight for the cause of Islam. Although drug use and cigarette smoking are not mentioned in the Qur'an, the Prophet would have certainly discouraged these, as recent fatwa against such practices testify to.

The research indicates that health behaviors are much better in Muslims who follow Islamic teachings. Alcohol and drug use, cigarette smoking, and extramarital sexual activity are all much less common among those who are devoutly religious. Sharia law helps to enforce Islamic teachings across Muslim-majority countries, which increases their influence on health behaviors. There is less consensus, however, with regard to exercise, diet, and weight, even among the more religious (especially with regard to diet and weight in more affluent Islamic societies). Cultural influences also have their effect on health behaviors, and these may not always line up with the core teachings of Islam and the lifestyle of the Prophet.

For example, the traditional diet in Middle Eastern countries prior to 40 years ago was characterized by high-fiber content, low in fat and cholesterol, and high in vegetables and fruit. That has changed with Western cultural influences that have brought a diet high in fat content, sugar, sodium, and cholesterol to this region of the world. According to one report, daily per capita fat intake has increased in most Muslim-majority countries during the past four decades, ranging from 14 % in the Sudan to 143 % in Saudi Arabia (Musaiger 2002).

Physical Health

The source of the power in Islam for enhancing physical health is belief in and submission to God (Allah) (Fig. 12.1). This gives rise to devout beliefs that foster human values, affect daily decisions and lifestyle choices, influence health behaviors, promote positive emotions and social relationships, and help to prevent negative emotions and mental disorders. The effects of Islamic beliefs and practices on physiological systems, physical health, and longevity are largely indirect, acting through psychological, social, and behavioral pathways. Because they are indirect, these effects are more difficult to demonstrate than are the effects that Islam has on psychological and social health. There is a rapidly growing research base, however, that is now demonstrating how emotions, social relationships, and health behaviors can directly affect basic physiological systems responsible for maintaining physical health or responding to injury and disease. This body of research provides plausible explanations for how Islamic beliefs and practices could influence physical health, and those mechanisms can be studied and better understood through research methods in the social and behavioral sciences.

Ideas about how thoughts, emotions, and social behaviors can influence the body are not new. The possibility that psychosocial factors can affect physical health has been a consistent belief throughout the history of Islam. Many early great Islamic physicians were "interactionalists," i.e., believed that the mind interacted with the body and vice versa in causing disease. This view contrasted with the prevailing Greek and Roman scientific views of the time (see Chap. 2). Islamic physicians, in fact, foresaw the development of psychosomatic medicine, which has now become a mainstream part of modern medicine throughout the world. The influence of emotional and psychological factors on physiological systems is thought to be one of the key mechanisms by which religious involvement influences physical health and longevity.

Psychosocial Influences. Physiological processes most likely to be influenced by psychological and social factors are the immune, endocrine, and cardiovascular systems. The latter systems are known to be essential for preventing disease, maintaining physical health, and enabling recovery from illness. As noted above, a vast amount of observational and experimental research documents the effects that psychological and social factors have on physiological processes (see Chida and Steptoe 2008; Steptoe et al. 2009, for reviews of this area). We know, for example, that positive psychological states predict a slower progression of HIV/AIDS (Ironson and Hayward 2008) and improve cardiovascular disease outcomes (Kubzansky and Thurston 2007; Tindle et al. 2009; Hoogwegt et al. 2014). Likewise, depression, stress, and negative emotional states contribute to the development of heart disease and predict worse cardiac outcomes (Krantz et al. 2000; Orth-Gomer et al. 2000; Das and O'Keefe 2006; Ziegelstein 2007). Greater social support and stronger social network are also known to have a positive influence on physical health and predict greater longevity (House et al. 1988; Cohen et al. 2000; Uchino 2009; Pantell et al. 2013). This research has resulted in a rapidly expanding field that has

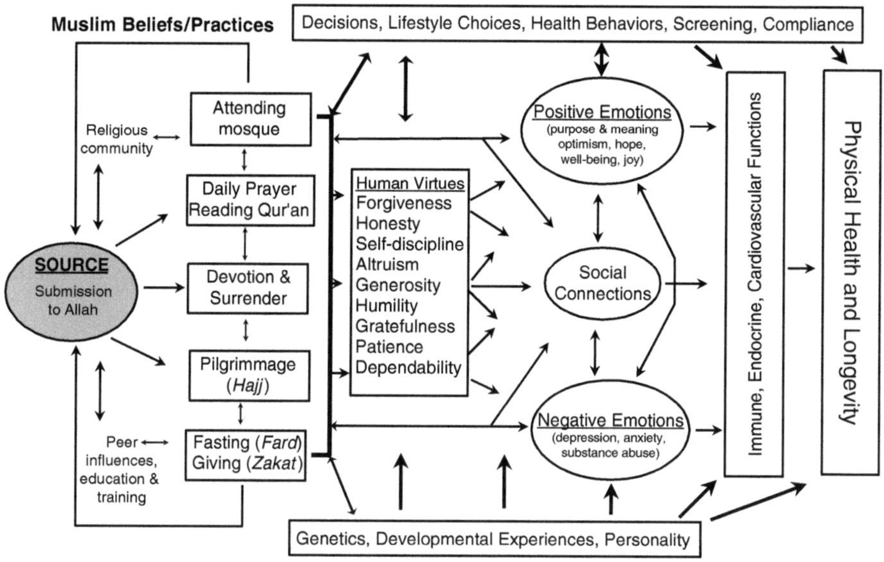

Fig. 12.1 Theoretical causal model explaining Islam's effects on health (adapted from Koenig et al. 2012)

been variously called psychoneuroimmunology, psychosomatic medicine, or mind–body medicine. If greater religiosity among Muslims is related to better coping with stress, less emotional distress, more positive emotions, and better social connections, then the devoutly religious should also have better physical health.

Lifestyle and Behavioral Influences. Besides being influenced by psychological and social influences, physical health is also directly affected by lifestyle choices and other health-related behaviors. As noted in Chap. 10, research has documented that regular exercise, a healthy diet, maintaining an ideal body weight, and avoiding cigarette smoking have the potential to reduce chronic diseases by as much as 80 % and extend the life span by more than a decade (Ford et al. 2009; Lee et al. 2009; Kvaavik et al. 2010). Based on the latest meta-analyses of prospective studies, research has now confirmed the positive effects of exercise on longevity (Woodcock et al. 2011), the negative effects of cigarette smoking on heart disease (Huxley and Woodward 2011), and the role that obesity plays in early mortality (Flegal et al. 2013). There can be little doubt that living a healthy lifestyle can have a huge impact on physical health and longevity.

Our research review found that religiosity in Muslims was associated with less cigarette smoking in 70 % of studies and less risky sexual behaviors in nearly 80 % of studies (Table 12.2). Almost no research, however, has examined religiosity and exercise, diet, and weight in Muslim-majority populations, although the little research now available is not particularly positive. When comparing Muslims and non-Muslims (rather than examining effects of religiosity in Muslims), Muslims are less likely to smoke cigarettes (38 % of studies) and are less likely to engage in risky sexual behaviors outside of marriage (67 % of studies). The majority of studies also show that Muslims tend to have a lower body weight (except in wealthy Muslim countries), despite having a worse diet in some studies. Exercise is less common in Muslims compared to non-Muslims in two-thirds of studies, which places Muslims at somewhat greater risk of poor health. Nevertheless, if Muslims adhere to the teachings of their faith (which encourage exercise, discourage overeating, discourage cigarette smoking, and emphasize sexual relationships only within marriage), then we would expect Muslims to live longer and healthier lives. Of course, this assumes that everything else is equal (i.e., safe living conditions, access to healthcare, preventive services, screening, etc.), which is seldom the case.

Genetic and Environmental Influences. Genetic factors also play a role in the relationship between religiosity and health in Muslims, particularly in terms of vulnerability to disease that may be increased by a high prevalence of consanguinity. In one study from Jordan, nearly 50 % of all marriages involved some level of consanguinity, with marriage to a first cousin being present in about one-third of cases (Khoury and Massad 1992). However, there is nothing in the Qur'an that encourages consanguineous unions (Hussain 1999). In fact, there is a Hadith that says the Prophet discouraged cousin marriages (although the Prophet did marry his daughter Fatima to Ali, his paternal first cousin, setting a precedent that some might follow and justify on those grounds). The physical health of Muslims might also be affected by moral prohibitions against abortion, even when significant fetal anomalies are present as a result of consanguineous marriages. Thus, there are multiple ways that genetic factors could influence the physical health of Muslims, often in the direction of worse health outcomes.

Environmental factors also have their influences, both in Muslim-majority countries and in Muslim immigrants to Western countries. Environmental factors that affect health include physical safety from war; adequate income to ensure necessary water, food, and living accommodations; community efforts to prevent disease (i.e., vaccinations against communicable diseases, efforts to ensure safe water and food supplies, and so forth); and access to healthcare when needed. Many Muslims live in developing or war-torn countries where none of these can be guaranteed. Environmental influences also affect the health of Muslim immigrants to Europe, Canada, and the USA, although often in a different way. Poor health may result from immersion in a liberal Western lifestyle, including the consumption of high-calorie high-fat foods; exposure to "progressive" views on dress and sexual behavior via TV, movies, and music; and a culture based on relative moral values rather than those that are absolute. Retaining a strong Muslim religious faith may help to combat many of these negative environmental influences.

Other Influences on Physical Health. There are also factors besides those that are psychological, social, behavioral, genetic, or environmental that can influence health and longevity, the most important of those being early disease detection, timely seeking of medical care when sick, and compliance with medical treatment once a disease is diagnosed.

Disease Detection. We know that if people receive regular medical care and undergo screening for common illnesses, then they will have diseases detected earlier and treated before illness has a chance to advance and worsen. How might Islam beliefs affect health by increasing or decreasing screening for disease? Islamic beliefs that encourage respect and care for the physical body would be expected to increase disease detection through screening. Likewise, greater involvement in faith community activity at the mosque might increase the flow of health information that could alert people to the need for high blood pressure, diabetes, and prostate cancer screening in men or breast and cervical cancer screening in women. Alternatively, belief in destiny and the supremacy of God's will might discourage disease screening and thereby allow disease to take its natural course. Modesty among Muslims who are more devout might also play a role, especially with regard to screening procedures for cervical and breast cancer. Furthermore, economic factors and access to healthcare might be confounding factors that reduce disease screening in Muslims, especially those in developing countries.

Only limited research exists on disease screening in Muslim populations, although the findings support the complexity of these interacting factors. For example, in a study of breast cancer screening in a random sample of 568 Arab women ages 20–60 living in Israel, Azaiza and Cohen (2006) compared Muslims, Christians, and Druze in this regard. The primary outcome was clinical breast exam (CBE) and mammography. Religiosity was assessed using a single question that asked participants to self-rate themselves as secular, mildly religious, or very religious. Other predictors included demographics, family history of cancer, perceived susceptibility to breast cancer, perceived severity of breast cancer, benefits of and barriers to CBE and mammography, and health motivation. Results indicated that Muslims and Druze were significantly more likely than Christians to never have had a CBE (66 % Muslims and Druze vs. 44 % in Christians). Muslims and Druze were also significantly more likely to report either never having had mammography or not having it within the past 5 years (73 % Druze and 58 % Muslims vs. 40 % Christians). Barriers to CBE and mammography were also much higher among Druze and Muslims. Finally, even after statistically controlling for these factors (barriers, physician recommendation, and history of breast cancer), researchers found that Muslims and Druze women were still less likely than Christians to engage in early detection practices for breast cancer, and greater religiosity was related to less frequent CBE. Researchers concluded that religious beliefs influence women's likelihood of engaging in breast cancer screening practices.

Timely Medical Care. Once symptoms of disease appear or a disease is detected through screening, prompt medical attention is necessary in order to limit the negative consequences on health. As noted in Chap. 3, the Prophet Muhammad encouraged his followers to seek medical care when they became sick and he himself sought medical attention when necessary (perhaps even from Christian and Jewish doctors). The Qur'an emphasizes the value of life and the importance of staying healthy so that a person can serve God and share their faith. There is no excuse, then, for Muslims not to seek medical care when necessary or to delay it unnecessarily. The fact that some of the greatest contributions to medical science were made by Islamic physicians is no accident.

Compliance with Treatment. Health outcomes can also be affected by the extent to which Islamic beliefs and practices influence compliance with medical treatment. However, almost no systematic research exists on the effects of religiosity in Muslims on compliance with treatment. Again, adherence to Islamic beliefs that promote care for the physical body and the preservation of life should result in greater compliance with medical treatments among Muslims who are more religious. However, religion and medicine might also conflict in certain cases, and the result might be a reduction in medical compliance. In the last chapter, for example, we found that fasting during Ramadan takes precedence over recommendations from the doctor even among those with serious illnesses such as diabetes (Gaborit et al. 2011). Changes in use of inhaled medications among patients with asthma have likewise been documented in Muslim patients during Ramadan, prompting experts to recommend careful monitoring (Erkekol et al. 2006). The presence of forbidden substances that make up the inert ingredients of prescribed medication (i.e., pork products) might also reduce compliance among devout Muslims (Sattar et al. 2004). Nevertheless, while much speculation exists on the potential negative impact of religiosity on compliance among Muslims (particularly as a result of fasting during Ramadan), little research documents such negative effects (see Chap. 11).

Summary and Conclusions

There are many plausible explanations for why religiosity in Muslims might be related to better mental, social, behavioral, and physical health. Islamic beliefs and practices help people to cope better with stress and trauma (decreasing depression, suicide, and anxiety). They provide healthy guidelines for both individual and communal living (reducing alcohol and drug abuse, delinquency, crime, and marital instability and increasing social capital and social engagement). Islamic beliefs also encourage a healthy lifestyle (discouraging overeating, extravagant living, risky sexual behaviors, and cigarette smoking, and promoting exercise and productive activity). There are also other factors that affect the emotional, social, and physical health and longevity of Muslims, including genetic factors, environmental factors, and issues related to disease detection, timely seeking of medical care, and complying with medical treatment. Nevertheless, we would argue that the power of religious faith to influence health and well-being lies in the willingness of Muslims to submit to God and to live a surrendered, devout, moral life.

References

Azaiza, F., & Cohen, M. (2006). Health beliefs and rates of breast cancer screening among Arab women. *Journal of Women's Health, 15*(5), 520–530.

Bradshaw, M., Ellison, C. G., & Flannelly, K. J. (2008). Prayer, God imagery, and symptoms of psychopathology. *Journal for the Scientific Study of Religion, 47*, 644–659.

Chida, Y. C., & Steptoe, A. (2008). Positive psychological well-being and mortality: A quantitative review of prospective observational studies. *Psychosomatic Medicine, 70*, 741–756.
Cohen, S., Underwood, L. G., & Gottlieb, B. H. (2000). *Social support, measurement, and intervention: A guide for health and social scientists*. New York: Oxford University Press.
Das, S., & O'Keefe, J. H. (2006). Behavioral cardiology: Recognizing and addressing the profound impact of psychosocial stress on cardiovascular health. *Current Atherosclerosis Reports, 8*(2), 111–118.
Erkekol, F. O., Balik, G. E., Kaskin, C. E., Gullu, E., Mungan, D., & Misirligil, Z. (2006). Fasting: An important issue in asthma management compliance. *Annals of Allergy, Asthma & Immunology, 97*, 370–374.
Flegal, K. M., Kit, B. K., Orpana, H., & Graubard, B. I. (2013). Association of all-cause mortality with overweight and obesity using standard body mass index categories: A systematic review and meta-analysis. *Journal of the American Medical Association, 309*, 71–82.
Ford, E. S., Bergmann, M. M., Kroger, J., Schienkiewitz, A., Weikert, C., & Boeing, H. (2009). Healthy living is the best revenge: Findings from the European prospective investigation into cancer and nutrition-Potsdam study. *Archives of Internal Medicine, 169*, 1355–1362.
Gaborit, B., Dutour, O., Ronsin, O., Atlan, C., Darmon, P., Gharsalli, R., Pradel, V., Dadoun, F., & Dutour, A. (2011). Ramadan fasting with diabetes: An interview study of inpatients' and general practitioners' attitudes in the South of France. *Diabetes & Metabolism, 37*, 395–402.
Hoogwegt, M. T., Versteeg, H., Hansen, T. B., Thygesen, L. C., Pedersen, S. S., & Zwisler, A. D. (2014). Exercise mediates the association between positive affect and 5-year mortality in patients with ischemic heart disease. *Circulation, 129*, e295–e298.
House, J. S., Landis, K. R., & Umberson, D. (1988). Social relationships and health. *Science, 241*, 540–545.
Hussain, R. (1999). Community perceptions of reasons for preference for consanguineous marriages in Pakistan. *Journal of Biosocial Science, 31*, 449–461.
Huxley, R. R., & Woodward, M. (2011). Cigarette smoking as a risk factor for coronary heart disease in women compared with men: A systematic review and meta-analysis of prospective cohort studies. *Lancet, 378*, 1297–1305.
Ironson, G., & Hayward, H. (2008). Do positive psychosocial factors predict disease progression in HIV-1? A review of the evidence. *Psychosomatic Medicine, 70*, 546–554.
Khoury, S. A., & Massad, D. (1992). Consanguineous marriage in Jordan. *American Journal of Medical Genetics, 43*, 769–775.
Koenig, H. G., King, D.E., Carson, V.B. (2012). Handbook of Religion and Health, 2nd edition. NY, NY: Oxford University Press.
Krantz, D. S., Sheps, D. S., Carney, R. M., & Natelson, B. H. (2000). Effects of mental stress in patients with coronary artery disease: Evidence and clinical implications. *Journal of the American Medical Association, 283*(14), 1800–1802.
Kubzansky, L. D., & Thurston, R. C. (2007). Emotional vitality and incident coronary heart disease: Benefits of healthy psychological functioning. *Archives of General Psychiatry, 64*(12), 1393–1401.
Kvaavik, E., Batty, G. D., Ursin, G., Huxley, R., & Gale, C. R. (2010). Influence of individual and combined health behaviors on total and cause-specific mortality in men and women: The United Kingdom health and lifestyle survey. *Archives of Internal Medicine, 170*, 711–718.
Lee, C. D., Sui, X., & Blair, S. N. (2009). Combined effects of cardiorespiratory fitness, not smoking, and normal waist girth on morbidity and mortality in men. *Archives of Internal Medicine, 169*, 2096–2101.
Musaiger, A. O. (2002). Diet an prevention of coronary heart disease in the Arab Middle East countries. *Medical Principles and Practice, 11*(suppl 2), 9–16.
Orth-Gomer, K., Wamala, S. P., Horsten, M., Schenck-Gustafsson, K., Schneiderman, N., & Mittleman, M. A. (2000). Marital stress worsens prognosis in women with coronary heart disease: The Stockholm Female Coronary Risk Study. *Journal of the American Medical Association, 284*(23), 3008–3014.

Pantell, M., Rehkopf, D., Jutte, D., Syme, S.L., Baines, J., & Adler, N. (2013). Social isolation: A predictor of mortality comparable to traditional clinical risk factors. *American Journal of Public Health 103*(11), 2056–2062.
Sattar, S. P., Ahmen, M. S., Majeed, F., & Petty, F. (2004). Inert medication ingredients causing nonadherence due to religious beliefs. *Annals of Pharmacotherapy, 38*, 621–624.
Steptoe, A., Dockray, S., & Wardle, J. (2009). Positive affect and psychobiological processes relevant to health. *Journal of Personality, 77*(6), 1747–1776.
Tindle, H. A., Chang, Y. F., Kuller, L. H., Manson, J. E., Robinson, J. G., Rosal, M. C., Siegle, G. J., & Matthews, K. A. (2009). Optimism, cynical hostility, and incident coronary heart disease and mortality in the women's health initiative. *Circulation, 120*(8), 656–662.
Uchino, B. N. (2009). Understanding the links between social support and physical health. *Perspectives on Psychological Science, 4*(3), 236–255.
Woodcock, J., Franco, O. H., Orsini, N., & Roberts, I. (2011). Non-vigorous physical activity and all-cause mortality: Systematic review and meta-analysis of cohort studies. *International Journal of Epidemiology, 40*, 121–138.
Ziegelstein, R. C. (2007). Acute emotional stress and cardiac arrhythmias. *Journal of the American Medical Association, 298*(3), 324–329.

Chapter 13
Future Research Needs on Islam and Health

There is great need and opportunity for researchers to conduct systematic studies on almost every aspect of Islam and health. Indeed, the research possibilities in this area are almost endless. Based on our systematic review of research on religion and health around the world up through mid-2010, only 3 % of quantitative studies (103 out of 3,141) were conducted in Muslim-majority countries (see Table 12.1). The influence of religiosity on every aspect of health—psychological, social, behavioral, and physical—needs further study. Given the dominant influence that Islamic beliefs and practices have on the lives of over 1.6 billion Muslims, the effect that these religious influences have on health can no longer be ignored by psychosocial, behavioral, and medical scientists. Besides having mainstream researchers begin to examine the effects of religiosity on health in Muslim populations, we also hope that young investigators just beginning their academic careers will become interested in and focus some of their research in this area. We review here research topics that should be of highest priority in the future, dividing them up into mental, social, behavioral, and physical categories. Besides scientific priority, we also consider feasibility and cost, given the difficulty of finding research funding to support such projects. For a more in-depth discussion, see Koenig (2011).

Mental Health

Much of the past research on religiosity and health in Muslims has focused on mental health. However, many more studies are needed in Muslim-majority countries, and in particular, the research designs used in future studies need improvement.

Of the 153 studies we identified in (1) our 2010 systematic review, (2) current review of studies missed by that review, and (3) review of studies conducted since 2010, there were a total of seven randomized clinical trials (RCTs) and two prospective studies. All the rest (94 %) were cross-sectional in design, and two-thirds of

H.G. Koenig and S. Al Shohaib, *Health and Well-Being in Islamic Societies: Background, Research, and Applications*, DOI 10.1007/978-3-319-05873-3_13,

those did not statistically control for any other factors that might have influenced the relationships found. Furthermore, of the seven RCTs, six were conducted in a way that subjects in the intervention group received additional psychotherapy (compared to controls). This makes it impossible to determine whether it was simply the additional time spent with the therapist or the religious nature of the therapy that resulted in better outcomes. Thus, there is an urgent need for studies in this area to improve on study design.

First, future cross-sectional studies need to statistically control for potential confounding variables that could otherwise explain the relationships found. Second, there is a tremendous need for prospective studies that follow participants over time and seek to determine whether religiosity at baseline predicts future changes in mental health (two prospective studies are simply not enough). Third, future RCTs need to be designed in a way that the control groups receive the same amount of therapist attention as the religious intervention groups, so that results can be interpreted in a meaningful way. These design issues are common to all areas where further research is needed. We now discuss highest priority areas of research that need further study in Muslims.

Common Mental Disorders. Emotional disorders such as depression, anxiety, and even substance abuse are common among Muslim populations and need further study. These are among the most disabling conditions in the world, equivalent to the disability caused by heart disease (Lopez and Murray 1998). Only one prospective study to date has examined how religiosity affects these conditions (Hamdan and Tamim 2011). Thus, we have almost no information on whether greater religiosity precedes changes in these emotional disorders and so either prevents them from developing or affects their outcome. The same is true for religiosity and alcohol or drug use or abuse, on which only six studies have been published, all cross-sectional and only three in adult populations. Also needed are intervention studies (RCTs) designed in a way to truly test whether integrating Islamic beliefs and practices into psychotherapy results in more rapid and more sustained improvement in emotional disorder (including substance abuse disorders) compared to an equivalent secular therapeutic intervention. Not needed is another cross-sectional study in college students, although the studies done thus far in student populations have been very important in establishing a baseline. Unfortunately, prospective studies and RCTs are difficult to conduct and can be very expensive to conduct well. Therefore, researchers in some of the more wealthy Muslim (or Western) countries, where funding support is available, should probably take the lead.

Chronic Mental Disorders. There is a tremendous need for research on the effects of religiosity on chronic mental or psychiatric disorders, including bipolar disorder, schizophrenia, and other chronic psychotic disorders. We could locate only three studies that examined religiosity in Muslim psychiatric patients (Salib and Youakim 2001; Suhail and Ghauri 2010; Amr et al. 2013). All were cross-sectional, and two out of the three found that psychiatric illness was significantly worse in those who were more religious. Thus, we have no information on how these relationships came about over time, i.e., did religious involvement cause a worsening of the psychiatric illness, or did these patients turn to religion for comfort and hope in the midst of their suffering? Again, prospective studies are needed to sort out the order of effects and provide information about the direction of causality.

Emotional Disorders in Older Adults. Although most Muslim-majority countries have relatively young populations, this is changing fast. As these countries are improving public health measures and availability of medical care, their populations are already beginning to age. With advancing age comes chronic illness and challenges related to loss of loved ones and friends and loss of the ability to work and contribute, and to increasing dependency on others, and this, in turn, can lead to lack of meaning and purpose in life. In developed countries such as Saudi Arabia, for example, one national study of adults over age 60 found that 39 % experienced significant depressive symptoms (Al-Shammari and Al-Subaie 1999). Older adults are particularly likely to find comfort in their religious beliefs. However, only one study in the entire scientific literature has examined the relationship between religiosity and depression or suicide in older Muslims (Chaaya et al. 2007). Likewise, only one study has examined religiosity and anxiety in Muslims where a majority of the sample was over age 60, and this study was conducted in Israel (a non-majority Muslim country) (Azaiza et al. 2010). Both studies above were cross-sectional, and both studies reported a significant positive relationship with religiosity (i.e., lower depression/suicide and lower anxiety in those who were more religious).

Happiness and Well-Being. The seeking of positive emotions is what drives almost everything that humans do. Research in adult populations is needed that examines the role of religiosity in generating positive emotions such as happiness, well-being, joy, meaning and purpose, optimism and hope, and other experiences that make life worth living. Again, prospective studies are especially needed to determine whether Islamic beliefs and practices might actually increase positive emotions over time. All studies so far have been cross-sectional in design.

Response to Treatment. Studies are needed that examine how religiosity influences treatment response in those with mental or emotional disorders. Do those who are more religious improve more quickly to conventional therapies and does that response last longer? For example, do depressed religious patients treated with antidepressant medication respond more quickly to the medication than do nonreligious depressed patients? Similarly, do conventional or secular psychotherapies for anxiety disorder resolve anxiety more quickly in those who are religious compared to those who are not? There is some evidence that this is true in Christian patients (Bowen et al. 2006), but no studies have yet examined the interaction between conventional therapies and religiosity in Muslim patients. This kind of study would not cost much. A brief measure of religiosity could be administered at baseline in a RCT conducted for some other purpose (i.e., examining the effectiveness of a conventional medication or psychotherapy), and then the effects of the intervention could be compared in religious and nonreligious patients. "Piggybacking" religious measures onto existing studies is one of the most cost-effective ways of conducting research on religion and health.

Social Health

Social health involves high levels of social support from family and friends, marital stability, low rates of crime/delinquency, and high social capital as indicated by robust levels of community engagement and trust. Social health is crucial for both individual and community health. A total of 32 studies (31 cross-sectional in design) have now examined religiosity and social health in Muslims. Although the vast majority reports positive findings, we still don't really understand what these findings mean. The only prospective study performed thus far was conducted in adolescents aged 13–15 (French et al. 2011), so we know nothing about how religiosity influences social health over time in Muslim adults. Given the importance of social health to the stability and flourishing of communities and nations, especially during this time of social unrest ("Arab spring"), studies are needed to determine how religiosity affects social health over time. Does greater religiosity increase or decrease social trust and community engagement? No well-designed prospective studies have yet been conducted that would allow us to even speculate in this regard (beyond adolescence).

Behavioral Health

There are several areas of religion and behavioral health that need more intensive study in Muslim populations. First, our research found that compared to non-Muslims, Muslims tend to be less physically active and may not always consume a healthy diet and maintain a healthy body weight, factors which could influence physical health and susceptibility to disease, especially chronic disease (see Table 12.2). Second, research thus far suggests that religiosity if anything is associated with less physical exercise, worse diet, and mixed findings with regard to body weight (see Table 10.1). Thus, given the impact of these health behaviors on maintaining health as people age, research is urgently needed to better understand why these patterns exist. Future cross-sectional and prospective studies are needed that carefully control for confounding variables (age, ethnicity, gender, education, socioeconomic status) and then determine if these findings continue to persist. Once more information about these associations is known, then faith-based interventions might be developed to educate religious communities about the importance of diet, exercise, and maintaining an ideal body weight for both physical health and spiritual health. Failure to reverse this trend, as Muslim populations age and poor health behaviors contribute more and more to the development of disabling chronic illnesses, could have dramatic effects on the cost of health services in the future.

Of particular importance are studies that examine the effects of religiosity during youth on preventing the development of cigarette smoking, alcohol or drug use, sexual immorality, and unhealthy habits involving food consumption and sedentary lifestyles. As Western influences permeate the youth culture through the Internet, movies, videos, and popular music, and traditionally Islamic countries begin to "modernize" and secularize, how will the decline in religious beliefs, behaviors, and values influence the health habits of young people in Islamic societies? Research studies are needed to document and track these changes so that preparations can be made to deal with the consequences (or efforts made to alter these health behaviors through education and public policy changes).

Physical Health

Perhaps the area of highest priority where future research on religiosity needs to focus is on physical health. With regard to the research on religiosity and physical health up through 2013 that we reviewed in Chap. 11, only 46 studies were identified (see Table 10.1). Of those studies, 27 (59 %) were on the effects of Ramadan, leaving only 19 studies in the world literature that examined the effects of religiosity per se on heart disease, inflammation/coagulation, hypertension, cerebrovascular disease, dementia, diabetes, cholesterol, immune function, endocrine function, cancer, self-rated health, and mortality. To our knowledge, only one study each has been conducted on religiosity and heart disease, diabetes, cholesterol, dementia, and overall mortality, whereas no studies at all have examined religiosity and cerebrovascular disease, immune function, endocrine function, or cancer in Muslims. Given the importance of Islamic beliefs and practices to mental, social, and behavioral health, factors known to influence physical health and longevity, how can this area of research remain unexamined in Muslims around the world? This is a huge research gap that needs filling. We discuss here only studies with the greatest relevance to public health, although given the lack of research in the area more generally, almost any study on religiosity and physical health would make a significant contribution.

Heart Disease. Heart disease is the number one killer and greatest cause of disability worldwide. Research that examines the effects of religiosity on this disease in Muslims, then, should receive immediate attention. Many questions need answering. First, is religiosity associated with more or less heart disease, and what aspects of religiosity in Muslims are most likely responsible? The only study to date by Burazeri and colleagues (2008) is a case–control study, and while that study is a place to start, more needs to be done. Similar cross-sectional studies are needed in large population-based samples to confirm the positive relationships reported by that research group, and these should be followed by prospective studies that allow researchers to determine whether religious involvement is serving to reduce heart disease risk or vice versa. Information from these observational studies will help to predict the need for health services in the future as the effects of modernization and secularization are increasingly felt. Ultimately, the goal is to identify and test religious interventions (educational or otherwise) that might reduce the risk of heart disease or improve its course over time, including its impact on disability.

Metabolic Disorders. Given the high prevalence of diabetes and lipid disorders in Muslim populations and their strong relationship to cardiovascular and cerebrovascular disease, further research is needed on the impact of religiosity on the development of diabetes and on its management. We already noted in Chap. 11 that the rate of diabetes among older adults in Saudi Arabia has increased from 18.7 % in 1982 to 26.0 % in 1997 among women (nearly a 40 % increase) and from 11.0 to 22.0 % in men (a 100 % increase) (Nielsen 1999). Poor lipid profiles (high cholesterol and triglycerides) are also thought to be responsible for the high rate of cardiovascular disease in East Asians living in the UK (McKeigue et al. 1991) and in Arabs immigrating to the USA as their diets have westernized. For these reasons, understanding the role of religiosity in the development and management of metabolic disorders such as diabetes and hypercholesterolemia in Muslim populations is of crucial importance.

Cancer. As noted in Chap. 11, cancer is the second leading cause of death in high-income countries after heart disease. The same kinds of studies described for heart disease and metabolic disorders are needed for religiosity and cancer, especially cancers that are likely to be influenced by psychosocial factors and health behaviors. These include cancers of the lung, pancreas, stomach, breast, and colon and possibly cancers of the blood or immune system (leukemia, lymphoma). Since not a single study in Muslims has yet examined the relationship between religiosity and any aspect of cancer (development, course, or treatment), these studies are a high priority.

Neurological Disorders. According to the World Health Organization (2011a), cerebrovascular diseases such as stroke and stroke-related dementia are the second most common cause of death and disability worldwide, having only slightly less of an impact than ischemic heart disease. In fact, these disorders are the most common cause of death and disability in upper middle-income countries. No studies have yet examined religiosity and stroke in Muslims, and only one study has examined religiosity and dementia (and only within the past year, i.e., Inzelberg et al. 2013). Again, as Muslim populations age, disabling diseases like these will become more and more prevalent, requiring younger people to stay home and care for them rather than work outside the home. There is every reason to think that devout religious involvement in Muslims may help to prevent or slow the progression of dementia or cognitive decline with aging, as numerous prospective studies in Christians have shown (see Chap. 6).

Immune System Disorders. Medical disorders associated with either an underactive immune system (i.e., HIV/AIDS) or an overactive one (i.e., rheumatological diseases) are widespread in both developing and developed countries. This is especially true for HIV/AIDS in low-income countries, where this disease is the second most common cause of death worldwide (World Health Organization 2011b). Research in Christian populations suggests that not only does religiosity help to prevent HIV/AIDS (by influencing sexual behavior), but it also affects the progression of the disease (see Chap. 6). Although some studies have found that religious Muslims are less likely to contract HIV/AIDS (due to safer sexual practices), no studies have yet examined the effects of Islamic beliefs and practices on the progression of HIV/AIDS once it has developed. With one exception (Yilmaz et al. 2008), studies on religiosity and rheumatological diseases are also lacking in Muslim populations, and such research will become increasingly important as Muslim populations age and inflammatory disorders (e.g., rheumatoid arthritis, osteoarthritis, psoriasis, connective tissue diseases) become more prevalent and disabling.

Other Stress-Related Diseases. Stress-related diseases other than those mentioned above include conditions such as asthma, peptic ulcer disease, inflammatory bowel disease, chronic fatigue syndrome, and other diseases that psychological and social factors are known to influence. These conditions are prevalent in Muslim populations and cause much suffering and distress. Religious involvement likely has positive influences on psychological and social factors that underlie or exacerbate these diseases, although no research to our knowledge has examined this possibly in Muslims.

Physical Disability. If a person lives long enough, increasing physical disability and dependency is the result of many disorders discussed above. As noted earlier, caring for chronically ill disabled populations in the future has the potential to bankrupt many developing and developed Muslim countries, causing a tremendous drain on already scarce resources. However, the actual level of disability and a person's perception of their disability may not always be the same. People who are anxious, depressed, and/or have no meaning or hope often perceive their disability as much greater than it actually is, resulting in greater dependency and increased use of health services. Research in Christian populations has found that religious involvement may actually reduce the perception of disability and help to prevent the progression of disability that occurs with increasing age and chronic disease. To our knowledge, however, no studies in Muslims have examined this effect of religious activity.

Mortality. One of the best ways to demonstrate that religious involvement has an effect on health is to determine if religious people live longer. A big surprise in our current review of the research was that only one study has examined the effects of religiosity on mortality in Muslim populations, and that study (Lerch et al. 2010) only compared those with and without a religious affiliation in Switzerland. There is vast opportunity, then, to examine whether or not Islamic beliefs and practices influence longevity. What is needed is a prospective study that assesses religious involvement at baseline, along with factors such as age, gender, education, ethnicity, and other characteristics related to both religiosity and mortality, and follows individuals over time until a significant proportion of the sample has died. Over 120 such studies have been conducted thus far in Christian populations, with the vast majority (especially the higher-quality studies) finding lower mortality among those who are more religious (see Chap. 6).

Interactions with Biological Treatments. We already noted the importance of examining how religiosity influences responses to current mental health treatments. The same applies to how religion affects responses to medication, surgery, radiation therapy, and other biological therapies used to treat a wide range of medical diseases. For example, to what extent (if any) does a Muslim's religious faith influence the speed at which an infection responds to antibiotics, a cancer responds to chemotherapy, high blood pressure responds to antihypertensive agents, or coronary artery disease responses to agents use to prevent or treat it. Almost no research exists in either Christian or Muslim populations on this interaction, despite its importance.

The speed at which an infection responds to antibiotics or a wound heals after surgery/trauma depends on healthy immune and cardiovascular systems, both of which are influenced by psychosocial stress. If religious involvement helps to reduce stress and improve coping, then it might also lead to a more rapid healing response. Religiosity may also decrease the side effects of biological treatments such as chemotherapy, as some research in Christian populations is beginning to show (Lissoni et al. 2008a, b). Again, there are numerous clinical trials now going on in many Muslim countries, and it would be very inexpensive to simply add a few questions on religiosity to the baseline evaluation. No additional resources would be needed, except the time to analyze the data and write up the results.

Faith-Based Interventions. Given problems with obesity, poor diet, sedentary activity, and late detection of treatable diseases such as hypertension, diabetes, and cancer in the USA, faith-based interventions within religious communities are a growing phenomenon in this and other Western countries. Such programs rely heavily on health education that takes place in religious congregations during or after worship services. The programs often involve members of the congregation exercising together while praying or perhaps dieting as a group (and holding each other accountable for eating habits). These programs have become particularly widespread in minority communities where health disparities are a serious problem. Researchers are now beginning to study and refine such faith-based interventions (see *Handbook of Religion and Health*, Koenig et al. 2012, pp. 918–923). With few exceptions (Al-Krenawi and Graham, 1997), such programs have yet to be developed or tested in Muslim congregations, although there is no reason why this could not be done.

Other Research Areas. There are many other potential research studies needed and, while of lower priority than the studies described above, are nevertheless important for the development of our understanding of how religiosity may impact health in Islamic societies.

Physiological Functions. No studies have examined religiosity and immune, endocrine, or other physiological functions in Muslim populations. Indicators of immune function of particular interest are natural killer cell activity, lymphocyte proliferation, t-lymphocyte cell numbers, pro- and anti-inflammatory markers (cytokines), and responses to immunization. Unfortunately, many of these immune indicators are expensive to measure, with the exception of cytokine levels in blood. Similarly, stress hormones such as cortisol, epinephrine, norepinephrine, growth hormone, and prolactin, as well as centrally acting neurotransmitters such as serotonin and dopamine, are known to modulate immune and cardiovascular responses and to be influenced by psychological and social stressors. Several of these substances can be measured in urine or saliva at relatively low cost. Other physiological markers of interest are those related to cardiovascular health, and include C-reactive protein and fibrinogen (predictors of coronary artery disease), endothelial function (predictor of vascular disease in general), heart rate variability, blood pressure reactivity (predictor cardiovascular and cerebrovascular outcomes), and carotid artery thickness (associated with risk of stroke and dementia). A major reason for doing these studies is to identify biological mechanisms to explain religion's effects on health. If physiological mechanisms can be established, then it is much more likely that mainstream scientists in the Islamic world will begin to study religiosity (or the lack thereof) as a standard risk factor for disease. This would contribute immensely to the field in general and research on Islam and health in particular.

The Aging Process. As emphasized over and over again here, Islamic societies are rapidly aging due to improvements in healthcare and public health measures. For example, in Saudi Arabia the life expectancy at birth was 74 years in 2010. Population projections indicate that persons over age 60 will increase from 5 % of the population in 2010 to nearly 20 % by 2050 (Mirkin 2010). Even a wealthy country like Saudi Arabia is not prepared to deal with the healthcare needs that will be required by this demographic. There is growing evidence from Western countries, however, that psychosocial stressors and negative emotions may actually affect the aging process itself, speeding up aging at the cellular level (measurable by assessing telomere length) (Epel et al. 2004). Positive emotions, on the other hand, may have the opposite effect. Research in Christian populations has shown that religiosity is related to lower levels of inflammatory cytokines, which ordinarily increase with age, increase a person's susceptibility to age-related diseases, and speed the rate at which cells age (Koenig et al. 1997; Lutgendorf et al. 2004). Thus, there is solid rationale for expecting that devout Islamic beliefs and regular religious practices might help to slow down the aging process and decrease the risk of age-related chronic disease.

Genetic Influences. Genetic factors are now known to influence the onset and course of many medical illnesses, and research in genomics is now one of the hottest areas of research around the world. Regulator genes are known to turn genes on and off and thereby increase or decrease the production of proteins necessary for organ functioning and human survival. Different forms of these regulator genes (called polymorphisms) exist within the population. In psychiatry, the most well-known polymorphism is that of the promoter region of serotonin transporter gene. Individuals with one or two copies of the short form of this gene are more susceptible to depression in the presence of stressful life events (Caspi et al. 2003). Given the relationship between religiosity and survival, certain gene polymorphisms may have been selected over time that make persons more prone to become religious. While largely theoretical at this time, there is some evidence that religious involvement may be influenced (not determined, but influenced) by genetic factors (Dew and Koenig 2013).

No research has been conducted in Muslim populations to determine whether certain genetic polymorphisms might influence either the likelihood of devout religious involvement or the susceptibility to mental disorders such as depression or physical disorders such as diabetes. Furthermore, nothing is known about how Islamic beliefs and practices might delay or prevent the switching on or off of genes responsible for chronic diseases common in Muslims. These are cutting-edge areas of research in molecular biology for which funding support may be available, at least for traditional genetic research. However, it would be easy and very inexpensive to piggyback religious variables onto such studies by including them in baseline questionnaires.

Summary and Conclusions

Thus far, research has barely scratched the surface of the relationship between religiosity and health in Muslim populations. The result is that there are limitless opportunities for researchers to make seminal contributions in this area. Many aspects of religiosity and health that are crucial to the survival and flourishing of Islamic societies remain completely unexplored. For example, no studies have examined the relationship between religiosity and chronic mental disorders such as bipolar disorder in adults or attention deficit disorder in children. Only one study has examined the relationship between religiosity and heart disease. Only one study has explored how religiosity affects the development or course of diabetes in Muslims. Only one study has analyzed how religiosity affects survival and only in the most rudimentary way. No studies exist today on religiosity and cancer. Muslims today with the research training and academic position to conduct cutting-edge research on religiosity and health have not done so. Perhaps this is because their professional training has taught them to keep their religious beliefs and professional lives separate. We hope that this volume will help excite and prepare investigators to begin focusing more attention on this highly promising and potentially beneficial area of research that could affect the lives of Muslims worldwide.

References

Al-Krenawi, A., & Graham, J. R. (1997). Nebi-Musa: A therapeutic community for drug addicts in a Muslim context. *Transcultural Psychiatry, 34*, 377–391.

Al-Shammari, S. A., & Al-Subaie, A. (1999). Prevalence and correlates of depression among Saudi elderly. *International Journal of Geriatric Psychiatry, 14*, 739–747.

Amr, M., El-Mogy, A., & El-Masry, R. (2013). Adherence in Egyptian patients with schizophrenia: The role of insight, medication beliefs and spirituality. *The Arab Journal of Psychiatry, 24*(1), 60–68.

Azaiza, F., Ron, P., Shoham, M., & Gigini, I. (2010). Death and dying anxiety among elderly Arab Muslims in Israel. *Death Studies, 34*, 351–364.

Bowen, R., Baetz, M., & D'Arcy, C. (2006). Self-rated importance of religion predicts one-year outcome of patients with panic disorder. *Depression and Anxiety, 23*(5), 266–273.

Burazeri, G., Goda, A., Roshi, E., & Kark, J. D. (2008). Religious affiliation and acute coronary syndrome: A population-based case-control study in Tirana, Albania. *European Journal of Public Health, 18*(3), 329–334.

Caspi, A., Sugden, K., Moffitt, T. E., Taylor, A., Craig, I. W., Harrington, H., et al. (2003). Influence of life stress on depression: Moderation by a polymorphism in the 5-HTT gene. *Science, 301*, 386–389.

Chaaya, M., Sibai, A., Fayad, R., & El-Roueiheb, Z. (2007). Religiosity and depression in older people: Evidence from underprivileged refugee and non-refugee communities in Lebanon. *Aging & Mental Health, 11*(1), 37–44.

Dew, R. E., & Koenig, H. G. (2013). Religious involvement, the serotonin transporter promoter polymorphism, and drug use in young adults. *International Journal of Social Sciences Studies* 2(1), 98–104.

Epel, E. S., Blackburn, E. H., Lin, J., Dhabhar, F. S., Adler, N. E., Morrow, J. D., & Cawtrhorn, R. M. (2004). Accelerated telomere shortening in response to life stress. *Proceedings of the National Academy of Sciences, 101*, 17312–17315.

French, D. C., Purwono, U., & Triwahyuni, A. (2011). Friendship and the religiosity of Indonesian Muslim adolescents. *Journal of Youth and Adolescence, 50*, 1623–1633.

Hamdan, A., & Tamim, H. (2011). Psychosocial risk and protective factors for postpartum depression in the United Arab Emirates. *Archives of Women's Mental Health, 14*, 124–133.

Inzelberg, R., Afgin, A. E., Massarwa, M., Schechtman, E., Israeli-Korn, S. D., Strugatsky, R., Abuful, A., Kravitz, E., Lindsay, A. F., & Friedland, R. P. (2013). Prayer at midlife is associated with reduced risk of cognitive decline in Arabic women. *Current Alzheimer Research, 10*(3), 340–346.

Koenig, H. G. (2011). *Spirituality and health research: Methods, measurement, statistics, and resources*. Conshohocken, PA: Templeton Foundation Press.

Koenig, H. G., Cohen, H. J., George, L. K., Hays, J. C., Larson, D. B., & Blazer, D. G. (1997). Attendance at religious services, interleukin-6, and other biological indicators of immune function in older adults. *International Journal of Psychiatry in Medicine, 27*, 233–250.

Koenig, H. G., King, D. E., & Carson, V. B. (2012). *Handbook of religion and health* (2nd ed.). New York: Oxford University Press.

Lerch, M., Oris, M., Wanner, P., Forney, Y., & Dutreuilh, C. (2010). Religious affiliation and mortality in Switzerland, 1991–2004. *Population, 65*(2), 217–250.

Lissoni, P., Messina, G., Balestra, A., Colciago, M., Brivio, F., Fumagalli, L., Fumagalli, G., & Parolini, D. (2008a). Efficacy of cancer chemotherapy in relation to synchronization of cortisol rhythm, immune status and psychospiritual profile in metastatic non-small cell lung cancer. *In Vivo, 22*(2), 257–262.

Lissoni, P., Messina, G., Parolini, D., Balestra, A., Brivio, F., & Fumagalli, L. (2008b). A spiritual approach in the treatment of cancer: Relation between faith score and response to chemotherapy in advanced non-small cell lung cancer patients. *In Vivo, 22*(5), 577–582.

Lopez, A. D., & Murray, C. C. (1998). The global burden of disease, 1990–2020. *Nature Medicine, 4*, 1241–1243.

Lutgendorf, S. K., Russell, D., Ullrich, P., Harris, T. B., & Wallace, R. (2004). Religious participation, interleukin-6, and mortality in older adults. *Health Psychology, 23*(5), 465–475.

McKeigue, P. M., Shah, B., & Marmot, M. G. (1991). Relation of central obesity and insulin resistance with high diabetes prevalence and cardiovascular risk in South Asians. *Lancet, 337*, 382–386.

Mirkin, B. (2010). Population levels, trends and policies in the Arab region. Challenges and opportunities. United National Development Programme, Regional Bureau of Arab States, Arab Human Development Report (p. 33). Retrieved October 6, 2013, from http://www.arab-hdr.org/publications/other/ahdrps/paper01-en.pdf

Nielsen, J. V. (1999). Diabetes in the Arab world: Prevalence and risk factors. *Practical Diabetes International, 16*(3), 82–86.

Salib, E., & Youakim, S. (2001). Spiritual healing in elderly psychiatric patients: A case-control study in an Egyptian psychiatric hospital. *Aging & Mental Health, 5*(4), 366–370.

Suhail, K., & Ghauri, S. (2010). Phenomenology of delusions and hallucinations in schizophrenia by religious convictions. *Mental Health, Religion & Culture, 13*(3), 245–259.

World Health Organization (2011a). World health rankings: Stroke. Retrieved October 6, 2013, from http://www.worldlifeexpectancy.com/cause-of-death/stroke/by-country/

World Health Organization (2011b). The 10 top causes of death. Retrieved October 6, 2013, from http://who.int/mediacentre/factsheets/fs310/en/

Yilmaz, S., Kart-Koseoglu, H., Guler, O., & Yucel, E. (2008). Effect of prayer on osteoarthritis and osteoporosis. *Rheumatology International, 28*(5), 429–436.

Part III
Applications

In this section we begin to explore the practical applications of the research reviewed in earlier chapters. The following chapters are of great importance in that they illustrate why such research on religiosity and health is important for Muslims. In the first chapter, we focus on implications for the care of Muslim patients in healthcare settings such as hospitals, outpatient clinics, and long-term care facilities. In the second chapter, we speculate on what the research reviewed here means for the health and well-being of Muslims living in Islamic societies throughout the world. We also discuss the importance of Muslim–Christian relations on human survival and economic progress more generally. Some applications described here can and should be implemented immediately, whereas others will depend on further discussion and future research to help guide the next steps.

Chapter 14
Applications in Clinical Practice

Based on the research reviewed on religiosity and health in Muslim populations and on extrapolations from what is known about the importance of spiritual needs during illness in Christian populations, we discuss practical applications to the care of Muslim patients in healthcare settings. The focus is on why and how to integrate spirituality into the routine care of patients with physical or mental illness. We first provide the rationale for doing so and then describe how such integration might be accomplished. We now switch our terminology from talking about "religion" to discussing issues in terms of "spirituality." First, however, we explain the reasons for this change in language.

The Language of Spirituality

Much of the research in previous chapters was discussed using the term religion, since most of the interpretable research conducted thus far has been measuring religious beliefs and practices. This is especially true for research focused on religion and health in Muslim populations (see definitions, Chap. 6). When applying this research, however, we switch from the language of religion to that of *spirituality*. The primary reason for doing so is that spirituality today is understood in much broader terms than religion. When addressing these issues with patients coming from a wide range of different religious traditions (even within Islam), it is important to use a more neutral language that everyone can relate to. For most Muslims, spirituality and religion will mean the same thing, so when health professionals speak about spiritual needs or take a spiritual history, patients will usually know what they are talking about and can apply it to their specific religious tradition.

We have learned a lot from mistakes trying to integrate spirituality into healthcare within Christian populations, where patients come from a wide range of religious traditions, even more so than in Islam. One lesson learned is that the process of integrating spirituality into patient care must begin with the patient. In other

H.G. Koenig and S. Al Shohaib, *Health and Well-Being in Islamic Societies: Background, Research, and Applications*, DOI 10.1007/978-3-319-05873-3_14,

words, the word "spiritual" means whatever the patient wants it to mean (which may differ from what the health professional means by spirituality). The task of the health professional is to learn how the patient understands this term and then address the patient's spiritual needs from that perspective. Indeed, given the highly personal nature of religious beliefs, there is no other sensible way to integrate spirituality into patient care in pluralistic healthcare settings where both patients and providers may come from different faith traditions (or have different views within the same faith tradition). Indeed, integrating spirituality is like the health professional and the patient engaged in a ballroom dance and in this dance, the patient always leads.

Why Integrate Spirituality

Many reasons exist for integrating spirituality into patient care, whether the illness is physical or mental. We describe seven reasons below:

1. *Many Patients Are Religious*. Most Muslim patients are religious and might wish their beliefs to be considered in their healthcare. For devout Muslims, Islamic beliefs and practices determine their worldview and serve as a guide for how they will act and will expect to be treated when they become sick. Spiritual beliefs will determine the kinds of treatments that are acceptable and those that are not. For example, a Muslim patient may not wish pain medication if he or she believes the pain and suffering is serving a higher purpose (either as a test of their faith or a way to purify their spiritual life). Likewise, Muslim patients may want to practice their religious faith when sick, and health professionals are obligated to create a healthcare environment in which this is possible. Religious activities may involve praying five times daily, reading and reciting the Qu'ran, or having an Imam or Islamic faith healer visit and perform healing rituals at the bedside. There are many religious and cultural practices that influence how Muslim patients wish to be cared for. Health professionals (particularly non-Muslim) must become knowledgeable about these practices and accommodate the healthcare environment to take them into account (see Koenig 2013, pp 265–268). Spiritual needs related to illness may also surface at this time, including spiritual struggles that can adversely affect physical health and response to treatment (Pargament et al. 2001). Not only do unmet spiritual needs decrease quality of life, they may significantly increase the cost of healthcare, particularly among those with advanced disease or terminal illness (Balboni et al. 2011).
2. *Religion Used to Cope*. When illness or misfortune strikes, as noted in Chap. 7, the vast majority of Muslims—whether adult patients, children, family members, trauma survivors, or even medical students—turn to religion to cope. Those who do so report that Islamic beliefs and practices help them to cope better, feel less sad, relieve anxiety, and enable them to relax and worry less. Given the adverse effects that depression and anxiety have on physiological functions (immune, endocrine, cardiovascular), effects known to adversely affect the healing

process, anything that helps patients to cope better and prevents or lessens emotional distress will improve their response to medical treatments. Thus, when health professionals support a Muslim patient's religious faith, this may have a direct bearing on the recovery process itself, as well as improve the bond of trust between patient and healthcare provider (Kristeller et al. 2005).

3. *Religion Affects Patients' Decisions.* The religious beliefs of Muslim patients often influence their medical decisions, may conflict with the views of the medical team, and could affect whether or not patients comply with treatment. Health professionals who are not open to discussing a patient's religious beliefs are at a distinct disadvantage, since they are forced to make medical decisions without knowing whether or not the patient will accept the treatment. The important role that religious beliefs play in medical decision-making has been well documented in Christian populations in the USA, particularly among patients with serious medical illness (Koenig 2013, pp 32–34). Research has shown that one of the most common reasons why patients (even adolescents) want to discuss their religious beliefs with physicians is because those beliefs impact decisions about their care.

4. *Religion Affects Physicians' Decisions.* The religious beliefs of physicians also influence decisions made about the kind of medical care they are willing to provide to patients, and this is often not acknowledged. This applies to many areas, including prescribing medication for pain or birth control, writing do-not-resuscitate (DNR) orders, withdrawing life support, referring patients for abortion, and, in some cases, even referring patients for organ transplants. Conservative religious beliefs influence many physician decisions that involve ethical or borderline ethical procedures. These beliefs are seldom discussed openly with patients and family members since religion is *supposed to be* kept separate from medicine (which is not possible to do in real practice). Furthermore, it may be quite important for some Muslim patients—especially those being treated for mental health issues—to know that their health professional shares their religious beliefs (Al-Solaim and Loewenthal 2011). Open discussion of such issues, then, becomes essential.

5. *Religion May Affect Health.* As noted in Part II of this book, Islamic beliefs and practices are related to a wide range of mental, social, behavioral, and physical health outcomes. To fail to address spiritual issues in clinical practice, then, ignores a major factor influencing patient health. This includes the medical outcomes of patients experiencing traumatic injuries or undergoing surgery, since psychological factors have a major influence on the speed of wound healing and susceptibility of the wound to infection (Kiecolt-Glaser et al. 1996). If religious beliefs were unrelated to health, then there would be no need for health professionals to address them. The research, however, shows otherwise.

6. *Religion Influences Support.* Islamic beliefs influence the amount and kind of support that Muslims receive from family members and the broader community. Devout beliefs (or more important, lack thereof) may affect how well Muslim patients are integrated within their family and wider support network. This could

influence the willingness of others to offer emotional support and even physical care to the patient when needed. Having a supportive community will ensure that medical care is provided in a timely fashion and that treatments will be complied with once prescribed (due to increased monitoring of the patient by family and friends). Health professionals, then, need to know whether patients have religious supports available to them when discharged back into the community.

7. *Meeting Healthcare Standards*. In the USA, the accreditation of healthcare organizations (hospitals, clinics, nursing homes, home health agencies) requires that patients' cultural and spiritual beliefs are respected and honored. Fulfilling this requirement is necessary for payment of services and is increasingly being monitored by government agencies (Koenig 2013, pp 43–45). This is especially true for areas of healthcare involving acute hospitalization, substance abuse treatment, and hospice care. The requirement that health professionals provide culturally competent care is also increasingly being implemented in Muslim countries (Al-Shahri, 2002). Providing culturally competent care is impossible without assessing religious beliefs that may be influencing that care.

How to Integrate Spirituality

How do health professionals integrate spirituality into patient care? This is relatively simple and not nearly as time-consuming as some might fear. Indeed, the two main barriers that keep health professionals from assessing and addressing spiritual issues are concerns about the extra time this will take and the lack of training on how to do so. Time is much less of an issue when health professionals know how to proceed.

Take Spiritual History. The most important task of the health professional is taking a spiritual history. Many spiritual history measures are available and have been used successfully in clinical practice. We recommend a spiritual history that gathers the information needed in as brief a time as possible and has the respect of other medical professionals. The spiritual history recommended here involves five short questions and has been published in the *Journal of the American Medical Association* (Table 14.1) (Koenig 2002). A spiritual history need not be taken on all patients. Those with a time-limited medical condition who are being treated as outpatients for minor trauma, a limited infection, minor procedure, or prenatal exam do not need a spiritual history. However, a spiritual history should be taken on patients being seen for the first time (initial evaluation), those being seen for a wellness visit (where time is often reserved to address family and psychosocial issues), patients being admitted to the hospital for serious medical illness or to a long-term care facility, patients with any chronic disabling illness, and those who are terminally ill. All psychiatric patients should have a spiritual history taken, given the relevance of religious issues to many psychiatric conditions (either helping patients to cope with the condition or contributing to the pathology itself). The best time to take a

Table 14.1 The spiritual history

1.	Do your religious or spiritual beliefs provide comfort and support or do they cause stress?
2.	How would these beliefs influence your medical decisions if you became really sick?
3.	Do you have any beliefs that might interfere or conflict with your medical care?
4.	Are you a member of a religious or spiritual community and is it supportive?
5.	Do you have any spiritual needs that someone should address?

Source: *Journal of the American Medical Association,* 288(4), p 490 (Koenig 2002)

spiritual history is during the social history, when the physician or nurse asks about whether the patient has family members and other sources of support.

At least one randomized clinical trial has examined the effects of taking a spiritual history. This study found that the spiritual history increased the length of the visit by about 2.1 min, was well received by both patients (mostly Christian) and physicians (two Christians, a Hindu, and a Sikh), and benefited both the doctor–patient relationship and the patient's quality of life (Kristeller et al. 2005). No research, to our knowledge, has examined the effects of taking a spiritual history with Muslim patients.

The spiritual history should be conducted by the physician in charge of the patient's care (primary care physician or the physician who admits the patient to the hospital), since the information gathered is necessary for making medical decisions. Physicians seldom read the notes of other providers like nurses or chaplains, so the spiritual history cannot be deferred to those health professionals. Besides providing information related to healthcare and medical decision-making, the spiritual history communicates to the patient that this is an area that he or she can discuss with the physician when necessary or relevant to healthcare. In the USA, only about 10 % of physicians regularly take a spiritual history from patients (Curlin et al. 2006). As a result, the task often falls to nurses or other health professionals. Consequently, this information almost never gets communicated to the physician. When a spiritual history is taken by nurses or other health professionals, the information typically acquired is seldom useful to the physician. Today in the USA, the spiritual history usually consists of checking a few boxes that indicate the patient's religious denomination and whether they wish to see a chaplain. This is not adequate, since it ignores the beliefs of patients related to coping with illness, medical decisions, or identification of spiritual needs that may be present.

Finally, before taking the spiritual history, the health professional should prepare the patient so as not to surprise him or her by these questions. Otherwise, such inquiry may unintentionally send the patient into a panic. In the past, the subject of religion or spirituality was only brought up when the patient was terminal and nothing else could be done and the clergy had to be brought in. Therefore, patients may misinterpret such questions to mean that they are extremely sick or dying. To avoid this, the health professional should state that these questions are routine and have nothing to do with the patient's medical condition or how serious it is, but rather is an attempt to be sensitive to religious or cultural factors that might influence the patient's care.

Document. Once the spiritual history is taken, it needs to be communicated to other healthcare providers so that they do not repeat the history. A brief note in the medical record should indicate that the spiritual history has been taken and that there are no issues relevant to the care of the patient or, alternatively, that spiritual needs have been identified and referral to a chaplain or pastoral counselor has been made.

Orchestrate Resources. After the spiritual history, the health professional will need to do something with the information learned. If unmet spiritual needs are present, then the health professional should ensure that those spiritual needs are addressed by someone. Examples of spiritual needs of Muslims might be the need for a prayer rug, information on the direction of Mecca, a copy of the Qu'ran, an Imam or Islamic healer contacted, or more complex spiritual needs that might involve spiritual struggles or doubts about their faith. In the latter case, Muslim patients would be referred to a chaplain or pastoral counselor (preferably Muslim) who is trained to address these issues. The non-chaplain health professional seldom has the knowledge or skill to address spiritual needs of this kind and should not attempt to do so.

Refer to Chaplain. The chaplain is a highly trained healthcare professional who in the USA is often considered a member of the healthcare team. After receiving the referral, the chaplain will conduct a comprehensive spiritual assessment (more detailed than the brief spiritual history the health professional takes) and will develop a treatment plan to address spiritual needs that are present. In some cases, the treatment plan will be documented in the medical record or shared with the medical team less formally (i.e., during medical rounds or during case presentations). The hospital chaplain may also develop a plan for addressing the patient's spiritual needs after discharge back home (especially if spiritual needs are not resolved at the time of discharge). The patient's Imam or other member of the religious community should not be contacted until after the chaplain has obtained explicit consent from the patient to do so. It is always important for the chaplain to honor the medical privacy of the patient.

Support Spiritual Beliefs. When taking the spiritual history, the health professional should do it in a manner that supports the patient's religious or spiritual beliefs, whatever those beliefs are. This is true even if beliefs appear to conflict with the treatment plan. This is not a time to try to change the patient's spiritual beliefs or argue with them over whether their beliefs are correct or not. The health professional's goal is to understand the patient's spiritual beliefs from the patient's perspective, and the spiritual history helps him or her to do that. If there is conflict with the medical plan, then the health professional should work with the chaplain to develop a plan to address the issue in a sensitive and nonconfrontational manner.

Supporting patients' beliefs can be done in several ways. First, all spiritual beliefs should be taken seriously, since these may be vital to the patient's coping and emotional stability. Second, when taking the spiritual history, the health professional should listen carefully and display physical signs of interest. This often involves nodding of the head and positive responses to what is being said, perhaps repeating or rephrasing what the patient has communicated so that it is clear that the health professional understands. Asking questions to learn more about the patient's beliefs (not challenge them) often indicates support and interest.

Consider Spiritual Intervention. The only time a spiritual intervention should be considered is if requested by the patient. For example, the Muslim patient may wish the health professional to join them in performing one of the five daily prayers. This is acceptable if it appears that such an action will bring comfort to the patient. In some instances, the patient may even wish the health professional to pray out loud for them at the bedside or in the office (more common for Christian patients). Such requests for prayer will likely be less common from Muslim patients, where intercession to God by the health professional may not be acceptable. Alternatively, a Muslim patient might request that the health professional read a verse or ayah from the Qur'an, one that is encouraging or has healing properties (as the Prophet would recite when he was sick—see Chap. 3). However, the health professional should not agree to any such request until a thorough spiritual history has been taken. In the unlikely event that a Muslim patient asks for prayer, the health professional should always inquire about what the patient wants prayer for, so that prayers can be directed as the patient wishes. Likewise, if asked to recite a verse from the Qur'an, the health professional should ask the patient to choose the verse. If the health professional feels uncomfortable praying with the patient or reading a verse from the Qur'an, then one alternative is to ask the patient to pray or to read the verse while remaining with the patient in a supportive manner. Such spiritual interventions can be very powerful but also should be done carefully and according to guidelines. For a more detailed discussion, see Koenig (2013, pp 88–94).

Work with Religious Community. Health professionals can also volunteer to provide health education to local religious communities. This accomplishes several goals. First, it will help to educate persons in the faith community about common health problems and important screening tests and provide information about diet and exercise to identify and prevent future health problems. Second, such education will inform members of the religious community when it is necessary to seek healthcare services themselves and when to encourage loved ones to do likewise. Third, it will provide guidance to members of the faith community on how to support and care for patients with medical problems after they return home from the hospital. Such interactions will help to optimize the health of religious community members and ensure that those who are sick receive adequate monitoring and follow-up.

Limitations

There are also limitations in what health professionals should do when taking a spiritual history or addressing patients' spiritual needs. We would encourage all health professionals to avoid the following, which may violate a patient's human rights because of the psychological vulnerability that patients experience when ill.

Prescribe Religion. Although much research has found a positive association between Islamic beliefs or practices and health, health professionals should never prescribe religion to nonreligious patients, attempt to convert patients to their own religious beliefs, or try to change or alter patients' religious beliefs. As indicated earlier, this is true even when religious beliefs conflict with medical care. This is a highly sensitive area, especially for Muslims who take their religion seriously, so health professionals should always respect and honor these beliefs. This includes honoring the absence of religious beliefs as well if patients should indicate that this is not an important area of their lives.

Force a Spiritual History. Never force a spiritual history if it is clear that the patient is not religious and has no interest in religion. When that becomes evident, the health professional should engage the patient in a broader discussion of what gives life meaning and purpose in the setting of his or her medical illness. Further discussion of spiritual or religious issues should not be pursued. However, if the patient is being treated for mental health problems, the mental health professional may later come back to the topic after a therapeutic relationship has been established. The reason is because religious issues are often related to the mental health problem. When readdressing the issue, especially if the patient has shown resistance or discomfort when asked before, the mental health professional should proceed gently, sensitively, and be guided by cues from the patient.

Coerce Patients to Believe or Practice. There are no circumstances in which health professionals should coerce or force nonreligious (or even religious) patients to believe or practice, or argue with patients about religious issues. In rare instances, the health professional may gently suggest that religious practices could be helpful to the patient, particularly when conventional treatments have been ineffective and the patient has previously shown interest in religion (determined from the spiritual history). However, if the medical patient shows any resistance or discomfort to such suggestions, the subject should be dropped and not pursued further.

Pray with Patients Unless Asked. Health professionals should not pray with or conduct any spiritual intervention with patients (recite from the Qur'an, refer to a religious professional, provide other religious resources, etc.) unless the patient initiates the request. Physicians or nurses should not ask patients if they want to pray, because if not wanted, patients may not feel free to refuse prayer or other religious activity with a health professional who they depend on for healthcare. When it is clear from the spiritual history that the patient is religious and that prayer is important, the health professional may gently inform the patient that he or she is willing to pray, recite the Qur'an, or do other religious activity with patients if this is something the patient wants. In that case, the patient can *later* initiate a request for prayer (or other acceptable Muslim religious practice) if desired.

Spiritually Counsel Patients. Unless health professionals have specific religious training (i.e., is a chaplain or pastoral counselor), they should usually not counsel or provide advice to patients regarding Islamic beliefs or practices. Such advice should always be left up to religious professionals. In some cases, however, patients may be reluctant to talk with a religious professional or refuse referral to a chaplain, yet may be struggling with spiritual issues that someone needs to address. In those circumstances, the health professional should either convince the patient to see a chaplain or, if necessary, take a little extra time with the patient to listen and try to understand the patient's spiritual struggle, without trying to fix it by offering advice. Health professionals should realize that simply listening to patients verbalize their religious struggles is immensely helpful and by itself makes it easier for patients to work through these issues on their own.

Any Activity Not Patient Centered. In general, the health professional should not attempt to implement any spiritual interventions that are not patient centered and patient directed. The patient needs to feel safe and be in complete control of such activity. As emphasized previously, instead of controlling and directing, health professionals should seek to *understand*, relying on the patient to inform them. Recall what we said earlier. Assessing and addressing spiritual issues with patients is like a dance, where the health professional lets the patient lead the dance and tries not to step on their toes.

Health professionals who follow the above guidelines will seldom run into trouble when addressing spiritual issues with patients. Instead, they will find that doing so is a personally rewarding experience and is often of great benefit to patients. For a more in-depth discussion of integrating spirituality into patient care, the reader is referred elsewhere (Koenig 2013).

Summary and Conclusions

Both common sense and growing evidence from research suggest that health professionals should assess Muslim patients for religious or spiritual needs, particularly those with serious, chronic, or terminal illnesses, and ensure that those needs are addressed by someone. Islamic cultural and religious beliefs influence the type of healthcare that Muslims wish to receive when they are sick. Health professionals should take a brief spiritual history, identify spiritual needs related to illness, and mobilize resources to meet those needs. Honoring and respecting patients' religious beliefs is essential, even when there is conflict between those beliefs and medical treatments. When complex spiritual needs are present, Muslim patients should be referred to a chaplain or pastoral counselor (preferably Muslim) who is trained to address these issues. The goal of the health professional is to try to understand and appreciate the role that patients' religious beliefs play in their illness, which usually involves taking the time to listen. There are also clear boundaries across which health professionals should not step. A good rule of thumb is that any activity by health professionals in this sensitive area should be patient centered and patient directed. Finally, we emphasize that the recommendations made here must be adapted to the particular Islamic beliefs and practices of patients, and these will vary from country to country and even from region to region within each country.

References

Al-Shahri, M. Z. (2002). Culturally sensitive caring for Saudi patients. *Journal of Transcultural Nursing, 13*(2), 133–138.

Al-Solaim, L., & Loewenthal, K. M. (2011). Religion and obsessive-compulsive disorder (OCD) among young Muslim women in Saudi Arabia. *Mental Health, Religion and Culture, 14*(2), 169–182.

Balboni, T., Balboni, M., Paulk, M. E., Phelps, A., Wright, A., Peteet, J., et al. (2011). Support of cancer patients' spiritual needs and associations with medical care costs at the end of life. *Cancer, 117*(23), 5383–5391.

Curlin, F. A., Chin, M. H., Sellergren, S. A., Roach, C. J., & Lantos, J. D. (2006). The association of physicians' religious characteristics with their attitudes and self-reported behaviors regarding religion and spirituality in the clinical encounter. *Medical Care, 44*(5), 446–453.

Kiecolt-Glaser, J. K., Marucha, P. T., Malarkey, W. B., Mercado, A. M., & Glaser, R. (1996). Slowing of wound healing by psychological stress. *Lancet, 346*(8984), 1194–1196.

Koenig, H. G. (2002). An 83-year-old woman with chronic illness and strong religious beliefs. *Journal of the American Medical Association, 288*(4), 487–493.

Koenig, H. G. (2013). *Spirituality in patient care* (3rd ed.). Conshohocken, PA: Templeton Foundation Press.

Kristeller, J. L., Rhodes, M., Cripe, L. D., & Sheets, V. (2005). Oncologist Assisted Spiritual Intervention Study (OASIS): Patient acceptability and initial evidence of effects. *International Journal of Psychiatry in Medicine, 35*(4), 329–347.

Pargament, K. I., Koenig, H. G., Tarakeshwar, N., & Hahn, J. (2001). Religious struggle as a predictor of mortality among medically ill elderly patients: A two-year longitudinal study. *Archives of Internal Medicine, 161*, 1881–1885.

Chapter 15
Implications for Public Health

With few exceptions, Islamic beliefs and practices are associated with better mental health, including less depression, lower anxiety, less substance abuse, greater well-being, and higher life satisfaction. They are likewise associated with better social health, such as more social support, greater marital stability, and less delinquency or crime. Several positive health behaviors, including less cigarette smoking and more conservative sexual practices, are more common among Muslims who are more religious. Finally, Islamic beliefs and practices are related to better physical health, such as less heart disease, lower blood pressure and, in some studies, less cognitive impairment and lower mortality.

Should future research confirm and extend these health benefits of religious practice, such findings will have important implications for Islamic societies—serious implications that bear on the future health and productivity of many Muslim-majority countries. We now speculate on what these implications might be at the population level.

Positive Implications

The findings presented in this book should be encouraging to those who devoutly adhere to Islamic beliefs and practices and should affirm what people have instinctively known and passed down from generation to generation over literally thousands of years. Furthermore, the research reviewed here and research in the future may help to identify spiritual interventions that complement conventional treatments in medicine and psychology. The result could be more effective and more cost-efficient healthcare that addresses the needs of the mind, body, and spirit, with benefits for both patients and healthcare providers. This research may also provide important information for those who are religious but not devout practitioners of the Islamic faith, who may value and respect the latest findings from scientific studies, studies that seek to objectively examine these relationships. Such individuals may

H.G. Koenig and S. Al Shohaib, *Health and Well-Being in Islamic Societies: Background, Research, and Applications*, DOI 10.1007/978-3-319-05873-3_15,

be striving to live fuller, more satisfying and meaningful lives and are open to new ideas and direction. This research may even be relevant to those who are completely secular causing them to pause and reconsider whether religion really has no value or place in society. If the research accomplishes any of these goals, then an important result may be that sacred traditions are maintained and societies flourish as the advances of modern medicine add to (rather than replace) the rich cultural and religious heritage that Islamic societies now possess.

Negative Implications

If these research findings are ignored and not followed up on by future studies that examine the health benefits and risks of devout Islamic belief and practice, then this too may have consequences. The relatively young Islamic societies in the world today will continue to age over time, with each generation of youth living longer than the previous generation as medical care and public health measures improve. This means that many young Muslims today could live well into their 70s and 80s and will have to deal with age-related illnesses that cause increasing disability and loss of independence. Secular trends, as occurring in Europe and the West, will also likely influence Islamic societies over the ensuing decades. Increasing secularization means that the potentially "protective" effects of Islamic beliefs and practices on psychological, social, behavioral, and physical health may gradually decrease as the populace takes on modern values and beliefs. If—as we have found—religious beliefs and practices preserve health and enhance the flourishing of Islamic societies, then their decline and loss of influence may have the opposite effect: increasing drug/alcohol use and abuse, delinquency and crime, marital instability, sexually transmitted diseases, and less self-care and self-control resulting in more chronic illness. One might easily imagine increased costs needed to maintain social order (previously provided naturally by religious values and commitments). Likewise, increased costs might result from the need to provide healthcare to an aging chronically ill population suffering the consequences of smoking, drinking, drug dependence, a sedentary slovenly lifestyle, sexual promiscuity, and other unhealthy behaviors that religious traditions have long discouraged.

Healthcare costs could also be affected by an increasing number of older adults being single and without family support due to broken marital relationships, as increasingly now seen in the West, where the two-parent family is becoming less and less the norm. According to the National Marriage Project (2012), in 2011 less than two-thirds of children in the USA had two parents living with them in the same household (compared to 85 % in 1960). Similarly, over 40 % of babies were born out of wedlock (compared to 5 % in 1960). Finally, only about 50 % of adults aged 15 or older were married (compared to closer to 70 % in 1960), and most couples are now choosing to have only one or two children. In Europe, according to Eurostat (2013), extramarital births now account for the majority of live births in Estonia (58 %), Slovenia (57 %), Norway (57 %), Sweden (54 %), France (56 %), and Iceland (65 %). Single-parent homes often result in the government having to pay for the care these children need through expensive social service programs. It is no secret that European countries are now experiencing serious financial problems as they attempt to support aging populations in an increasingly secular society.

Economic resources will have to come from somewhere to provide social control (pay for more police, build more prisons), pay for healthcare of the chronically ill, and support children and their single-parent caregivers. Most likely, these financial resources will be diverted from budgets for defense, research and development, and other key government programs necessary to keep a nation strong and competitive in the world marketplace. None of these pressures will come on suddenly, but rather will build up slowly over time as absolute moral values are replaced by relative values and as religiously conservative lifestyles are replaced by liberal lifestyles with few limitations or boundaries. Islamic countries should prepare for this if they allow the slow decline of sacred religious traditions that for centuries have held the social fabric of society intact.

The above considerations should cause pause for thought, if not incentive for the populations (and governments) of Muslim countries to make efforts now to preserve their Islamic beliefs, practices, and values and continue to instill them in their youth from an early age onward. Otherwise, where will the motivation come from to care for the poor, the elderly, and those less fortunate? Sacrificing one's own pleasures for the benefit of others does not come naturally and is difficult to legislate, especially when survival of the fittest is the primary rule that guides a people. Modernization does not always mean progress, particularly when the underlying moral and value structures of a society are the victims of such change.

Faith-Based Initiatives

Instead of allowing secular influences to dominate society and consume human and economic resources, why not utilize religious organizations to prevent illness and build social capital? Faced with rising crime and drug and alcohol abuse, deteriorating neighborhoods, and escalating costs of healthcare, the US government has now begun to use faith communities to improve social control, prevent disease, and reduce healthcare costs. Such programs could easily be developed in Muslim countries as well. With the opening of the Office of Faith-Based and Neighborhood Partnerships, originally established in 2001, the US government has begun to provide modest support for efforts by faith communities to provide social services and develop health programs. Although some have objected to this program, the aims of such partnership make perfect sense—to harness the power of faith communities to help maintain the health of members; to decrease rates of crime, delinquency, and drug use in surrounding communities; and to reduce health disparities between racial and ethnic groups (Sager 2010). Here are five examples of faith-based programs described in the literature that are relevant to the health problems that many Muslims struggle with:

1. *Weight Loss*. A faith-based program, called the Baltimore Church High Blood Pressure Program, was initiated over 20 years ago to help women control their

weight and reduce blood pressure (Kumanyika and Charleston 1992). In that program, 188 female church members participated in 8 weekly 2-h counseling and exercise sessions. Before and after measurements of weight and blood pressure were taken. Results indicated that women lost an average of 6 lb. Furthermore, those who were taking antihypertensive medication dropped their mean systolic/diastolic blood pressure by 10/6 mmHg, and those not needing antihypertensive medication decreased their average systolic/diastolic pressures by 5/3 mmHg ($p < 0.001$ for pre–post comparisons). As a result of the program, 74 % of women had a final systolic blood pressure that was under 140 mmHg (compared to 52 % initially), and 92 % had a diastolic blood pressure that was under 90 mmHg (compared to 65 % initially). On 6-month follow-up of 74 participants in the original sample, 65 % maintained or exceeded the weight loss achieved while in the program. Faith aspects were vital to the success of the program. Not only were all sessions held in church, but because participants were members of the same church involved in choir rehearsal, prayer, and Sunday services, fellow church members provided spiritual support to help each other exercise and lose weight.

2. *Breast Cancer Screening*. Many Muslm women do not adhere to breast cancer screening guidelines, resulting in preventable morbidity and mortality. After a brief period of training, members of churches in Los Angeles County conducted telephone peer counseling to encourage women in their churches to obtain mammograms for breast cancer detection (Duan et al. 2000). A clinical trial format was used to test the effectiveness of this telephone counseling program in 437 women. Thirty churches were randomized either to the telephone counseling or to a control group that received no counseling. Follow-up 1 year later revealed that mammography nonadherence was reduced from 23 to 16 % in those who received the telephone counseling. Researchers concluded that "partnerships between the public health and faith communities" were effective for maintaining and increasing cancer screening. Other educational programs in churches have reported even greater increases in mammography screening, especially in rural areas (one such study achieving a 38 % increase in screening) (Powell et al. 2005).

3. *Smoking Reduction in Youth*. Churches and other faith-based organizations in Mississippi implemented a program titled Students Working Against Tobacco to prevent students from taking up cigarette smoking (Reinert et al. 2003). This involved a partnership between faith-based groups, the community, and public schools. Churches were responsible for conducting five education sessions on tobacco use prevention to groups involving 35–50 youth each. These were specifically targeted at children in grades 4 through 7. Although the effectiveness of the program was not assessed, a published report describes how the program worked in two churches and makes recommendations on how to design future faith-based programs to address youth smoking.

4. *Improve Nutrition, Increase Exercise*. A faith-based Internet-based program called Guide to Health was administered in churches with the goal of improving nutrition by decreasing dietary fat; increasing dietary fiber, fruits, and vegetables; and increasing exercise (measured by steps taken per day using a pedometer)

(Winett et al. 2007). The program was conducted in 14 churches in the Virginia area. Assessments (questionnaires, along with weight and height measurements) were conducted in the churches at baseline and follow-up. Besides health education, participants received support in church to boost the effects of the intervention, including prompts and reminders from their ministers, posters throughout the churches, and a competition between participating churches. Some churches increased motivation by giving award badges to those meeting their step count and nutrition goals for the week. Results indicated that participants in the program significantly increased fruit, vegetable, and fiber intake, level of exercise, and amount of weight lost, compared to the control group.

5. *Diabetes Prevention.* This report describes the development, implementation, and results of a 16-session diabetes prevention program conducted over 4 months in a rural African-American church in Georgia (Boltri et al. 2008). Those in the church at high risk for diabetes ($n=26$) were identified through screening and then recruited into the program. This program was administered at the church in a group format and focused on nutrition, physical activity, and behavior change. Participants were assessed at baseline and followed up at 4, 6, and 12 months. Those involved in the program experienced a significant reduction in weight, blood pressure, and fasting blood sugar.

Other faith-based programs have been developed to increase prostate cancer screening, support families of those with chronic mental illness, complete advanced directives (instructions on what medical care they wish to have when they are dying and unable to respond), improve adult vaccination, increase seat belt use, and treat cocaine dependency (Koenig et al. 2012). All of these faith-based programs were conducted in the USA and involved Christian churches. The principles and lessons learned in the development and implementation of these programs could help guide Muslim communities who may wish to develop similar programs. Of course, programs like these will have to be designed to fit the particular needs and circumstances of Muslims within their specific religious and cultural environments. The great promise of faith-based programs, however, is that they may help to prevent disease and thereby reduce healthcare costs for hard-to-reach groups with less access to healthcare resources and education.

Implications for Muslim–Christian Relations

Based on a comprehensive and systematic review of the scientific literature, we have found that, in general, greater religious involvement is related to better mental health, better social health, and better physical health in both Christian and Muslim populations. These research findings also have implications for the relationship between Muslim and Christian societies. If devout beliefs and practices in each of these faith traditions lead to better health and greater human flourishing, then this should give us a clue about the intentions of a perfect, merciful, and unimaginably good God with regard to Muslim–Christian relations.

For the past millennium, but especially the past 25 years, animosity has been widespread between Muslims and Christians in many parts of the world. Consider the conflicts today in Nigeria, Egypt, Lebanon, and Kenya, to name just a few examples, not to mention the burning of mosques in New York City and Missouri or the Qur'an burnings in Florida. Many Christians view the terrorist attacks on the World Trade Centers and on the US Pentagon that occurred September 11, 2001, as an attack on Christianity, whereas many Muslims view the US interventions in Iraq and Afghanistan and efforts to help Israel as a direct attack on Islam. There are fundamental differences in belief between Christians and Muslims that cannot be reconciled. These create conflict and are often used to justify war and terrorism.

Nevertheless, there are also many areas of the world where Muslims and Christians live peacefully side by side as warm neighbors who cooperate and support one another. For example, prior to the American invasion of Iraq, it was not uncommon to see Muslims praying in Christian churches and Christians praying in mosques (Anderson 2011). Likewise, consider the Russian republic of Tatarstan, where Muslims, Orthodox Christians, and Roman Catholics live together in harmony respecting each other's traditions (Kishkovsky 2008). Until recent times, Christians and Muslims also lived together without conflict in Lebanon (Khoury 2010) (as well as in Nigeria and Ethiopia). There continue to be efforts around the world today to return to such peaceful coexistence. Consider that Muslims in the Dallas/Fort Worth area are going out of their way to invite Christians to visit their mosques, attend post-Ramadan fast dinners, and engage in real dialogue (Hunt 2010). These are just a few examples of Muslims and Christians living together and making efforts to get to know one another. No doubt, there are many other examples that we are not aware of.

How can such efforts be justified? While there may be irreconcilable differences between Muslims and Christians, there are also plenty of similarities, especially among devout adherents (see Chap. 5). Indeed, it is the Qur'an that says that Christians and Muslims are the closest of all religions:

> "You [Prophet] are sure to find that…the closest in affection towards the believers are those who say, 'We are Christians,' for there are among them people devoted to learning and ascetics. These people are not given to arrogance, and when they listen to what has been sent down to the Messenger, you will see their eyes overflowing with tears because they recognize the Truth [in it]. They say, 'Our Lord, we believe, so count us amongst the witnesses. Why should we not believe in God and in the Truth that has come down to us, when we long for our Lord to include us in the company of the righteous. For saying this, God has rewarded them with Gardens graced with flowing streams, and there they will stay: that is the reward of those who do good" (5:82–85).

We think that Jesus would have totally agreed. There are over 1,600 million Muslims and over 2,100 million Christians who now live on our planet. Together, Muslims and Christians make up over 50 % of the world's population. Although each religion would like to convert the other to its own belief system, the fact is that most Muslims alive today are going to die Muslim and most Christians alive today are going to die Christian. From a theological standpoint, it would seem to us (a devout Muslim and a devout Christian) that God must have a plan for both Muslims and Christians, and that plan does not include sending one group en masse to hell for all eternity. There are verses in both the Bible and the Qur'an backing up this statement (see Chap. 5). If that is true, then there are going to be a lot of Muslims and Christians in heaven, where Somebody is going to force us to get along as brothers and sisters. It would seem wise, then, for us to start trying now.

The scientific world is a great place to begin this effort. Muslim and Christian researchers almost always attend the same national meetings in their scientific fields. The research world encourages objective examination, without the inflaming rhetoric characteristic of politicians, unscrupulous religious leaders, news agencies, or radical groups with their own agendas that are seldom consistent with the fundamental teachings of either the Qur'an or the Bible. Scientific progress necessitates cooperation and dialogue so that new ideas can build one upon the other. This type of cooperation was nowhere more evident than in the Islamic Golden Age, when Islamic scientists translated Greek and Roman texts into Arabic and made their own original discoveries that were later translated into Latin and English. Likewise, this was a time when Christian physicians treated Muslim caliphs and Christian chapels were widely present in Muslim hospitals. We believe that there can be another Golden Age in the future, a Golden Age of Muslim–Christian cooperation, which could lead to an explosion in knowledge and scientific advancement, rather than to the other kind of explosions we are seeing today that have the potential to destroy our world and end life as we know it.

Summary and Conclusions

The implications of the research findings for public health are vast. If acknowledged and responded to positively, then sacred Islamic beliefs and traditions will be supported and will continue to exert positive influences on health, complementing advances made by modern medicine and healthcare. Likewise, if Muslims–Christian relationships improve with increasing recognition of the many similarities in beliefs, practices, and values that bond these two faith traditions together, this may stimulate cooperation between government and religious leaders, social scientists, and medical researchers in efforts to maximize individual and community health. Alternatively, if this research is ignored, then this too will have consequences. A "perfect storm" is now brewing, as several sociodemographic and cultural trends are beginning to merge. The first is the aging of populations in Muslim-majority countries over the next 30 years, where many who would have otherwise died young will survive into later life because of advances in healthcare and public health measures. The second is the increasing burden of chronic illness that these aging populations will face. The third is a trend toward increasing secularization, as Islamic societies begin to modernize and take on more liberal worldviews toward traditional Islamic beliefs, practices, and values. As religious influences lessen, so too will their protective effects on mental, social, behavioral, and physical health. To compensate for this, additional resources for social control and healthcare services will have to be redirected away from defense, technology, and economic growth, affecting the security and stability of Islamic societies worldwide.

References

Anderson, B. (2011, March 8). Iraq Muslims, Christians wish to live together in peace again. *National Catholic Reporter*. Retrieved October 5, 2013, from http://ncronline.org/news/global/iraqi-muslims-christians-wish-live-together-peace-again

Boltri, J. M., Davis-Smith, Y. M., Seale, J. P., Shellenberger, S., Okosun, I. S., & Cornelius, M. E. (2008). Diabetes prevention in a faith-based setting: Results of translational research. *Journal of Public Health Management & Practice, 14*(1), 29–32.

Duan, N., Fox, S. A., Derose, K. P., & Carson, S. (2000). Maintaining mammography adherence through telephone counseling in a church-based trial. *American Journal of Public Health, 90*(9), 1468–1471.

Eurostat (2013). European Social Statistics, 2013 edition. Eurostat European Commission (Luxembourg: Publications Office of the European Union). Retrieved October 5, 2013, from http://epp.eurostat.ec.europa.eu/portal/page/portal/product_details/publication?p_product_code=KS-FP-13-001

Hunt, R. A. (2010, August 17). Can Muslims and Christians live together in peace? *Patheos: Hosting the conversation on faith*. Retrieved October 5, 2013, from http://www.patheos.com/Resources/Additional-Resources/Can-Muslims-and-Christians-Live-Together-in-Peace.html

Khoury, Y. (2010, December 30). Who says Christians and Muslims can't live together? *The Guardian*. Retrieved October 5, 2013, from http://www.theguardian.com/commentisfree/belief/2010/dec/30/christians-muslims-can-live-together

Kishkovsky, S. (2008, November 28). Catholics, Orthodox, and Muslims live peacefully together in Tatarstan. *New York Times*. Retrieved October 5, 2013, from http://www.nytimes.com/2008/11/28/world/europe/28iht-kazan.4.18239617.html?pagewanted=all&_r=0

Koenig, H. G., King, D. E., & Carson, V. B. (2012). *Handbook of religion and health* (2nd ed., pp. 918–923). New York: Oxford University Press. see Appendix.

Kumanyika, S. K., & Charleston, J. B. (1992). Lose weight and win: A church-based weight loss program for blood pressure control among Black women. *Patient Education and Counseling, 19*, 19–32.

National Marriage Project (2012). *The State of our Unions, 2012: Marriage in America* (pp. 65, 94). Charlottesville, VA. Retrieved October 5, 2013, from http://nationalmarriageproject.org/reports/

Powell, M. E., Carter, V., Bonsi, E., Johnson, G., Williams, L., Taylor-Smith, L., et al. (2005). Increasing mammography screening among African American women in rural areas. *Journal of Health Care for the Poor and Underserved, 16*(4 Suppl A), 11–21.

Reinert, B., Campbell, C., Carver, V., & Range, L. M. (2003). Joys and tribulations of faith-based youth tobacco use prevention: A case study in Mississippi. *Health Promotion Practice, 4*(3), 228–235.

Sager, R. (2010). *Faith, politics, and power: The politics of faith-based initiatives*. New York: Oxford University Press.

Winett, R. A., Anderson, E. S., Wojcik, J. R., Winett, S. G., & Bowden, T. (2007). Guide to health: Nutrition and physical activity outcomes of a group-randomized trial of an Internet-based intervention in churches. *Annals of Behavioral Medicine, 33*(3), 251–261.

Chapter 16
Summary and Conclusions

This volume is the first comprehensive and systematic examination of health and well-being in Muslim populations. First, we provided a historical background, then reviewed the research on religiosity and health, and finally discussed applications at the bedside for health professionals and implications for public health. In the section on historical background, we described how Islamic beliefs and practices emerged out of Arabia and rapidly spread across the known world. Centuries before modern medicine appeared in the West, rapid advances were being made in science, medicine, and pharmacology in Muslim territories, ultimately leading to the Islamic Golden Age. This time of extraordinary scientific progress was followed by a period of decline, as war and political conquests began to reverse the gains that had been made. With this historical context, we then reviewed the core beliefs and teachings of Islam and of Christianity, examined their similarities and differences, and explored how religious beliefs influenced healing and health practices in each of these faith traditions. We found that distinct differences in belief exist between these two faith traditions, but that the number of similarities is also staggering and often underestimated, especially the common values and moral practices.

After briefly reviewing research on religiosity and health in Christian populations, we then focused on research in Muslim populations, examining relationships between religiosity and mental, social, behavioral, and physical health. Given the relatively few quantitative studies in Muslim-majority populations, we carefully described each study so that the quality of the research could be judged and the findings evaluated. We also reviewed research that compared Muslims and non-Muslims in each of these health domains. In general, the results of this review revealed that, as in Christian populations, the vast majority of studies examining Islamic beliefs and practices found that they were associated with better health.

Positive findings were especially evident for mental health, where religious involvement was related to fewer negative emotions and mental disorders (less depression, less suicide, less anxiety, less substance abuse) and more positive emotions (greater well-being, more purpose in life, greater optimism, and higher self-esteem). The findings regarding hope and sense of personal control were less consistent,

H.G. Koenig and S. Al Shohaib, *Health and Well-Being in Islamic Societies: Background, Research, and Applications*, DOI 10.1007/978-3-319-05873-3_16,

although few studies had examined these topics. With regard to personality traits, religiosity in Muslims was associated with being more conscientious and agreeable, the same traits found in deeply religious Christians. We also found better social health among devout Muslims, who experienced higher social support, greater marital stability, and lower rates of delinquency and crime in more than 80 % of studies. Social capital (community trust and engagement), while associated with greater religiosity in five of ten studies examined, was also related to lower religiosity in two reports, making the findings less consistent than for other indicators of social health.

Religiosity was less consistently related to behavioral health in Muslims. Although the vast majority of studies did find less cigarette smoking and fewer high-risk sexual practices among those who were more religious, this was not true for exercise, diet, and weight, based on the few studies that examined relationships with religiosity in Muslim populations. The link between religiosity and health behaviors, then, is in great need of further research.

A relative absence of systematic research on religiosity and physical health in Muslims was also found and perhaps most disturbing. The limited research to date, however, suggests positive relationships in a number of important health domains. Religiosity was associated with lower rates of acute coronary syndrome (myocardial infarction) in the only study published to date on the topic. Likewise, religious commitment was associated with both lower systolic and diastolic blood pressure in two of three studies. Cognitive impairment was also found to be less common among Muslim women who reported praying regularly during middle age. Finally, in the only study to examine overall mortality, Muslims in Switzerland experienced greater longevity than those with no religious affiliation. Other associations were not as positive. For example, religiosity was associated with a greater likelihood of having diabetes among Muslims in Israel, no association was found between prayer and cholesterol level in a single study in Turkey, and self-rated health was found to be significantly lower among more religious Muslims in Kenya.

No research whatsoever in Muslims has examined religiosity and cerebrovascular disease, immune function, endocrine function, or cancer. In fact, most research on religious practices and physical health in Muslims has focused on Ramadan fasting, which appears to have both positive and negative effects on health, with few consistent findings. Some research shows that the effects of Ramadan fasting are mostly positive (i.e., reduces heart disease risk factors such as pro-inflammatory markers, improves diabetic control, lowers serum cholesterol), some reports are mixed (i.e., higher or lower blood pressure, better or worse endocrine function), and the rest show little or no effect (i.e., heart disease, stroke, immune function). Regardless of the particular findings, the effects of Ramadan fasting do not appear particularly dangerous, although for those with certain medical illnesses (such as diabetes), education and careful monitoring during Ramadan fasting is recommended.

We also examined differences between Muslims and non-Muslims (primarily Christians, Jews, and Hindus). With regard to mental health, some studies reported that Muslims were worse off than non-Muslims. For example, anxiety was more common among Muslims in six of seven studies and optimism was lower in two of three studies. Possible reasons for these findings were discussed. Other studies, however, found better mental health in Muslims compared to non-Muslims. For example, psychosis was less common among Muslims than non-Muslims in both studies that examined this relationship; alcohol use/abuse was less common in 9 of 12 studies; and drug use/abuse was less common in three of six studies (the other three reporting no difference). The research findings were also mixed in terms of social health. Both studies examining social support found greater support in Muslims compared to non-Muslims and two of three studies also found significantly less delinquency or crime in Muslims. Marital stability was found to be significantly higher in one study, but a second study found that physical abuse was more common in Muslim than non-Muslim marriages in Syria. Studies of social capital were also mixed, with two studies reporting higher social capital in Muslims compared to non-Muslims, and two studies reporting significantly lower social capital in Muslims.

The findings on health behaviors in Muslims compared to non-Muslims also varied between studies. Note, however, that health behaviors are heavily influenced by socioeconomic status (i.e., availability of food, time for exercise) and cultural factors (i.e., obesity being a sign of success). Despite the fatwa against smoking, no difference in cigarette smoking was found between Muslims and non-Muslims in four of eight studies, whereas smoking was less common in Muslims in three studies and more frequent in one study. Exercise was significantly less frequent among Muslims in four of six studies, but was more common in one study and either higher or lower in the final study depending on how exercise was measured. Diet was worse among Muslims compared to non-Muslims in two of four studies, and the findings regarding weight were mixed (four of seven studies found lower weight in Muslims, whereas the remaining three studies reported heavier weight in Muslims). More consistent was lower extra-marital sexual activity, where 8 of 12 studies favored Muslims in this regard.

A number of studies have also compared Muslims and non-Muslims on physical health. With regard to heart disease, four of ten studies found higher rates in Muslims (of serious concern), only one study found lower rates, and the remaining studies reported mixed findings or no difference. In contrast, blood pressure was significantly lower among Muslims in six of eight studies, and both studies that examined stroke found lower rates in Muslims (consistent with lower blood pressure). With regard to diabetes, the findings were less consistent, with two of six studies reporting less diabetes in Muslims, two studies finding more diabetes, and the last two studies finding no difference. Serum cholesterol levels, however, were significantly lower in Muslims compared to non-Muslims in two of three studies.

With regard to cancer, Muslims had lower rates in 7 of 19 studies, higher rates in two studies, and no difference was found in most of the remaining studies. Muslims were somewhat less likely to rate their health as good compared to non-Muslims (four of eight studies). Differences in mortality were also mixed, with 6 of 14 studies finding lower mortality in Muslims and five studies reporting higher mortality (most examining child mortality, which is heavily dependent on availability of healthy food, access to health care, vaccinations, etc.).

In summary, *religiosity* in Muslim populations is generally related to better health, no matter what domain of health is measured. The only exceptions are health behaviors such as exercise, diet, and weight, although the research here is very sparse. We presented a theoretical model explaining the mechanisms by which religiosity could influence health in Muslims. These pathways appear similar to those found in Christians. Nevertheless, many more studies are needed on religiosity and health, especially those with research designs that account for other factors (socioeconomic influences, education, etc.) that could explain the health benefits or risks associated with greater religiosity. The research comparing *Muslims and non-Muslims* is more mixed. On the one hand, anxiety is higher, health behaviors generally worse, heart disease more common, and in some countries such as Saudi Arabia, diabetes is increasing. On the other hand, psychosis, alcohol and drug use/abuse, and delinquency/crime are all less common and social support higher, and both hypertension and stroke are less common in Muslims. Few studies, however, have controlled other important risk factors. Given the existing findings, several areas of health need improvement in Muslims, including attention to exercise, diet, and maintaining an optimal weight, especially in Muslim regions where food resources are abundant.

Because of the few well-done research studies in this area, there is an unlimited opportunity for conducting research on religiosity and almost every aspect of health in Muslim populations (especially health behaviors and physical health). This will require a new generation of scientists who are adequately trained and funded to develop programs of research in this area.

The research findings reviewed here have many potential applications, both for the care of Muslim patients in clinical practice and for maintaining and improving public health in Muslim populations worldwide. With regard to clinical practice, numerous applications could be implemented immediately. Besides the growing research base that shows greater religious involvement in Muslims is related to improved coping with illness and better health outcomes, there are many other reasons for assessing and addressing the spiritual needs of Muslim patients in health-care settings. We recommended that health professionals (especially physicians) take a spiritual history from all patients with serious or chronic illness. The purpose is to identify spiritual needs related to illness and determine how religious beliefs might influence medical decisions and compliance with treatment. Once spiritual needs are identified, it is important to accommodate health care to support patients' religious beliefs and have trained clergy available to address those needs. In select circumstances, spiritual interventions by health professionals may also be indicated if requested by Muslim patients.

The implications of this research for public health are particularly important. This applies to all Muslim countries, both those that are developed and those that are developing, given that all are now being influenced by the forces of secularization. We speculated in the last chapter on how increasing secularization might impact the future health of Muslim populations and the economic resources needed for social control. If religious involvement helps to maintain health and well-being, increases social health, and promotes health-related behaviors, then a lessening importance of Islamic beliefs and practices has the potential to adversely affect health more generally, increasing the need for mental health services, for medical services, and for social control (expanded police forces and prisons). Such changes have the potential to drain Muslim countries of important economic resources that could otherwise be spent on economic development and infrastructure growth, resulting in a weakening and reduced flourishing of Islamic populations.

Based on the findings reported here, we recommended that Islamic countries make every effort to support and preserve religious beliefs, practices and traditions, while at the same time pouring resources into increasing the availability and effectiveness of modern medical and psychiatric care. We believe that these twin healing traditions—medicine and religion—*complement* each other, and that true health can only result when these are in equal balance, one supporting the other.

We also stressed the importance of Muslims and Christians getting along, given the many similarities in beliefs, practices, and values that they share. We recommended that one place to start might be in the area of science and medicine, where there are fewer political forces that drive people apart and where all are joined together in a quest for knowledge to improve the health and well-being of human populations. We believe that a new Golden Age is now within our grasp, but it will require Muslims and Christians to cooperate and respect each other's religious faith, working side-by-side as brothers and sisters submitted to one God. Failure to do so, on the other hand, will also have consequences for health both on the individual and the societal level.

Index

A
Acute coronary syndrome (ACS)
  in Albanians, 245
  religious affiliation, 245
Age of ignorance, 6
Aging process, 319
Agreeableness, 191
Alcohol use/abuse, Muslims
  binge drinking, 157
  Christian-majority countries, 114
  chronic "arrack", 156
  DSM-IV, 155
  multivariate analyses, 156
  regression model, 157
  religiosity, 155
  R/S, 155
Ancient religions and empires
  Egyptian and Persian, 4
  human civilization, 3
  Roman, 4
  Sassanid, 4
  Sumerian, Akkadian, Babylonian and Assyrian, 3–4
  Zoroastrianism, 4
A new Golden Age, 347
Anxiety, Muslims
  death apprehension theory, 148
  fluoxetine, 148
  GAD, 142
  Hamilton Anxiety Rating Scale, 142
  HAS, 147
  Islamic psychotherapy, 142
  multiple regression, 145
  OCD, 143
  PTSD, 147
  randomized clinical trials, 148
  RCP, 142
  religiosity, 144
  religious coping, 145
  risk factors, 146
  and R/S, 114
  SRI, 143
  S/R intervention, 147
  TAF-morality, 146
  Taoist orientation, 144
  weighing, good and bad, 141
Arabia
  early Islamic period, 8
  pre-Islamic times, 6–7
Arabic medicine
  Al-Razi, 17
  pre-Islamic, 9, 12
Ashipu, 5

B
Believers
  Jews, 102
  love and peace, 100
  Muslims and Christians, 98
  physical health, 106
Body mass index (BMI)
  college students, 230
  diabetics and nondiabetics, 229
  Muslim and Christian adolescent, 230
  Muslim dress, 229
  Muslims *vs.* non-Muslims, 229
Breast cancer screening, 338

H.G. Koenig and S. Al Shohaib, *Health and Well-Being in Islamic Societies: Background, Research, and Applications*, DOI 10.1007/978-3-319-05873-3,

C

CAD. *See* Coronary artery disease (CAD)
Cancer
  Bombay Cancer Registry, 275
  breast, 275
  cervical, 277
  CIN, 274
  death rates, 277
  epidemiology, 276
  head/neck, 274
  HPV18 infection, 274–275
  missed studies, 275
  Muslims, 277–278
  oral and pharyngeal, 275
  prognosis, Muslims, 273
  screening, 338
  social factors, 277
Cerebrovascular disease
  Muslims *vs.* non-Muslims, 258
  PMR, 258
  Ramadan fasting, 257
  stroke, 257
Chaplains, 330
Cholesterol
  physical health, 119–120
  and triglycerides (*see* Triglycerides)
Christian beliefs
  Day of Judgement, 64
  denominations, membership, 57, 58
  divine book, 65–66
  divisions, 57
  faith, 58
  god, 59–61
  the Gospel, 62–63
  heaven, 66
  hell, 66–67
  Jesus, 61–62
  Mary, 65
  Nicene Creed, 58–59
  original sin, 61
  Pew Foundation Research Center, 57–58
  prophets, 65
  range of, 77
  related to health, 57
  salvation, 63–64
Christian practices
  donation, 69–70
  fasting, 68
  media, 68–69
  pilgrimage, 69
  prayer, 67–68
  range of, 77
  reading scriptures, 68
  religious, 67
  services, religious, 69
  volunteer, 70
Christian values
  ethics, 70–71
  family, 72
  individualism, 71
  love, 71
  vulnerable individuals care, 72–73
  work, 71–72
Chronic mental disorders, 312–313
Comparison of Muslims and non-Muslims
  alcohol use/abuse, 155
  cigarette smoking, 218–219
  drug use/abuse, 157
  energy expenditure, 224
  hypertension/blood pressure, 253
  intrinsic religiosity, 133
  LOC, 182
  social support, 198
  suicide, 140
  well-being, 167
Compliance
  medical treatment, 306
  Muslims, 308
  religiosity, 308
Comprehensive and systematic examination
  beliefs and practices, 343, 347
  golden age, 343, 347
  health behaviors, 344
  implications, 346
  marital stability, 345
  mental health, 343–344
  Muslims and non-Muslims, 344–345
  physical health, 344
  religiosity and health, 343, 344
  research, 345–346
Conscientiousness, 190–191
Coronary artery disease (CAD), 243
Creation story, Christians and Muslims
  differences, 82
  similarities, 93

D

Daily spiritual experiences scale (DSES), 153
DAS. *See* Dyadic Adjustment Scale (DAS)
Day of judgement, 31–32
Decline of Islam
  Eastern Islamic empire, 23
  modern hospitals, 23
  Mongols, 21–22
  the Ottoman empire, 23
  Persia, 22
  Qajar dynasty, 22

scholars and doctors, India, 22
Sunni and Shia Muslims, 22
Treaty of Lausanne, 23–24
Turkish Ottoman empires, 22
Unani/Tibi medicine, 23
Western Islamic empire, Spain, 23
Definitions
religious coping, 112
spirituality, 112–113
Delinquency and crime
adolescents, 208
antisocial behavior, 205
crime prevention, 206
gross domestic product, 206
Islamic fundamentalism, 205
justifiability scale, 207
participant involvement, 207
political violence, 204
pro-social behavior, 208
regression analysis, 205
risk behaviors, 208
sense of community, 205
social determinants, 206
structural equation modeling, 205
Dementia/Alzheimer's disease
MCI, 259–260
Muslim-majority countries, 258–259
Muslims *vs.* non-Muslims, 259
Demons, 49–50
Depression, Muslims
anxiety, 131
Brief Symptom Inventory, 132
clinical trials, 130
EPDS, 134
Hamilton Depression Scale, 131
intrinsic religiosity, 133
mental disorders, 130
multidimensional child
and adolescent, 134
multiple regression, 132
psychotherapy, 130
religiosity, 131
and R/S, 113
standard care, 131
systematic review, 135
Diabetes
metabolic syndrome, 261–262
Muslims and Christians, 262
and religiosity, 260–261
Diet
child-hood and adult health, 227
diabetic risk factors, 227
eating patterns and food intake, 226
and exercise, 331, 346
fruits and vegetables, 228
halal meat, 226
health-promoting behaviors, 227
Muslims *vs.* non-Muslims, 227
nutrition, 338
Differences in beliefs
creation story, 82
divine books, 86
god, 82
holy spirit, 84
Jesus, 83–84
original sin, 82–83
Prophet Muhammad, 85–86
Qur'an, 104–105
salvation, 85
Disease prevention, 304
Divine book
Bible, 65–66
Christian beliefs, 65–66
Day of Judgement, 85
differences, 86
Islam, 31
Muslims, 31
Qur'an, 86
similarities, 95–97
Divinity of Jesus
differences in beliefs, 83–84
similarities in beliefs, 93–95
Drug use/abuse
cigarette smoking and illicit, 159
doping behavior, 158
family attachment, 159
majority populations, 160
marijuana use, 158
religiosity, 158
2010 systematic review, 158
DSES. *See* Daily Spiritual Experiences Scale
(DSES)
Dyadic Adjustment Scale (DAS), 199

E
Early Islamic period
Abbasid dynasty, 8
Fatimid dynasty, 8
Islamic law, 9
Prophet Muhammad, 7–8
Qur'an (Koran), 8
schools of law, 9
traditionists, 9
Umayyad dynasty, 8
Edinburgh Postnatal Depression Scale
(EPDS), 134
Emotional disorders, 312, 313

EMSP. *See* Extramarital sexual partnerships (EMSP)
Endocrine function
PBMC, 273
Ramadan fasting, 271–272
stress hormones, 271
Environment
factors, 306
and genetic influences, 306
health and longevity, 306
EPDS. *See* Edinburgh Postnatal Depression Scale (EPDS)
Ethical issues in medicine
abortion, 51
contraception, 51
suicide, 50–51
Ethics and values, 101
Exercise
adult-onset diabetes, 225
coronary heart disease, 225
description, 226
lifestyle, 225
Muslim countries and immigrant population, 224
Muslims and non-Muslims, 224–225
Palestinians and Israelis, 225–226
population-based sample, 224
"sexual excitement", 224
Extra-marital sex
Hindu and Muslim, 231
human papillomavirus, 232
Muslims *vs.* non-Muslims, 231
religiosity, 236
religious affiliation, 232
sexually transmitted diseases, 231
Extramarital sexual partnerships (EMSP), 236
Extraversion
description, 186–188
Eysenck Personality Inventory, 185
intrinsic religiosity, 186
IROS, 186
MARS, 185–186
personality scales and traits, 185–186

F
Faith-based initiatives
breast cancer screening, 338
communities, 337
diabetes prevention, 339
implementation, 339
nutrition and exercise, 338–339
programs, 337
religious and cultural environments, 339
secular influences, 337
smoking cessation, 338
weight loss, 337–338
Faith-based interventions, 318
Fasting
Christian practices, 68
differences, 87
physical health benefits, 37
Ramadan (*see* Ramadan fasting)
similarities, 99
stress, 87

G
Generalized anxiety disorder (GAD), 142
Genetics
and environmental influence, 306
factors, 306
GNP. *See* Gross national product (GNP)
God
Allah, 29
Christian beliefs, 59–61
differences in beliefs, 82
similarities in beliefs, 90–92
God's will
and destiny, 54
vs. seeking medical treatment, 49
Golden Age of Islam
caliph, 11–12
description, 11
House of Wisdom *(bayt al-hikmah)*, 12
the Middle East, 12
Good deeds
differences, 88–89
similarities, 99
The Gospel, 62–63
Gross national product (GNP), 283

H
Hadith, 28, 30, 31, 34, 35
Hajj, 28, 34, 37
Hamilton Anxiety Scale (HAS), 147
Happiness
feelings and experiences, 167
OHI, 170
regression model, 168
self-esteem, 193
HAS. *See* Hamilton Anxiety Scale (HAS)
HBP. *See* Health-based intervention (HBP)

HDL. *See* High-density lipoprotein (HDL)
Healing in Islam
  source, 48
  spiritual, 48
Healing in Qur'an
  Apostle of Allah, 46
  Hadith, 43, 46
  and health, 43, 44
  Sahih al-Bukhari, 43, 45
Health and healing
  abortion, 76
  beliefs, 74–75
  care, 72–73
  contraception, 76
  drugs, 76–77
  medical care, 74
  prayer, 74
  scripture, 74
  sickness, 73–74
  suicide, 75–76
Health-based intervention (HBP), 221
Health behaviors
  cigarette smoking (*see* Smoking)
  diet, 118, 226–228
  exercise, 118
  physical activity/exercise (*see* Exercise)
  sexual behavior (*see* Sexual behavior)
  smoking, 118
  weight, 118, 228–230
Healthcare seeking, 306, 308
Health practices
  alcohol, 53
  circumcision, 52
  exercise, 52
  and medical care, 48–49
  money spending, 53
  oral care, 52
  sleep, 52
  social relationships, 53–54
Health-related quality of life (HRQOL), 129
Heart disease
  ACS, 244–245
  CAD, 243
  CCU, 246
  CRP, 248–249
  EKG, 246
  Muslims *vs.* non-Muslims, 244
  Ramadan, 244
  religiosity, cardiovascular and neurological disease, 249–251
Hell and heaven, 98
High-density lipoprotein (HDL), 266
High priority studies, cancer, 316
Holy spirit
  Christian beliefs, 64–65
  differences in beliefs, 84
Hope
  description, 174–175
  Egypt and Hungary, 171, 173
  Muslim populations, 171
  PTG, 173
  religiosity/spirituality (R/S), 171
HRQOL. *See* Health-related quality of life (HRQOL)
Hypertension/blood pressure
  ED, 253
  Hindus, 256–257
  Muslims and non-Muslims, 253
  pain and anxiety scales, 256
  preeclampsia, 254
  regression analysis, 256
  religiosity, 255
  religious involvement, 252
  SRH, 255

I
Immune function
  fasting, 269
  missed studies, 269
  religiosity, 270–271
  religious involvement, 269
Immune system disorders, 316–317
Immunity. *See* Immune function
Importance of religiosity *vs.* Muslim/non-Muslim differences, 346–347
Infant mortality rates (IMR), 283
Insufficient research, 345–346
Integrating spirituality
  chaplain, 330
  coping, 326–327
  document, 329–330
  effects, patient health, 327
  faith community, 331
  healthcare standards meeting, 328
  history, 328–329
  intervention, 331
  Islamic beliefs, 326
  medical decisions, 327
  orchestrate resources, 330
  patient care, 326
  patients' beliefs, 330
  physicians' decisions, 327
  religious and cultural practices, 326
  struggles, 326
  supporting network, 327–328
IROS. *See* Islamic Religious Orientation Scale (IROS)

Islamic beliefs
  angels, 32
  in Arabic, 28
  day of judgement, 31–32
  description, 28–29
  destiny, 32–33
  divine books, 30–31
  in God/Allah, 29
  individual, 34
  intercession, 33–34
  life after death, 33
  in Prophets Muhammad, 29–30
Islamic medicine
  description, 12
  hospitals, 14
  medical knowledge, translation, 13
  pharmacology, 13–14
  physicians, 12
  surgery, 13
  Umar ibn Al-Khattab (634–644 CE), 14–15
Islamic physicians
  Al-Kindi, 16
  Al-Majusi, 19
  Al-Nafis, 21
  Al-Razi, 17–19
  Al-Ruhawi, 16–17
  Al-Tabari, 16
  Al-Zahrawi, 19
  Hunain ibn Ishaq, 15
  Ibn Sina, 19–20
  medicine, 16
  Tabib/Hakim, 15
  treatment records, 16
Islamic practices
  description, 34
  fasting, 36–37
  Hajj, 37
  prayer, 35
  zakat, 35–36
Islamic Religious Orientation Scale (IROS), 186, 190
Islamic values and attitudes
  adultery, 39
  ethical, 38
  family, 38–39
  polygamy, 39
  positive attitudes, 38
  work, 39–40
Islamic views on the body, 46
Islam influences health
  behavioral, 303
  mental and social (*see* Social and mental health)
  mental, social, behavioral and physical, 295, 298
  physical, 303–308
  religiosity and health, Muslim populations, 295–297

J
Jesus, 61–62

K
Kaaba/al-Ka'bah, 6

L
Language of spirituality, 325–326
LDL. *See* Low-density lipoprotein (LDL)
Limitations, health professionals
  coerce/force nonreligious patients, 332
  counseling, 332–333
  patient-centered, 333
  prayer, 332
  prescribe religion, 331–332
  spiritual history, 332
Locus of control (LOC)
  Arabs and Jews, 182
  business managers, PWE, 182
  description, 174–175, 184
  diabetes, cancer/heart disease, 183
  internal and external, 181
  Islamic identification, 183
  marketing and accounting, 183
  Muslims *vs.* Christians, 184
  Muslims *vs.* non-Muslims, 182
  orientation and depressive symptom, 184
  personality traits, 185
  psychological factors, 182–183
  Punishing God Reappraisal, 183–184
  religious coping, 183
  Rotter's Locus of Control Scale, 181
Low-density lipoprotein (LDL)
  cholesterol, 268
  and VLDL, 268

M
Makkah, 6
Marital stability, Muslims
  community organizations, 204
  DAS, 199
  divorce rates, 199, 202
  PAIR scale, 202–203
  physical abuse, 204
  regression analysis, 202
  RRFS, 203
  spouse selection, 203

Marriage, Muslims
DAS, 199
physical abuse, 204
Mary
Christian beliefs, 65
Christians and Muslims, 95
and saints, 60
Meaning and purpose
life, Muslims, 177
religion and positive emotions, Muslims, 177
Mechanisms
health behaviors, 121
mental and physical health, 121, 122
and pathways, 295
psychological and social, 295
religious faith, 121
religious involvement influences, 304
R/S effects, 121–122
Media
Christian practices, 68–69
religious, 68
social, 117
Medicine of the Prophet
Al-Jauziyah, physicians, 10
As-Suyuti, 10
description, 9–10
Islamic orthodoxy, 10
pre-Islamic Arabic, 9
Mental health
chronic/psychiatric, 312–313
control, 312
emotional disorders, 312, 313
happiness and well-being, 313
negative, 113–114
positive, 114–115
prediction, 312
research designs, 311–312
R/S beliefs and practices, 113
social (*see* Social and mental health)
terrorist attacks, 113
therapist attention, 312
therapy, 312
treatment response, 313
Metabolic disorders, 315–316
Miracles, 49
Mortality
Bangladesh Fertility Survey, 282
GNP, 283
Hindus, 282–283
IMR, 283
Muslims and Hindus, 282
Muslims *vs.* non-Muslims, 285–286
religion *vs.* no religion, 284–285
religiosity, 282
risk factors, 283
socioeconomic, ethnic and cultural factors, 284
MRPI. *See* Muslim Religiosity-Personality Inventory (MRPI)
Muslim beliefs
description, 27
Qur'an, 28
Sunni and Shia, 27–28
Muslim–Christian relations, 339–341
Muslim Religiosity-Personality Inventory (MRPI), 212
Muslims
alcohol use/abuse, 155–157
anxiety, 141
chronology, 126
delinquency and crime, 204–209
depression, 130–135
drug use/abuse, 158–160
health policy decisions, 125
marital stability (*see* Marital stability, Muslims)
psychosis, 150–154
religiosity and mental health, 125–126
religious coping (*see* Religious coping)
social capital, 209–213
social support, 197–199
strengths and weaknesses, 125
suicide (*see* Suicide)
2010 systematic review, 126
Muslims *vs.* non-Muslims
BMI, 229
Christian participants, 233–234
diet/nutritional intake, 227
HIV infection, prevalence, 234
Pentecostals, 234
physical activities, 224, 226
"primary" and "secondary" abstinence, 235
regression models, 234
sexual knowledge, attitudes and behaviors, 234
smoking, 218–219

N

Negative mental health
alcohol, 114
anxiety, 114
depression, 113
drug use/abuse, 114
psychosis, 114
relationships, 113
suicide, 114
Neurological disorders, 316

Neuroticism, 116, 189–190
Nicene Creed, 58–59
Nutrition and exercise, 338–339

O
Objective
reasoning, 105
religiosity, 282
religious practice indicator, 159
scientific method, 105
and systematic manner, 106
Obsessive compulsive disorder (OCD), 143
OHI. *See* Oxford Happiness Inventory (OHI)
Optimism
adults, Algeria, 176
American *vs.* Kuwaiti college students, 176
Arabic Scale of Optimism and Pessimism, 173, 176
Jordanians and Americans, 176
Muslim populations, 174–176
Original sin
Christian beliefs, 61
and god, 82–83
Oxford Happiness Inventory (OHI), 168–170

P
PAIR scale. *See* Personal Assessment of Intimacy in Relationships (PAIR) scale
PAS. *See* Physician-assisted suicide (PAS)
Patient-centered, 333
Personal Assessment of Intimacy in Relationships (PAIR) scale, 202–203
Personality
agreeableness, 116
conscientiousness, 116
description, 116
extraversion, 116
Eysenck Personality Inventory, 185
MARS, 185–186
neuroticism, 116, 189
openness, experience, 116–117
schizotypal and authoritarianism, 192–193
spiritual experiences, 185
Physical disability, 317
Physical health
aging process, 319
biological treatments, 317–318
cancer, 120, 316
cerebrovascular disease, 119
cholesterol, 119–120
compliance, treatment, 308
dementia/Alzheimer's disease, 119
diabetes, 119
disability, 317
disease detection, 307
endocrine function, 120, 318
faith-based interventions, 318
genetic and environmental influences, 306
genetic factors, 319
heart disease, 119, 315
hypertension, 119
immune function, 120, 318
immune system, 316–317
Islam's effects, 304–305
lifestyle and behavioral influences, 305–306
markers, 318–319
metabolic disorders, 315–316
mortality, 121, 317
neurological disorders, 316
psychosocial influences, 304–305
and religiosity, 315
research areas, 318
self-rated, 121
stress-related diseases, 317
timely medical care, 307
Physician-assisted suicide (PAS), 141
Pilgrimage
Christian practices, 69
differences, 88
Hajj, 37
Jerusalem, 69
Mecca, 7
religious, 69
similarities, 99–101
Portional mortality ratio (PMR), 258
Positive and negative health effects, 343–344
Positive and negative implications
conventional treatment, 335
cost, health care, 335–336
health benefits and risks, 336
Islamic beliefs and practices, 335
measure, 336
modern medicine, 336
motivation, 337
social control, 337
Positive and negative influences
anxiety, 301
attitude, women, 301
delay treatment, 302
justice, mercy, 302–303
psychosis, 301–302
sick, 302
worsen guilt, 301
Positive emotions
agreeableness, 191

conscientiousness, 190–191
description, 167
extraversion, 185–188
hope, 171, 173
meaning and purpose, 177
neuroticism, 189–190
openness, experience, 192
optimism (*see* Optimism)
self-esteem (*see* Self-esteem)
sense of control (*see* Locus of control (LOC))
well-being, 167–171
Positive mental health
description, 114
meaning and purpose, 115
optimism, 115
R/S and hope, 115
sense of control, 115
well-being, 115
Posttraumatic growth (PTG), 173
Post-traumatic stress disorder (PTSD), 147
Practices of Christians and Muslims
divinity of Jesus, 104–105
fasting (*see* Fasting)
good deeds (*see* Good deeds)
pilgrimage (*see* Pilgrimage)
prayer (*see* Prayer)
Qur'an, 105
reading scripture, 87, 98–99
religious services, 87–88
Prayer
Christian practices, 67–68
differences, 87
similarities, 98
Pre-Islamic times, 6–7
Pre-marital sex
daily prayers, 235–236
extramarital sex, 236–237
Malaysian and Indonesian adolescents, 233
Muslims *vs.* Christians, 233–234
Prophets Muhammad, 29–30
Psychosis
alcohol and drug use, 153, 154
antipsychotic medication, 151
delusional themes, 152
DSES, 153
hallucinations, 153
Islamic faith healing, 152
qualitative analyses, 151
R/S, 153
schizophrenia, 150
spiritual healing, 151
WHO, 153
Psychosocial influences
HIV/AIDS, 304
psychoneuroimmunology, 304–305
PTG. *See* Posttraumatic growth (PTG)
PTSD. *See* Post-traumatic stress disorder (PTSD)
Public health
faith (*see* Faith-based initiatives)
Muslim–Christian relations, 339–341
positive and negative implications, 335–337
Purpose of illness, 47

Q
Quantitative studies, Muslims
hemodialysis, 130
HRQOL, 129
intrinsic religiosity, 128
psychometric properties, 129
regression analyses, 129
religious coping, 129
systematic review, 128
Qur'an, 28–36, 38–40

R
Ramadan fasting
cerebrovascular disease, 257
cholesterol and triglycerides, 266
diabetes, 261, 263
endocrine function, 272
heart disease, 244
hypertension/blood pressure, 252
RCP. *See* Religious-cultural psychotherapy (RCP)
Reading Qur'an, 331, 332
Religion and early medicine
ancient Egypt, 4
financial resource, 5
magi/physician, 6
Mesopotamian, 5
Persia, 6
physical body and soul, 5
scorpion sting/snakebite, 5
temple sleep, 5
Religion and physical health, Muslims
cancer, 273–278
cerebrovascular disease, 257–258
cholesterol and triglycerides, 264–268
dementia/Alzheimer's disease, 258–260
description, 243
diabetes, 260–264
endocrine function, 271–273

Religion and physical health, Muslims (*cont.*)
heart disease, 243–252
hypertension/blood pressure, 252–257
immune function, 269–271
mortality, 282–286
SRH, 278–281
Religiosity/spirituality (R/S), 155
Religious coping
qualitative studies, 126
quantitative studies, 128–130
reports, 127–128
2010 systematic review, 126
Religious-cultural psychotherapy (RCP), 142
Research methods
acculturation, religious intolerance and self-esteem, 180
adult-onset diabetes, 225
agreeableness, 191
behavioral, 314–315
college students, 230
community-dwelling adults and nursing home patients, 179–180
conscientiousness, 190
coronary heart disease, 225
diabetes, cancer/heart disease, 183
diabetic risk factors, 227
discrimination, 180
Egypt and Hungary, 171
HBP, 221
intrinsic-extrinsic religiosity, 170, 186
Islamic identification, 183
Islamic Religiosity Scale, 169
Jordanians and Americans, 176
lifestyle, 225
LOC, 182
meaning and purpose, 177
mental (*see* Mental health)
multi-item scales, 169–170
Muslim immigrants, USA, 180
Muslims (*see* Muslims)
Muslims *vs.* Christians, 184
Muslims *vs.* non-Muslims, 227
neuroticism, 189
non-Islamic group, 221
non-pregnant women, 230
obesity, prevalence, 229
openness, experience, 192
orientation, LOC and depressive symptom, 184
Palestinians and Israelis, 225–226
personality scales, 186
physical (*see* Physical health)
PTG, 173
Punishing God Reappraisal, 183–184
relationship, 320
religiosity and dietary behavior, 228
religiosity and health, 311
Religious affiliations, 230
religious attitude scale, 220
religious coping, 183
smoking, Muslims *vs.* non-Muslims, 218
social isolation, 170
"social norms", 171
spirituality, 180
survival and flourishing, 320
well-being, 181
Western dress, 229
Revised Religious Fundamentalist Scale (RRFS), 203
R/S. *See* Religiosity/spirituality (R/S)

S

Sahih al-Bukhari, 30, 33
Salvation
Christian beliefs, 63–64
good deeds, 63
Protestant and Catholic Christians, 63
Scale of religious index (SRI), 143
Seeking healthcare
purpose of illness, 47
sick person, role, 47
sick, visiting, 47
Self-esteem
acculturation and religious intolerance, 180
adolescents, 178
adults and nursing home patients, 179–180
Bedouin Arabs, 177
community-dwelling Pakistanis, 178
description, 174–175, 181
discrimination, 180
Indonesia, adolescents, 178–179
Intrinsic religiosity, 178
Muslim immigrants, USA, 180
Pakistani Muslims, 178
practices, 178
psychological well-being, 179
sociodemographic and health characteristics, 178
spirituality, 180
SWB scale, 179
well-being, 181
Self-rated health (SRH)
immigrant and host adolescents, 281–282
missed studies, 279
Muslim Arabs and Jews, 278
Muslims *vs.* non-Muslims, 279
religiosity, 279

religious services, 280–281
and sociodemographic factors, 280
Sexual behavior
AIDS, 231–232
Arab Muslims, 232
Christian participants, 233–234
college students, 231
cross-national data, 236
daily prayers, 235–236
EMSP, 236
extramarital sexual activity, 236
foreplay/sexual intercourse, 233
Hindu and Muslim, 231
human papillomavirus, 232
knowledge, attitudes and behaviors, 234
logistic regression model, 232
Malawi Diffusion and Ideational Change Project, 232
Malaysian and Indonesian adolescents, 233
masturbation, 233
Muslims *vs.* non-Muslims, 231, 233
Pentecostals, 234
prevalence, HIV infection, 234
"primary" and "secondary" abstinence, 235
regression models, 234
sexually transmitted diseases, 231
"Sujda", 235
Shari'ah law, 28, 39
Shia, 27, 28, 31
Similarities in beliefs
angels, devil and demons, 97–98
believers, 98
creation story, 93
Day of Judgement, 98
divine books, 95–97
god, 90–92
hell and heaven, 98
Jesus, 93–95
Mary, 95
the prophets, 95
Qur'an, 104
values (*see* Values)
Smoking
Buddhist Thai adult smokers, 218
cessation, 338
college students, Jordan, 220
description, 221–223
"fatwa", 217
HBP, 221
high school students, Mostar, 220
Muslim-majority populations, 217
Muslims *vs.* Non-Muslims, 218–219
Non-Islamic Group, 221
pregnancy, 220
quantitative study, 218
randomized clinical trial, 221
regression model, 218
religious attitude scale, 220
religious influence, 219
teachers, 218
Social and mental health
fostering generosity, 300–301
healthy decision-making, 300
meaning and purpose, 299
positive worldview, 295, 298, 299
psychological integration, 299
satisfying answers, 300
social support, 300
tools, cope, 299
Social capital, Muslims
civic engagement, 211
community health, 209
engagement and community trust, 211
interpersonal/institutional trust, 213
MRPI, 212
multivariable logit model, 211
religious affiliation, 212
social disorganization, 210
WVS, 210
youth religion, 209
Social health
capital, 117
delinquency and crime, 117
marital stability, 117
support, 117
Social support, Muslims
correlational analysis, 198
psychological-spiritual, 198
religious commitment, 197
risk factors, 197
secular, 198
Spiritual healing, 10–11, 48
Spiritual interventions, 331
Spirituality
integrate (*see* Integrating spirituality)
language, 325–326
limitations, 331–333
recommendations, 333
religious beliefs, 333
research literature, 333
Spiritual medicine
abdominal pain, drugs, 11
definition, 10
Khawass al-Qur'an, 10
SRI. *See* Scale of religious index (SRI)
Stress-related diseases, 317

Stroke, 257
Subjective well-being, 167–169, 179
Suicide
  adolescents, 135
  bipolar disorder, 139
  ideation scale, 137
  mortality data, 138
  other violent deaths (OVD), 138, 139
  PAS, 141
  psychiatric facility, 139
  psychopathology, 138
  religiosity, 135
  researchers, 140
  secular education, 135
  Taoist orientation, 138
  WHO, 140
Sunni, 27, 28, 30, 31
Supernatural beliefs
  demons, 49–50
  miracles, 49
Supporting beliefs, 330–331
Systematic examination. *See* Comprehensive and systematic examination
Systematic research
  definition, religion, religious coping and spirituality, 111–113
  health behaviors, 118
  mechanisms, 121–122
  mental health (*see* Mental health)
  personality, 116–117
  physical health (*see* Physical health)
  social health (*see* Social health)
Systematic review
  agreeableness, 191
  anxiety, 141
  cigarette smoking and religiosity, 217
  delinquency and crime, 204
  depression, 130
  drug use/abuse, 158
  exercise/physical activity, 225
  Google Scholar, 126
  marital stability, 199
  neuroticism, 189
  optimism, 173
  PAS, 141
  psychosis, 150
  religion and health, 126
  religiosity and extramarital sexual behavior, 231
  religiosity and well-being, 169
  religiosity/spirituality (R/S) and hope, 171
  religious coping, 126–130
  self-esteem, 181
  social capital, 209

T

Taking spiritual history, 328–329
Triglycerides
  HDL, 266
  LDL, 267
  lipid levels, 268
  religiosity, 264–265

V

Values
  concern, poor, 102–103
  destiny, 89
  in early Islam, 46
  ethics, 101
  individualism, 89
  intoxication and behaviors, 104
  Islamic (*see* Islamic values)
  Muslim–Christian relationships, 102
  physical body care, 103
  pro-life, 103–104
  social relationships, 101–102
  spiritual, 49
  traditional family, 101
  women's rights., 89–90
  work, 103

W

Weight
  BMI, Muslim countries, 228
  college students, 230
  extravagance, 228
  Muslims *vs.* non-Muslims, 229
  non-pregnant women, 230
  physical activity, 228–229
  prevalence, obesity, 229
  Ramadan fasting, 230
  religious affiliations, 230
  religious rituals and social events, 228
  Western dress, 229
Weight loss, 337–338
Well-being
  description, 171, 172
  happiness/life satisfaction, 167
  intrinsic-extrinsic religiosity, 170
  mental and physical health, 168
  multi-item scales, 169–170
  Muslims *vs.* non-Muslims, 169

OHI and life satisfaction, 168–169
pain, anxiety and sleep quality, 169
religiosity and happiness, 168
social isolation, 170
"social norms", 171
SWB, 179
work satisfaction, 167–168

Women's rights, 89–90
World Health Organization (WHO), 153
World Values Surveys (WVSs), 210

Z
Zakat, 28, 34–36

MIX
Papier aus verantwortungsvollen Quellen
Paper from responsible sources
FSC® C105338

If you have any concerns about our products,
you can contact us on
ProductSafety@springernature.com

In case Publisher is established outside the EU,
the EU authorized representative is:
Springer Nature Customer Service Center GmbH
Europaplatz 3, 69115 Heidelberg, Germany

Printed by Libri Plureos GmbH
in Hamburg, Germany